'The most cool-headed and penetrating account yet of recreational drug use, and its pioneers and profiteers through the ages'

The Face

'Without doubt the best so far to straddle the territory of sociology, medicine and informative, informed journalism . . . not a crusading book, but it does a magnificent job'

Steve Grant, Time Out

'Each chapter takes in the historic, political and economic fortunes of the chemicals very systematically . . . can be safely recommended as a definitive work'

Blitz

'Eminently readable, being devoid of slang and technical terms. At the equivalent cost of four pints of lager or 50 cigarettes, I think it is extremely good value'

Community View

'The quality of the contents match the blurb on the cover . . . "for drug workers, drug users, teachers, parents, for everyone who needs or wants to know about drugs and drug-taking". Buy it'

The Standing Conference on Drug Abuse

About the Author

Andrew Tyler is a freelance journalist who for several years was a special correspondent for *New Musical Express* on social and political issues. He has since contributed to *Time Out*, *New Statesman*, *The Observer*, *The Independent*, *The Guardian* and others. He has extensive experience as a youth worker. He is married and lives in North London.

Street Drugs

Andrew Tyler

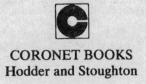

CORONET BOOKS
Hodder and Stoughton

For Sara, Davy, Oskie, Penny, Reggie,
Stanley, Fritzy and Liam

First published in Great Britain in 1986, and fully revised and
updated in 1988, by Coronet paperbacks as a paperback original.
This fully revised and updated edition published in 1995 by
Hodder and Stoughton, a division of Hodder Headline PLC.

A Coronet paperback

17

British Library Cataloguing in Publication Data

Tyler, Andrew
Street Drugs. – 2Rev.ed
I. Title
615.78

ISBN 0-340-60975-3

Typeset by Hewer Text Composition Services, Edinburgh
Printed and bound in Great Britain by
Mackays of Chatham plc, Chatham, Kent

Hodder and Stoughton
A division of Hodder Headline PLC
338 Euston Road
London NW1 3BH

CONTENTS

ACKNOWLEDGEMENTS

I have had a great deal of generous help and guidance in compiling this and previous editions of Street Drugs. Many thanks to the following (and apologies for anyone I've left out as a result of brain fatigue). Mary Treacy, Harry Shapiro, Mike Ashton, Pat Lenehan, ASH and Alcohol Concern for looking over all or some of the draft text. Lorraine Hewitt, Kevin Flemen, Eddie Modu, Sean Blanchard, Helen Fletcher, June Taylor, Willie McBride, Crew 2000, Narayn Singh, Denise Williams, Joan Keough, Mary Hepburn, Charles Medawar, Greg Poulter, Mike Goodman, the people at the Standing Conference on Drug Abuse, and that master librarian/archivist at the Institute for the Study of Drug Dependence John Witton. In fact thanks to ISDD – probably the world's best drug information resource – for being there.

INTRODUCTION TO
THIRD EDITION

It gives me a great deal of satisfaction to see *Street Drugs* still on the shelves ten years after it was first published, and to note that it still appears to be of use to a large number of people. Supportive comments regularly come my way from ordinary users, their friends and families, as well as from professional workers in the drugs field.

That there should be a third edition became inevitable given the fairly momentous changes that have occurred since *Street Drugs* Mark 2 was published in 1988. Crack, Ecstasy and anabolic steroids have all since become major phenomena. And there has been a substantial shift in the cultural landscape, with several senior figures from politics, the police and the media calling for a drastic rethink in terms of the way the War Against Drugs is being prosecuted.

I have done more than merely tack on bits to the pre-existing text. Following extensive recent travels around the country, talking to those involved in the scene; and after a consideration of literally thousands of specialist documents and media articles, I have reworked every chapter and created new ones. Sections relating to drugs' health impact, the cultural context, trafficking, the law and so on have all been thoroughly updated. Though some of the contents will be familiar from earlier editions, a great deal is new.

While I have not always refrained from offering an opinion on some matter or another, my principal objective – as before – has been to provide straightforwardly useful information for all those concerned with drugs and with those who use them.

London, January 1995

INTRODUCTION TO FIRST EDITION

In all parts of the world legally prohibited drugs are being consumed by increasingly large numbers of people who would otherwise consider themselves entirely average. This book aims to chart that phenomenon together with the great range of attitudes and postures that have risen to meet it. I explore the political and historical background to the substances – for it is from these sources rather than any pharmacological reality that drugs get their reputations. I also examine the style and mode of their use, their likely physical and mental impact, and offer self-aid tips, a guide to the law, to current policy, trafficking trends and include a list of support groups, agencies and clinics.

The whole area is an extraordinary one, studded with myth and falsehood. My ambition has been to circumnavigate it in language that is approachable without being facile, for there have been too many volumes that don't let the general reader through their thickets of technical jargon, and others that get just a little too sticky with tales of blood and vomit.

So what is meant by the term 'street drugs'? I admit it is not an especially satisfactory one since the substances are not only or even mostly trafficked and consumed on the streets: most are controlled under the Misuse of Drugs Act and so require discreet handling. But I stick with the term to differentiate between those substances handed out by doctors as medicines, and those taken recreationally for a good time. Having indicated the demarcation point, however, it has to be said that on both sides of the fence the distinction keeps breaking down. Recreational drugs quite often result not in fun but misery, while the physician's medicine can provoke bigger problems than those they were set against. Perhaps it is not well appreciated that the majority of the substances we now consider vanquishers of youth were in the first place dispensed by the medical profession. In fact, so often does a drug follow the route from wonder cure to deadly fix that

3

the rational person has to strain to avoid the conclusion that there is an amount of purposefulness to it all – if only by way of determined myopia.

No more powerful example exists than the case of the opiates. Modern medicine has always sought the safe, non-addictive painkiller-cum-sedative. Nature's own offering is the opium poppy (*Papaver somniferum*) and though not perfectly measuring up to the prescription, it is a plant of great utility. It was used in its simplest form in this country for some three hundred years before a combination of entrepreneurial activity and the fussing of a burgeoning medical lobby produced the first of a series of 'superior' alternatives. The first was morphine. Ten times more potent than opium, morphine was promoted not only as a more efficient painkiller, but as a 'cure' for those persons who, in the course of treatment, had become addicted to opium. How a substance actually derived from opium and so much more powerful could be expected to produce anything but a more vicious habit is to be wondered at; but the dislogic didn't end there. When it was finally recognised that morphine itself was leading to addiction, the newly-synthesised heroin began to be prescribed as an alternative that could both manage pain and overcome morphine addiction. But heroin is also largely derived from opium and is stronger still than morphine. Now that heroin has been unfrocked, a new substance called methadone is being issued by the state as a cure for the addiction heroin has brought about. Methadone is itself addictive and results in a withdrawal syndrome considered tougher and more protracted than heroin's.

Patterns of 'progress' like this have been repeated in other branches of the tree of psychoactive (mind-altering) medicines. For instance, the class of tranquillisers known chemically as the benzodiazepines (brand names Librium, Valium etc.) are presently being touted as comparatively safe substitutes for their discredited predecessors, the barbiturates. And yet one authority[1] estimates that some quarter of a million people in the UK are dependent on them – a dependence every bit as gripping as heroin's.

We can see that such dispensing trends demolish the idea that the medical profession is imbued with any special wisdom in the matter of psychoactive drugs. And this is as true of the present as for the past. The trends also underline the point that whatever alternative supply sources may have latterly sprung up, the original fount of most street drugs, heroin included, is the medical profession.

But this book adds up to more than a club with which to beat Big Brother medical profession and Big Sister government. Ordinary people, without any help, are quite capable of injuring themselves with drugs, either because they don't know enough about them or – if I may be pardoned a philosophical aside – they don't know enough about themselves. If power derives from knowledge, then weakness and debilitation derive from ignorance. People who know about and respect the potency of the drugs they use are capable of enjoying them for many years – as long as the law doesn't intervene. Those who treat their bodies like a pharmaceutical spittoon (or allow the drugs traders to) will harm themselves as well as all those around them. Getting the game right involves, in the current jargon, good personal management. And this, I suggest, means absorbing five basic lessons:

1. It is possible to become dependent on any mind-altering drug.
2. The impact of a drug is not fixed. It depends on dose, expectations, the mental and physical condition of the user and the setting in which it is taken.
3. Highly processed and concentrated substances (pills, powders, etc.) require more cautious use than their plant equivalents.
4. Hazards are greatly increased when the body's sealed circulatory network is invaded by the hypodermic syringe.
5. Heavy, prolonged use is like heavy, prolonged borrowing from the bank. The benefits don't come free. They are on loan from finite stocks. This is illustrated by the sensations experienced during withdrawal – invariably exactly the opposite to those which were sought from the drug itself. Thus, tranquilliser withdrawal leads to agitation, amphetamine withdrawal brings on exhaustion, and barbiturates (anti-convulsants and sleepers) lead to seizures and restless, often nightmarish sleep.

The above lend a curious equality to the mind alterers, for though it might be impossible to utter irrevocable statements of fact about any of them, the big, important rules apply across

5

the board. Looking at the way drugs have been perceived throughout history these straightforward formulae seem not to have been understood. In the pages that follow we will see how the status of a given substance has soared and plunged in line with the panics that were gripping society at the given moment. In the sixties, for instance, cannabis was seen as the comforter of an indolent, 'amotivational' breed of long-hairs. Yet three decades earlier in the United States it was linked with disaffected immigrant Mexicans who, it was believed, were made not indolent but violently mad by the drug. The reputation of cocaine has suffered even more extreme lurches. Though such movements have depended on society's topical panics, on a more fundamental level they have related to the climate created by powerful business and political interests. The opium wars prosecuted by Britain on the Chinese during the last century are an especially instructive case. So are the monumental manoeuvres down in South America with regard to the modern-day cocaine traffic.

If the generality of drugs tends towards a rough equivalence that has been unrecognised in history, then their specifics are also considerably different from what has been widely assumed. Right now we are seeing a stampede by 'concerned persons' in the direction of heroin. Yet the impact of the ever-popular amphetamine (speed) is being virtually overlooked: the problems incurred by speed's excessive use easily match those of heroin. Barbiturates are also underestimated. A straw poll of experienced drug agency workers would probably produce the consensus that barbs are the most intrinsically hazardous of all substances – easy to overdose on, painful to withdraw from, and liable, when injected without care, to result in appalling physical damage such as gangrene.

Then there is alcohol. Along with tobacco and caffeine this is one of society's un-drug drugs. We not only refuse to get outraged by alcohol, we scarcely notice the thousands killed and maimed on the roads due to its effects, or the hundreds of thousands who suffer more surreptitious mental and physical harm. And yet there is nothing inherently dangerous about a bottle of whisky. Drunk in manageable portions it can charge the spirit and leaven the atmosphere – which can be said to be the case for virtually every other drug examined in this book.

It would be idiotic to dismiss the media coverage of the past two or three years for heroin as being without foundation. Heroin does carry with it hazards, and its use is increasing markedly among an age range from the early teens to the mid-forties. But it should also be appreciated that a large part of the problem with heroin lies in society's jittery reaction to it, and that such a reaction generates distortions and falsehoods about the drug's true nature which exacerbate existing dangers. A lot of first-time users hate the stuff and never return. For those who do persist, it generally takes several weeks of fairly diligent use before a habit develops. Many users adopt avoidance tactics – spreading out their hits over a period (although many kid themselves addiction isn't happening to them when it is). Nor is heroin *per se* a killer drug. Addicts can go on using for decades, even via a needle, and remain comparatively healthy, as long as they can acquire an unadulterated solution, administer it hygenically at a cost they can afford, and avoid contact with the law. Given the drug's present status these conditions are virtually impossible to meet.

The truth about the pattern of drug taking we are now witnessing is that heroin is simply one politically dangerous drug we take with us into an uncertain technochip future. The fact that its use has increased indicates that more people want to get painlessly numb (for that is its principal pharmacological effect) in a UK that for many feels run down, divided, fearful and out of work. There are other important factors to our drug 'epidemic', not least among them being availability. A whole range of exotic drugs, quite simply, can now be purchased at an appropriate price everywhere, whether through the surgery or from a friend. And while the total volume might not have increased (for example, the UK's overall consumption of alcohol is about 80 per cent down on 1900[2]) the variety has. The public, unable to be sated any more with the traditional offerings of booze, fags, tea and coffee, is demanding a variety of materials. The great pity is that society lacks the maturity to handle these new drugs (which is why I reject the 'libertarian' idea of freely prescribed heroin as simpleton). It also lacks the basic user-friendly information. The old cultural networks of a couple of decades ago have broken up. In the present climate we find drug information books being prosecuted under the Obscene Publications Act. Teachers

7

and other professionals who dare to suggest cannabis is no more harmful than alcohol are being stripped of their jobs. Those who *know* drugs and might have something constructive to impart are forced on to the sidelines of the debate, as though they were extremists, which allows the air to get filled with the righteously ill-informed tut-tutting of those who know best; or else the language used to convey solid information is mordant and of no interest to those it is aimed at. This means young people (though not just the young) are coming to drugs knowing scarcely anything of them save what they have construed from the tabloid media. They will probably feel sordid, perhaps 'rebellious', and might well get a bad habit before they can set themselves right. For such people we must dispense with the fakery and the mystification and *inform* ourselves. Those who blame heroin for our damaged, rejected youth, for rising crime and poverty in already debased communities, are playing games of political evasion.

We must also create and properly fund a range of interconnecting services that don't over-concentrate on that dramatic ten-day Cold Turkey period. The struggle to regain self-respect and self-sufficiency goes on long afterwards and needs attending to. The disproportionate power in the hands of psychiatrists to decide and manage 'treatment' strategy should also be dissolved – a far bigger share going to the voluntary street agencies, to the mutual help groups and to the community services providing accommodation, education, job training and health care. It is with the help of these bodies that the problem user can discover that there is life without obsessive drug taking. And it is from them that s/he can receive the long-term bolstering that benefits us all. At the bottom line, though, there is just one person and his/her drugs. And that's where the determination lies.

London, April 1985

8

Notes

1 Malcolm Lader, 'The Rise of the Benzodiazepines', *MIMS Magazine*, 15.9.1983
2 *Beer Facts, 1983*, The Brewers' Society, Brewer Publications Ltd, London

THE BACKGROUND

What is a Drug?

The place to start is at the beginning and identify what we are talking about when we refer to *drugs*. Defining the term is not as easy as it sounds. Medical textbooks often say something like . . . a *drug is any substance that by its chemical nature alters the structure or functioning of a living being*.[1] This, though, would encompass not only heroin but table sugar – too much of the latter producing a bloated body and fluctuations in energy levels through its impact on the flow of insulin.

But heroin, it will be said, is a thousand times more potent and dangerous than sugar – to which the answer is *not always*. Someone who binges daily on cup cakes and sugary tea is being more self-destructive than a once-a-month moderate heroin snorter. The sugar-eater is also being more obsessive or, if you like, showing more obvious signs of addiction. Cut dead the sugar supply and that individual will probably suffer emotional distress and physical withdrawal symptoms.

The key to it is the intent and intensity of the using experience, as well as the amount consumed. The fact that some products, such as amphetamine and cocaine, are in a pure drug state (they are specially concocted to affect a change in mood) while others show a more innocent face (tea, a can of butane gas for refilling lighters) does not alter the basic reality. Neither does the source of the product nor its status in law. Tobacco's toll of dead and maimed is far greater than all the illegal drugs combined. And when it comes to addiction, it is not heroin or cocaine which have snared the largest number, but the benzodiazepine tranquillisers – a doctor-administered product that was for years avidly marketed as being free of such problems.

What is the Drug Problem?

If we are already struggling to identify what a drug is, defining 'the drug problem' presents several more layers of complexity. These are, in fact, boom times for sleuths and pundits who claim to have *the* angle on the nature of the predicament. Psychiatrists, criminologists, neurologists, music critics, naturopaths, historians, epidemiologists, style gurus . . . all offer their verdict.

I won't attempt to distil their ideas because it can't be done. Illicit drugs are used by every kind of individual for all kinds of purposes – from recreational fun use at one end of the spectrum to pain relief and suicide at the other. And while some onlookers are constitutionally pre-set to regard all drug-related activity as problematic, or at least as something to be tabulated and processed (the police, drug agencies, medical researchers), often all that is required is for people to be left alone.

Many consumers can't understand why they are free to feed their bodies a variety of plants and fruits but are prohibited from 'nourishing' their minds with the seeds, leaves, and resins of other plant products. Young dancegoers are aggravated by society's hostile response to their end-of-week sweat rituals. And yet, as any anthropologist knows, young people around the world and throughout time have sought some kind of feverish communal transcendence – often chemically and musically assisted. Adult society, in its resolute incomprehension, has not only made criminals of a good proportion of its youth, it has hardened the traditional, destructive divide between the generations.

Rather than a legislative assault on 'unauthorised' rave parties (the 1994 Criminal Justice and Public Order Act), young ravegoers have required sound information about the drugs they are taking from sources they can trust. They need up-to-date 'intelligence' on adulterants; on the latest 'miracle buzz'; tips on how to avoid heatstroke; a true assessment of the risks to their long-term emotional health (the most important and most neglected aspect of the Rave 'debate'); and they also require protection from spivvy club managers, some of whom – especially in the early days – switched off cold-water taps in toilets so as to boost bar sales of desperately needed liquids.

Some drug agencies (Manchester's Lifeline, for instance) are already providing this kind of support. Better still, there are instances of users themselves gathering together and offering help to their peers – simultaneously learning and teaching.

While many drug users need to be left alone or simply offered basic guidance, others find themselves drowning in their habit and dragging down those who matter most to them. The symptoms are visible everywhere: early mortality, drug-related theft and violence, physical illness, mental illness, and emotional anguish on the part of those who see no way of preventing those they love from destroying themselves. The scale on which these problems manifest themselves is heavily disputed, not only because precision is technically difficult to come by, but because prejudice and inter-disciplinary rivalry between professionals causes the figures to flip one way and then another. Even a so-called 'drug-related' death is not a clear-cut thing. A dead body with a high level of drugs in it didn't necessarily expire because of the drugs. 'Drug-related' sickness is more difficult still, since how are we to know that – for instance – it was cocaine which made an individual's heart beat with dangerous irregularity when that individual was also subjecting himself to all kinds of other insults in terms of caffeine consumption, lack of sleep, a ruinous diet, a sedentary lifestyle, tobacco, and the rest.

Many laboratory researchers produce their medical data by experimenting on animals. Apart from poisoning their subjects with extreme doses of the drug in question, these 'scientists' drive them screeching mad by use of electric shocks, starvation, and various mental torments. I make no apologies for expressing my emphatic abhorrence of such activities. Nor am I alone in regarding these works as the crudest form of bullying (doing to another what you wouldn't dare have done to yourself). The exercise is also bogus scientifically, because the information produced is irrelevant to human beings. Animal species are not only different from our own species in terms of their physical structure and chemical functioning, they are different from each other: a cat is not a monkey and a monkey is not a mouse. The sterile laboratory setting also confounds the outcome. Most people do not live in metal cages on a pelleted diet, devoid of any comfort.

Crime and drugs are no easier to correlate. In February 1994, the Labour Party's Tony Blair startled the nation by announcing that, according to a formula provided by Greater Manchester Police and data from official sources, around half of all the property crime committed in England and Wales was drug-related. People looking for cash to fund their habits were responsible for £1,999 million out of a £4,007 million total.

Blair's calculations worked on the assumption that 22,819 'notified' addicts were each consuming one gram of heroin a day priced at £80 a gram. This worked out at an annual consumption per addict of £30,000. Because stolen property can only be sold for around a third of its as-new value, the addicts each had to thieve not £30,000 worth of items but £90,000 worth.

The immediately apparent flaw in the Blair formula is that habitual users get money from all kinds of sources (social security, straight work, prostitution). Also, few consume a uniform amount; they'll cut back or quit from time to time. Against this, the near-23,000 addicts known officially to the authorities are probably only a fifth of the total.

Flawed or not, the problem the Blair figures posed for a Conservative government – apart from the obvious embarrassment caused by the spectre of runaway crime – was that they strengthened the hand of those arguing for decriminalisation of all or of some illegal substances.

The government's considered response came in an October 1994 strategy document[2] which crunched a heap more numbers to 'prove' that the maximum amount dependent heroin users needed to thieve each year was £864 million, while the minimum was £58 million; it all depended on how much they were paying for their fix and by how many times you cared to multiply the number of officially listed addicts.

Calculating how much drug use 'costs' in terms of pounds sterling was by now a burgeoning industry. *Time Out* magazine, in May 1994,[3] performed a number of complex sums to reveal that 'the total cost of London's drug problem was £517.9 million' – a figure embracing the cost of crime, medical treatment, education, and policing. This was nearly as much as total government spending in its anti-drugs war nationally, said the magazine.

The *Time Out* piece fell into the familiar trap of assuming that all drug-related expenditure is money that vanishes

14

from the economy. But when a police officer is hired to investigate a drug dealer, or an ad agency is commissioned to produce a government anti-heroin campaign, the money changing hands is all part of the grease that oils an economy and keeps people active. The real question relates not to how much cash and energy are expended but to who gets hurt as a result of drug use. When a family is burgled by an addict looking for drugs money, they pay a genuine price. They are distressed, they lose possibly irreplaceable objects, their insurance goes up, and their sense of security is reduced. The glazier who fixes their window pays no such price (unless their nervousness rubs off on him). This distinction is made not in a spirit of nit-picking abstraction but to indicate that we need to understand who loses and who gains from drug use and the war against it. A new substance panic can be good news for a research scientist looking for a hot item with which to attract funding for his/her department. The same might be said for a regional crime squad whose job is to chase the big dealers. According to one senior officer I spoke to, such squads 'want to go down the American road – which has failed. They want to get their hands on the drugs money they confiscate and reinvest it in more enforcement. My argument against this is that these squads then have a vested interest in the drug trafficker selling the stuff, because you can't buy new police cars and radios with a hundredweight of confiscated cocaine. You need it to be converted into money. Since you can convict a guy equally as well after he's sold the stuff as when he's in possession, you wait until he's sold and then you nick him and get the money [under the confiscatory powers of the Drug Trafficking Offences Act]'.

While my interviewee had no evidence that this was taking place, he told me that he had recently asked a senior officer formerly serving with the south-east regional crime squad if he thought it would be 'morally wrong' to tailor a bust with a view to the cash rewards on offer. His colleague answered, 'No, because it would be for the greater good.'

15

The Source of the Drug Problem

As governments throughout the industrialised world are now discovering, 'the drug problem' does not start and end with Third World producers of cocaine, cannabis, and heroin products.

Demand and supply

It's a rule of the market that demand and supply go hand in hand. A producer can artificially stimulate desire for a product but that desire cannot be sustained on a slogan or on the back of plentiful stocks. Drug use is increasing because people want to consume and, in turn, suppliers have succeeded in accommodating their appetites.

Why is demand rising? Firstly, because people enjoy taking drugs. Many don't fear or are not convinced by the messages they receive about the harm the products will do. Drug-taking, especially for youngsters who are new to it, can be an extraordinary, thrilling experience. It also unites them with their peers with whom they can make common cause against a disapproving adult world. This can be called the 'voluntary' end of the business. Some who start as voluntary users, however, are marked out – by reasons of their inherited temperament and/or their biology, or because of the circumstances in which they live – to slide into involuntary use.

This takes us into the sphere of politics and social science. The UK government, during the last several years, has sought to disprove any link between poverty and drug use – possibly a technically correct position since drugs are consumed by both the rich and the poor. But it is idiotic to argue that drugs are not used more destructively by those at the bottom of the social pile, or that drugs don't cause further serious degradation in already degraded communities.[4] Initiation rates into drug use might be remarkably constant across economic boundaries, noted the author of a 1993 British medical journal article, but 'abuse and dependence occur much more commonly among the poor and disenfranchised.'[5] A blindingly obvious statement to all but those who refuse to see it.

I have seen the evidence myself in places like East London, Hulme, Birkenhead, and the peripheral housing estates of Glasgow. Knots of young men who have never, and might not ever, see meaningful work hang around street corners spitting over the tops of their trainers, shoulders hunched against another pointless day. The ceremony of scoring, using and selling drugs might help the day go by but, for most of these young people, it ultimately proves to be a honey trap.

Joan Keough is founder of the Wirral-based Parents Against Drug Abuse (PADA). Two of her three sons got seriously caught up in heroin and, in seeking to retrieve them, Joan has travelled a long road from greengrocer's assistant to campaigner and lecturer on an international stage. She describes heroin's appeal like this: 'After they've left school and find out there's nothing for them to do, they also soon find out they can only stay in bed of a morning for so long. They can only watch television for so long. They get so depressed and somebody comes along and says, *well, just try this*, and they say, *Oh, I'm not touching that, it's addictive. Well, perhaps I'll just have it once but I won't have it any more*. They take it, then suddenly for five or six hours when they're up there, the world is as they want it to be. Then they've got to come down and face life again. Two months might go and they might start getting depressed again and they think, *I'll just have a bit of heroin to get me out of this*, and that's how it goes on, and they come closer and closer to using every day.'

She once blamed dealers for what happened to her sons: the lost years, many spent in prison. 'I thought they were murderers who should be locked up and the keys thrown away, or hung because it was all their fault. But over the years I've realised that every addict is a potential pusher and the majority of them do it to feed their own habit. They need help as much as anybody else. So my sympathies are with pushers as well.'

The licit sector

Several notches above the street-level dealers are the major traffickers. They fall into two main categories: licit and illicit. The first are the pharmaceutical companies and their physician agents who, historically, have been responsible for introducing and marketing most of the drugs now available on

17

the streets – heroin and cocaine included. While these two particular drugs are now also distributed via unauthorised channels, the licit sector still monopolises trade in the country's most heavily consumed mind-altering drugs of addiction (discounting alcohol): the benzodiazepine tranquillisers. If that verdict sounds unduly cynical in respect of the medical/pharmaceutical profession, I invite readers to study the benzodiazepines chapter and note the chronicle of high-level corruption and complacency that marks the history of these drugs.

But the tranks are merely the tip of the 'licit' iceberg. While still in our nappies, we are trained to believe that drugs can go most of the way to resolving our physical and emotional problems. We consume them in ever-greater quantities: £3.3 billion worth during 1992/93 in England alone – a 14 per cent increase in real terms on the year before.[6] Yet we are getting sicker. The government's own statistics show that the proportion of people suffering long-term illness increased between 1972 and 1992 by around 50 per cent. And it's not a case of lots more sick, elderly people distorting the general picture. The very young's health is failing quickest. Among nought- to four-year-olds, lingering illness has more than tripled (from 4 to 13 per cent).[7]

It is little wonder that, trained from birth, our assumptions and appetites for drugs should be carried over on to the street, along with all the damaging consequences.

The illicit sector

Like the pharmaceutical business, the trade in illega drugs is also a global commercial enterprise, yet more complex and dynamic because it must constantly outwit a vast enforcement effort designed to defeat it. That it has succeeded in meeting and/or stimulating an accelerating demand over the last two decades is due – according to one expert report – to at least four important factors:[8] a) the development of a vast and largely unregulated international market in industrial chemicals; b) easy availability of laboratory facilities and the expertise to run them; c) a transportation revolution, which has made it cheap and technically simple to shift products over great distances; d) the globalisation and deregulation of banking and financial markets, allowing the transfer of large

18

sums of money virtually unhindered. Added to these factors are two others that present any major player on the world scene with a cheap and deadly keen pool of labour. These are the enormous social and economic dislocations resulting from the implosion of communism, and the abysmally low standards of living experienced throughout much of the Third World.

The combination of all these ingredients has meant that 'over the last two decades there has been a Darwinian evolution of the entire industry in which the survivors have developed sophisticated and highly flexible organisations conducting worldwide commerce in their illicit products.'[9] This was the view of 100 experts brought together by the Washington-based Centre for Strategic and International Studies. Their solution, as reported in 1993, was to continue with the War on Drugs but apply more flexibility and co-operation between nations. Apply also a stronger focus on suppressing demand for the substances.

The fault with the CSIS report and others like it is that it assumes that drug trafficking is a semi-organised conspiracy against unsuspecting consumers whose appetites, once criminally aroused, must be suppressed. In fact, the drugs trade is peopled by as many small- and medium-scale operators as giant, killer syndicates. It flourishes because the product is popular. International regulatory authorities – however they 'enhance' their performances – stand as good a chance of seriously suppressing drug transactions as they do of curbing the trade in wood products or vegetables.

When the report points to the former communist bloc countries as an important new centre of activity, this is undoubtedly correct. Throughout 1993/94, the British public received press and television accounts of the flourishing trade in places like Poland and Russia and of the total ruthlessness of the 'mafia' gangs who were said to be commanding the business. Exaggerated or not, the drugs trade *is* a vast global enterprise that hooks together Andean peasant growers with dance-club snorters in Warrington and Milan. To pretend that it is a passing fancy or that it can somehow be successfully managed within the existing prohibitionist framework is an insanity.

My own view is that the world community must move – and fast – towards decriminalising the market so that it can assert some kind of control. If people are going to use drugs they might as well use unadulterated products made to an approved standard. They should also have access to balanced information about the pros and cons of what they are taking rather than not-very-well-camouflaged government warnings whose credibility is near zero. Similarly, no one is served when penniless Nigerian couriers, who have been paid a pittance to swallow ten condoms of cocaine, are slung into British jails for years at a time on the pretext that they are major traffickers. There is also little justice in hammering the growers, the couriers, and countless other individuals around the world who are simply servicing an established demand.

Writing as someone who has sampled most of the substances catalogued in this book, I personally have no interest these days in consuming drugs of any description. Perhaps it's a feature of my age (being no longer of the rave generation) but the world seems complicated enough without having to navigate it stoned. Nevertheless, for as long as people have the appetite, regulation within a legal context is the only way to reduce the harm being caused all down the line, from grower to consumer. If this basic principle were to be accepted, then the general public and/or the 'responsible' authorities could move on to answering questions relating to where and how different products might be dispensed (in pharmacies, pubs, corner stores?) and to which categories of people.

If we *were* to travel this road, no one would be happier than the pharmaceutical companies. For in that brave new future, it would be they who supplied all the cocaine, speed, heroin, Ecstasy, and the rest of the mind-altering pharmacopeia: their ultimate triumph. Government would benefit too. Instead of paying out hundreds of millions in enforcement money, they would collect a bigger sum in taxes. The drugged public would also be happier, or at least that proportion that wants its drugs delivered on a plate, free of any effort or drama.

Policy and Policing

The UK is not alone in being undecided as to whether it should treat, educate, or punish its drug users. It does a bit of all three, though without any staggering success. Total *war on drugs* spending now amounts to more than £500 million a year.[10] Seizures by police and Customs continue to rise. There are more convictions under the 1971 Misuse of Drugs Act, and – until the beginning of the 1990s – the state-supported drug treatment sector had seen virtually unchecked growth for more than twenty years. Yet despite such apparently promising indicators, more people are consuming a greater range of substances than ever before and are tending to start their using careers at an earlier age.

None of which is to say that drugs have received sustained political attention over the years. Much depends on the kind of threat to the majority of citizens the truly dangerous class of user has been thought to represent. Over the last thirty years this perceived menace has waxed and waned as youth has been seen, variously, as more or less dangerous; as racial tensions have grown and receded; and – especially – as AIDS established itself as the mother of all panics before falling down the agenda after the heterosexual, non-injecting majority concluded that they weren't in serious danger after all.

Community safety

The UK has a reputation for liberality in its conduct of drug policy but, in reality, it has tended towards a utilitarian approach: whatever was required to protect the majority from an errant minority has been done. The prevention of contagion has been the consistent objective, whether the infection has been of a subcultural nature (hippies in the 1960s, ravers in the 1990s) or viral (hepatitis and HIV). The latest contagion-fear is drug-induced crime, and the prescription for dealing with it is called 'community safety'.

Some regard community safety as old wine in a new bottle. It calls for a multi-agency, multi-disciplinary approach whose first priority, in the words of a major new government policy statement for England issued in October 1994, is 'to increase the safety of communities from drug-related crime' by way of 'vigorous law enforcement and a new emphasis on education and prevention . . .'

The document – designed to herald a period of consultation – was called *Tackling Drugs Together*,[11] and the jigsaw motif with which it was illustrated probably signified the still somewhat jagged alliance between the three government departments who authored it: Education, Health, and the Home Office.[12]

Education

Considered by some to be the most significant drugs policy statement in fifteen years of Conservative government,[13] the October 1994 document made it clear that no currently banned drug would be legalised or decriminalised – 'it would send totally the wrong signal.' But education in schools was rediscovered after years of fumbling and neglect. 'Drug misuse is an educational issue as much as a social evil,' noted the Department of Education. 'We have the responsibility to ensure that young people know the risks . . . and have the knowledge and skills to resist drugs.'

Resist? For years the government's bogeyman had been the pusher at the school gate. It was he who enticed youngsters on to the road that led to addiction. The October 1994 document marked an advance from that position but the government still couldn't stomach the idea that most young people use drugs because they want to, not because they succumb to unwelcome pressure from their friends. They select to use *in the company* of friends.[14]

Crime and punishment

On the crime front, the most significant policy move declared in the October 1994 report was the introduction of random drug testing of up to 60,000 prisoners every year. There would also be targeted testing of all inmates known to be users. Anyone coming up positive or refusing the test would be liable to a further twenty-eight days in jail, confinement to their cell, as well as loss of privileges and earnings.

'Drug-taking in prison', declared the Home Secretary, Michael Howard, 'can lead to violence, intimidation and disorder. This must be tackled with all the vigour at our command. Drug misuse in prisons will not be tolerated.'

If Howard was expecting cheers all round he didn't get it. Critics believed that extreme measures might indeed produce a reduction in the total volume of drugs circulating in prisons. But this would almost certainly force up the level of violence in what was already a volatile environment. It has been estimated that most of the roughly 100,000 UK drug injectors will end up in prison at some stage in their lives.[15] In 1993 alone, 12,000 were incarcerated within a system that is dangerously overcrowded, which offers no meaningful recreation or vocational training and precious little medical support for those who enter the system with a habit.

'Prison doctors refuse to give prisoners drug detoxification treatment which is standard in the outside community,' Michael Ross, a Bradford doctor experienced in the ways of prisoner addicts, told an April 1994 press conference.[16] 'As a consequence, prisoners are being forced back to heroin and to sharing needles.'

Health care guidelines allowed inmates one week of the heroin substitute methadone but, said Ross, seven weeks was the recognised minimum in the outside world, and some prison doctors refused to prescribe any meth. He warned that such short-sightedness placed prisons at risk of 'an HIV epidemic', whose consequences could spill over into the community at large. Two former inmates were on hand to support Ross's prognosis. A twenty-six-year-old, addicted for nine years, said that at Newhall women's prison there was one syringe going round a wing of thirty prisoners, of whom about a third were injectors. And a former resident of Armley jail declared that 'over 300 inmates were using the same needle. Only once in the last three years of rehabilitation have I relapsed and used heroin,' he declared, 'and that was due to the treatment I got in Armley.'

The Home Office's continuing refusal to provide clean syringes to prisoners was a decision supported by the Prison Officers Association, whose spokesman argued that by dispensing injecting equipment the authorities were, in effect, 'accepting drug-taking instead of fighting it. Needles can also be used as weapons.'[17]

A compromise option for the Home Office would be to make strong bleach available so that injecting prisoners can clean their works. But this would also signal *approval*. Instead, less efficient sterilisation tablets are sometimes issued, on the pretext that they are part of a general drive towards improving hygiene.

Many of the other proposals in the October 1994 government document related to reconstituting the existing bureaucractic treatment structures,[18] or called for more monitoring and the setting of 'performance targets' for agencies such as the police and Customs. Treatment centres were to make themselves more easily accessible, more cost-effective and 'appropriate' – a case of *this shall be done*, with little in the way of practical guidance on how any of it might be achieved.

Black users/women users

The contentious matter of the link between poverty and drugs was ducked, as were issues such as the demonstrable lack of responsiveness most treatment services extend to ethnic minorities and to women. It has long been recognised that women users delay coming forward for help because of the stigma that identification brings, and because those with families fear that their children will be taken from them. As a result, by the time they do seek help, their health and other problems are often far more intractable. Black users are also often reluctant attenders, partly through lack of effort to make them aware of what's on offer, partly because they seem to recognise that the UK drug treatment effort is directed mostly towards white male heroin users. This is not to say that blacks don't use heroin or that whites don't use cocaine/crack, but that structural prejudice and stereotyping block access to what might turn out to be useful support.

One experienced black worker in the field told me that he believed a 'treatment apartheid' was coming into being: all-black units and outreach teams catering for all-black clients. What he wanted to see were drug agencies reflecting the ethnic mix of a given area, with all staff trained in 'race awareness'.

Meanwhile, Home Office figures showed that black Londoners were five times more likely to be stopped and searched by the police than whites. Of 228,316 stopped in the Met area during 1993, a disproportionate 42 per cent were of ethnic background.[19]

The state fix

Methadone is the official state substitute for heroin. Over the past twenty-five to thirty years, the amount and duration of scripts on offer have been essentially a political decision. As noted above (see also heroin chapter), much has depended on how big a threat junk users were thought to present at any given time to the majority population. The new concern with community safety suggests that prescribers will be encouraged to loosen their grip and offer bigger methadone doses for longer periods. In this way, so the theory goes, users will not need to seek 'top-ups' from the street and, in any case, will be too mushy in the head to commit whatever crimes were necessary to pay for any extras.

If such a prescribing pattern does emerge, addicts will probably be obliged to make a trade-off: more methadone over a longer period, but the drug having to be taken at the clinic rather than – as has been the case to date – the script being 'cashed in' at a chemist and consumed at a place of the user's choosing.[20] In this way, it is believed, treatment 'compliance' would be guaranteed and the chances of licit meth reaching the street all but eliminated.[21]

Some people in the drugs field are fairly content to see intractable smackheads chemically *voided* by a state-issued fix.[22] In some parts of the country it is already happening, with a consequent high level of methadone overdose deaths. Advocates of the method see it as a way of preserving future generations of recreational drug users from a malign influence, and also as a way of enhancing the safety of the community at large. Opponents believe that treatment facilities should never be used to sacrifice and sideline patients for the apparent good of the majority. Such a policy, they contend, won't work anyway. People who are handled dishonestly are unlikely to roll over and make themselves quiet.

But the shape of treatment to come had still not been established at the time of writing. Cost will be a more important factor in a health service that is increasingly commercialised and in which the former generals of the drugs field – the consultant psychiatrists – are now outranked by price-conscious senior administrators. Another key to the future will be the contents of a detailed Department of Health treatment review due for publication in January 1996.

Scotland

Scotland is another story. Because of a number of intricate cultural reasons, as well as the sluggish manner in which support services have developed north of the border, Scotland has experienced far more drug-related harm than the rest of the UK. There are more Scottish injectors, who start at a younger age. In Glasgow, overdose deaths during the early 1990s were running at close to a hundred a year. In Edinburgh, the HIV infection rate – though stabilised by the early part of the decade – was still one of the highest in Europe.

This was the background against which a Scottish Ministerial Task Force, chaired by Lord Fraser, published a programme of action on the same day as English ministers were issuing their consultation document. The Fraser report[23] was more politically focused and more grounded than its English counterpart. The dire situation on the ground made that imperative. 'The Scottish task force's response to the pressing health issues before it was to opt for the "pragmatism" that has so far been the English way,' noted Mike Ashton, editor of the Institute of Drug Dependency's respected journal *Druglink*.[24] 'National political support for *harm reduction* appears to be waning in its English heartlands but flourishing in the previously hostile Scottish environment.'

Harm reduction

Harm reduction is a philosophy that recognises that some people will use drugs however fervently the *just say no* message is transmitted to them. This requires damage-limitation strategies, including the issuing of clean syringes, methadone, and guidance on how to use a given substance more safely – such information going out to school-age children if considered necessary. Whereas the October 1994 English document retreated from this harm-reduction message, Fraser's report specifically endorsed the approach, not least for young people. 'This is not to condone drugtaking but simply to acknowledge that it . . . take(s) place; and therefore the pragmatic response is to provide information and advice about minimising risks.'[25]

Wales

The best that can be said at the time of going to press is that the future policy direction for Wales has yet to be announced. No government document has emerged, though there were indications that a combined strategy was being developed for both alcohol and drug problems – two facets that have traditionally been treated separately.

Endpiece

So how looks the future? Two things, it occurs to me, are self-evident: 1) it is illogical to expect to see healthy drug use in a culture that is intrinsically unhealthy; 2) a society – and here I repeat myself – that trains its young to believe that drugs can solve their physical and emotional ills should not be amazed when those same young people subsequently choose to self-administer.

Self-help

What comes through clearly when we study the history of illicit drugs, and the policy and policing initiatives that have arisen to address their use, is a story of action without rational content. Sometimes the impulse to act comes from fear; other times from bemusement, cynicism, and plain prejudice. Having made an argument for the legalisation of the global drugs trade so that it can be properly regulated, I have to say that I don't expect the decision-makers to rush to compliance. Meanwhile, users and those who care for them will need access to untainted information and, in some cases, support and treatment.

Addicts are constantly reporting that the most powerful resource available to them is other users – so long as they are constructively motivated. The last ten years has seen the establishment of a few self-help groups, and some professional drug agencies have enlisted the services of current or ex-users (while not always paying them a fair return for the job).[26] Progress, however, has been slow, owing partly to a lack of sensitive support by the professionals in the field.

Helen Fletcher founded Manchester's Mainline in 1988, 'a service set up by drug users for drug users'. In a 1994 article directed at professional workers,[27] Helen argued that her group had 'dispelled many myths and reinforced the harm reduction message. We provided an alternative approach to service provision. We were at the forefront of being user-friendly, often being consulted by statutory services and professionals on how to reach the "hidden users".' Yet when it came to drawing up Manchester's community care plans, Helen complains that her service was not consulted, nor was it receiving secure funding.

Self-help and self-education are also of relevance to the recreational crowd, and here the Edinburgh-based Crew 2000 (ravers and drug users themselves) have shown what can be done by way of a series of unpretentious leaflets which they have circulated among their peers. They have also lectured at international drug conferences – gatherings of experts who too often know the pharmacological facts but lack current knowledge about how drugs are used in a constantly shifting scene. Where drugs are concerned, the context is (very nearly) everything.

Dangerous liaisons

Still on the subject of drug workers, I should like to sound a warning with their safety in mind. The field in which they function is a challenging, sometimes hazardous one. It requires contact with desperate people. Many workers of my acquaintance do their job with great integrity and a clear head. They are the best of people. But there is a tendency in some towards dangerous voyeurism. In meeting with suppliers and their 'enforcers', rules of engagement can end up being unclear – with potentially violent consequences. Even more reckless is a situation I came across in early 1994, which I'm sure is not unique. A small team of drug researchers were profiling an inner-city dealing scene through meetings with the main players. The body that commissioned the work was the city police force. Funding came from a major burger chain. With the intelligence collected by these means the police were able to launch a series of arrests and the area fell quiet – temporarily at least. But what would have befallen the researchers had their dealer contacts discovered during the course of the project that the information they were providing was not in the cause of disinterested sociological research but directed towards their own incarceration? I can see, literally, murder in the offing.

Drug futures

As to the substances we can expect to blow in and out of favour in future years – *smart drugs, mind machines, growth promoters, neurotransmitter-boosters, sex hormones* – the definition of a drug experience will become less easy to pin down as consumers succumb to the blandishments of a marketplace that will promise physical as well as mental transcendence. And from the very people who'll be designing and supplying these products – research scientists – will emerge promises of New Age cures for compulsive use. Drug-risk profiling will become *the thing* (for those who can afford it): drop-in shops, where people who harbour fears of innate weaknesses will be able to submit themselves or their offspring to brain scans, DNA profiling, psychological questionnaires, and life-history analysis. For those deemed to be high-risk, drugs will be prescribed to prevent them developing an appetite for drugs.[28] Ludicrous? Yes, but lucrative for the product suppliers.

(Grateful thanks to Mike Ashton, editor of Druglink, *the journal of the Institute for the Study of Drug Dependence, for helping me more fully appreciate a whole range of policy and enforcement issues. His assistance was invaluable. The views expressed, however, are mine alone.)*

Factfile

In no particular order, I offer the following possibly useful and interesting facts. They come mostly from government sources and the Institute for the Study of Drug Dependence.

- Money spent on government's response to drug use – around £500 million a year.

29

- Of this, £200 million is swallowed up by police and Customs.
- Estimated value of the UK black market in drugs – £3 billion.
- The cost of nursing a person with AIDS – £20,000 per year.
- The cost of supplying each addict with clean needles and syringes – £50 per year.
- The cost of supplying an addict with methadone for a year – £300.
- Value of property stolen to buy drugs each year – between £58 million (the lowest estimate by the Tory government) and £2 billion (the figure suggested by the Labour opposition).
- The number of drug addicts (old and new) notified to the Home Office during 1993 – 28,000 (a 13 per cent increase on the previous year).
- 56 per cent of this total inject their drugs.
- More than 1,400 drug-related deaths were registered in 1992 – a 4 per cent rise on the previous year. The number of mortalities arising from 'controlled drug abuse' in 1978 was 192.
- The number of premature deaths caused by alcohol – 28,000.
- Smoking-related diseases cause around 110,000 premature deaths each year in the UK. That's six times as many as the combined total caused by road accidents, suicides, homicides, fire, illicit drug use, and AIDS.
- Police and Customs made 72,000 seizures of controlled drugs in 1992 – a 3 per cent increase on the previous year. Eighty per cent involved cannabis.
- 56,000 people were 'dealt with' for drug offences during 1992, a 5 per cent rise on 1991. The number of 'offenders' has grown by between 10 and 13 per cent since 1981.
- In the UK as a whole, about 50 per cent of offenders were sentenced in court, the rest were cautioned or dealt with by compounding (fined by Customs, with the substance confiscated).
- In any one year, at least 6 per cent of the population take an illegal drug (some 3 million people).

- Among schoolchildren, 3 per cent of twelve to thirteen-year-olds and 14 per cent of fourteen to fifteen-year-olds admit to taking an illegal drug.
- Of young people living in inner cities, 42 per cent of sixteen to nineteen-year-olds and 44 per cent of twenty to twenty-four-year-olds have taken drugs at some time.
- 24 per cent of people aged sixteen to twenty-nine report long-term cannabis use. Among sixteen to nineteen-year-olds, 11 per cent have tried amphetamines, 9 per cent Ecstasy, and 8 per cent LSD.
- 97 per cent of twenty-five-year-old Londoners surveyed in 1993 by the listings magazine *Time Out* reported that they had tried cannabis.
- Less than 1 per cent in population samples report ever having used heroin, cocaine or crack. Inner-city samples of sixteen to twenty-five-year-olds suggest figures of 1 per cent having sampled crack, 2 per cent heroin, and 4 per cent cocaine.
- Rates of reported use of volatile substances (solvents) by young people are: twelve to thirteen-year-olds – 3 per cent; fourteen to fifteen-year-olds – 7 per cent; and fifteen to sixteen-year-olds – 6 per cent.
- 122 sudden deaths were caused by volatile substance sniffing in 1991.
- 60 per cent of all addicts notified in 1993 were in their twenties.
- The proportion of notified addicts under twenty-five has increased by 20 per cent since 1990.
- Between January 1987 and December 1993, courts in England and Wales ordered the confiscation of 'drug trafficking proceeds' totalling £51.5 million.
- Around 1,300 police officers and 5,100 Customs staff are directly involved in anti-drugs work.
- Between April 1993 and March 1994, Customs prevented drugs said to be worth nearly £2 billion from entering the UK.
- There were 660 alcohol-linked road deaths in 1991.

What drugs cost (mid-1994):

- heroin – £70–80 per gram
- cocaine – £60 per gram

- crack – £20–25 per rock
- amphetamine sulphate – £10 per gram wrap
- LSD – £2–5 per tab
- Ecstasy – £15–20 per tab
- cannabis resin – £13–15 per eighth of an ounce
- cannabis 'grass' – £15–20 per eighth of an ounce

1 D. Duncan and R. Gold, *Drugs and the Whole Person*, John Wiley & Sons, New York, 1982, p. 2.

2 *Tackling Drugs Together: A consultation document on a strategy for England 1995–1998*, HMSO, London, Annex B, p. 100.

3 'High society', in *Time Out*, 18 May 1994, p. 12.

4 For example, a four-city UK survey found that those of 'lower socio-economic status' used more frequently and resorted more often to injecting than those in the upper brackets. See 'Surveys suggest drug use has doubled in ten years; heavy use still rare', in *Druglink*, Institute for the Study of Drug Dependence (ISDD), January/February 1994, p. 6.

5 P. Robson, 'Preventing drug abuse', in *The Lancet*, Vol. 342, 11 December 1993, p. 1475.

6 *A Prescription for Improvement: Towards more rational prescribing in general practice*, Audit Commission report, 1994, pp. 3–4.

7 General Households Survey for 1990 (published 1992), HMSO.

8 'The Transnational Drug Challenge and the New World Order: The report of the CSIS project on the global drug trade in the post-Cold War era', Centre for Strategic and International Studies, Washington, DC, January 1993.

9 Ibid.

10 Source: ISDD.

11 HMSO, *Tackling Drugs Together*, op. cit.

12 Authored under the aegis of a government creation called the Central Drugs Coordination Unit.

13 M. Ashton, 'New drug strategies for England and Scotland', in *Druglink*, ISDD, November/December 1994, p. 6.

14 See N. Coggans and S. McKellar, 'Peer Pressure: A convenient explanation', in *Druglink*, ISDD, November/December 1994, p. 16.

15 Newsletter No. 3, Society Promoting AIDS-related Criminology (PO Box 3229, Birmingham B26 2SQ).

16 'Jail drug policies "foster HIV risk"', in the *Guardian*, 27 April 1993

17 'Prison AIDS scheme launch', in *Time Out*, 17 November 1993.

18 For instance, 100 new Drug Action teams were set up to 'tackle drug misuse locally'. They inherited the job of the old local drug advisory committees, which had brought together – under the aegis of health authorities – senior health, police, prison, and similar figures. With meetings often poorly attended, the advisory committees were generally considered a failure. Given that the new teams will be composed of half a dozen chief and

deputy chief executives from the same services, finding time to attend will continue to be a problem. Additionally, some pundits argue that such bodies should be more broadly based with, especially, solid community group representation.

19 'Stop and search race fury', in *Today*, 3 December 1994.

20 See 'ACMD calls for methadone maintenance American-style', in *Druglink*, ISDD, January/February 1994, p. 5.

21 This was the American model of methadone prescribing. The experience from the US, however, is that pharmaceutical methadone is still being diverted to the streets.

22 M. Gilman, 'Back to the future', in *Druglink*, ISDD, September/October 1993, p. 17.

23 *Drugs in Scotland: Meeting the challenge*, report of Ministerial Drugs Task Force, Scottish Home Office and Health Department, October 1994.

24 Ashton, op. cit.

25 Ibid.

26 For example, Void in Colchester, as well as Mainline in Manchester.

27 H. Fletcher, 'Users point the way to appropriate alternatives', *Newsletter*, Standing Conference on Drug Abuse, April/May 1994, p. 7.

28 See D. Concar and R. Mestel, 'Prisoners of pleasure', in *New Scientist*, 1 October 1994, p. 30.

ALCOHOL

Intro

Alcohol is our elixir and our poison. We have always known how well and badly we do from it. 'Wine maketh glad the heart of man,' sang the biblical poet (Psalms 104:15). But, a few pages later, the Proverbist asks: 'Who hath woe . . . who hath babbling? Who hath wounds without cause? Who hath redness of eyes? They that tarry long at the wine.' (Proverbs 23:29–30).

The bi-focal attitude continues. Here is a drug that can floor a full-grown man within half an hour; which kills and maims thousands on the roads every year; induces addiction, violence, disease and suicide; exacerbates an already desperate homelessness situation; and yet is freely available, freely advertised and dressed up not as a 'hard' drug but as a happy social lubricant.

Yet that, in part, is what it is. For we cannot repudiate a drug that has been a good companion to people all over the world for thousands of years, calming nerves, lifting spirits and conjoining groups in merry insobriety.

When we speak of alcohol we are referring to beverages that are for the most part concoctions of flavoured water, with the alcohol content of that water amounting to no more than 40 per cent in whisky and as little as a fraction of 1 per cent in low-alcohol beers. Consumed in this way, alcohol inevitably gets rated as less awesome a substance than it really is. The reputation is reinforced by the fact that neither ale, wine, nor spirits lend themselves to comfortable injection; the pure undiluted stuff never has been tried intravenously on a grand scale by even the most ardent users.

Alcohol's enormous attraction undoubtedly lies in its ability to unshackle normal behavioural restraints and cause an initial lift in spirits. But, fundamentally, it is a dulling, stupefying

35

substance that provokes no deep contemplation or dreaming experiences as do LSD and certain mushrooms. And therein lies some of the explanation as to why society tolerates it so well: alcohol is a status quo experience that might cause boisterousness and even aggression but is not associated with truly novel ways of thinking and acting. The rest of the reason why alcohol is culturally acceptable lies in the arbitrary nature of history. It found a niche and couldn't be dislodged.

Only Moslems are required to shun booze completely. Prohibition works – at some considerable cost – in the Islamic world, but elsewhere temperance and prohibition movements have succeeded only in modifying the drug's pattern of use. A fabric of rules and rituals has been created that makes mass use of the drug more manageable. Part of this process involves putting up the shutters on other strong intoxicants, except when used in a 'medical' context. The justification for such action is rooted in an elaborate lie which maintains that alcohol is less dangerous than it is, and other drugs much more so. It probably doesn't need to be stated again that alcohol is potentially as physically damaging, as addictive and as hazardous to withdraw from as practically any other intoxicant substance.

Because a whole range of drugs have seeped out on to the streets from the medical pharmacies and from 'Third World' growers, it is becoming virtually impossible to sustain the myth that alcohol is the one mass recreational drug in use, and that the new ones on the market – licit or not – are merely a temporary aberration whose ill-effects are amenable to a good dose of law and order. The game has been lost. It is like pretending that the motor car isn't really a major form of transport – that we are all still living in the horse age. For good or for ill, alcohol is now only one part of the story.

What is it?

Alcohol is a hydrocarbon compound derived from fermented sugar. The chemical polite people drink is *ethyl alcohol*, composed of the elements carbon, hydrocarbon and oxygen. More dispirited types resort to *methyl alcohol* whose legitimate uses are as a solvent in paint stripper and as an anti-freeze. The attraction of methylated spirits (a combination of methyl and ethyl alcohol) is that you can get drunk cheaper. A drawback is that the intoxicant rating is actually lower than regular drinking-alcohol. The methane in methyl alcohol (commonly called methanol) also upsets vision – sometimes in a total and permanent way. A third option for alcohol fanciers is *iso-propyl alcohol*, found in after-shave preparations and toilet waters. These are sometimes drunk down straight like a shot of Scotch, though this is considered less sophisticated than splashing it on the face.

So it is ethyl alcohol (otherwise called ethanol) which is the intoxicant factor in the beers, wines, spirits, liqueurs, etc. that we consume so abundantly.

Beer

There are three main types of beer – the traditional English ale, the heartier stout, and the light, bright lager that has long been the premier choice in most other parts of the world and, in recent years, has captured a little more than half the UK market. The major raw material in all these drinks is malted barley, made by soaking, heating and turning the grains from the barley ears until the plant's rich natural sugars are unlocked. Known as germination, the process is arrested by taking the grains to a kiln where they are heat-dried. The resulting malt is next milled into a powder, called grist, and mixed with hot water (known as 'liquor') so as to produce a sweet wort. The wort is boiled with hops, which not only add bitterness and aroma but preserve the brew and keep it free from infection. The hopped wort is now cooled and mixed with yeast. Fermentation – the conversion of the sugars into alcohol and carbon dioxide – is then allowed to proceed. 'Real ales' are those that are left to condition in the cask and are still alive when reaching the pub. The cleaned-up version is pasteurised, filtered and chilled to death in the breweries where it will be loaded into kegs, cans and bottles. Lager is a variation on the ale theme, calling for a different type of yeast and a longer, colder storage and conditioning period. Stout is a heavily hopped drink – a descendant of the richly flavoured London brew, known as porter, which dominated the market in the eighteenth and nineteenth centuries and helped create

37

the powerful commercial brewing companies. Today's stout, while not exceptionally strong alcoholically, is notable for its high hop rate and dark colouring. This is achieved by the use of more deeply coloured malt, or from the use of barley that is not malted at all, but roasted. Guinness is a notable example of the genre.

Vegetarians and vegans should note that animal-product 'finings' are used to produce cask or 'real' ale – usually a glutinous substance made from the swim bladders and other sticky materials of different fishes; sturgeon is preferred. Finings drag yeast cells and other particles to the bottom of the cask.

Cider and wine

Cider is made from fermented apple juice. Wines are fermented grape or other plant juice. Sparkling sorts, such as champagne, undergo a secondary fermentation during which the by-product, carbon dioxide, is retained in the bottle under pressure.

Fortified wines like sherry, port, Madeira and vermouth combine wines with either brandy or neutral (see below) spirits, as well as flavourings.

Spirits

The potency of spirits, as any adult from planet earth must know, is considerably greater than either alcoholic wine (which, on average, is 10 to 12 per cent alcohol) or beer (which runs from near-zero to 10 per cent).

Spirits range from 35 per cent of the total volume to 75 per cent in the case of certain highly inebriating rums. They are made by the literal 'spiriting' away of alcohol from the flavoured base in which they sit. Alcohol boils at a lower temperature than water, so if an already fermented liquid such as grape wine is heated in a vat, the alcoholic spirit will be released before the solution that contains it can evaporate. This spirit is then trapped and cooled. Its character will depend on the style in which it is boiled off. If done quickly in a continuous process, a neutral, featureless spirit will result, such as gin or vodka. Various flavourings can then be added to pep up the taste (juniper berries for gin) or it can be sold straight, as with vodka.

If the distiller wishes to preserve the special quality of the original fermented material (grape base for brandy, barley and corn for Scotch) then the boiling-up is done more slowly, and the result is a 'noble' spirit. After distillation, the noble ones must be aged in wooden casks for several years. Malt whisky is at its best only after ten years, and the best cognacs need fifty to peak. But since such fastidious methods cannot produce a beverage within the price range of the world's masses the distillers will eke out the precious noble nectars by mixing them with cheaper, mass-produced 'neutrals'.[1] French grape brandy, for instance, is made by mixing noble cognac with industrial alcohol distilled from the European Union's wine lake; while blended Scotch, like most Irish whiskies, takes the classier route of mixing pot-stilled malt with grain whisky that has been 'continuously' produced. Also falling between the noble and neutral traditions is bourbon whiskey, popular in the States, which is continuously distilled from legally specified grain and then aged in casks. Rum can be a straight neutral, through this too is sometimes aged in wood.

Liqueurs

Liqueurs are spirits buoyed up with various and usually secret combinations of herbs. In some cases the process starts with the fermentation of herbs in sugary water – a mixture that is then distilled. Sometimes the herbs are added to the spirit after it has been extracted. Their origins lie in herbal medicines concocted in the Middle Ages.

Congeners

Congeners are chemicals vital in determining the taste, smell and appearance of an alcoholic beverage. Present in tiny quantities in virtually all drinks, they are a natural part of the fermentation process. Among the most omnipresent are tannic acid, fusel-oil, ethyl acetate, various sugars, salts, minerals and B-group vitamins. While they play no part in getting you drunk they probably contribute to many of the typical hangover symptoms – headache, wobbly stomach, vacant brain. The amount of congeners in a given drink depends on its base material as well as the manufacturing process. The drink with the lowest rating is the neutral spirit vodka. Also low in congener ratings are gin and beer. Vastly more congener-loaded is bourbon, while wine falls somewhere in the middle range. But contrary to the notion that red wines hurt more than whites, it is the latter which contain the larger quantity of an especially noxious congener called acetaldehyde.

Potency

There are three popular methods of specifying the potency of drinks: the Unit system, the proof system, and by indicating the percentage of alcohol the flavoured drink contains.

The Unit system was introduced in the 1980s as an attempt to establish a rough equivalence between different types of drinks. This work out as follows: one half-pint of ordinary beer or lager equals a single measure of spirits, which is the same as a medium glass of wine or a small glass of sherry, vermouth or aperitif. Each is said to contain one Unit of alcohol, and a 'relatively safe' weekly intake is 21 Units for men and 14 for women.

Life at ground level is more complicated, especially in these times of no- and low-alcohol wines, and knock-you-dead 'export' lagers. A more precise method of calculating the inebriating factor is via the 'alcohol by volume' (ABV) system. Check bottle and can labels for ABV numbers and accompanying percentage signs. The higher the number, the more potent the drink. If a beer is described as being 4 per cent ABV, that means in every 100 ml of its liquid there is 4 per cent of alcohol. So, half a pint (284 ml) of it will contain 11 ml of alcohol. To convert this last figure into Units, divide it by 10. Thus, the half-pint drink in question will contain 1.1 Units of alcohol. If working that out makes you dizzy consider the proof system.

This dates back to the days when spirits were graded against gunpowder. Water and gunpowder will not ignite, but alcohol and gunpowder will. When gunpowder is soaked in mixtures of alcohol and water there is a point at which enough alcohol has been added to the solution to enable it to blow up. When it reaches this point the solution has 'proved' itself and is known as 100 degrees proof (100°). This has been found to be at 57.15 per cent alcohol. However, it is possible to produce spirit drinks in excess of 100° proof as well as below it. Typical British whisky is 70° proof, which means the alcohol content is about 40 per cent of total volume. To complicate matters, the American proof system rates differently from the British. It has nothing to do with gunpowder; every 2 degrees of proof equals 1 per cent alcohol.

Sensations

Aldous Huxley had a high-minded angle on what drunkenness was all about when he wrote, 'Sobriety diminishes, discriminates and says No. Drunkenness expands, unites and says Yes. It is in fact the great exciter of the Yes function in man . . . The drunken consciousness is one bit of the mystic consciousness and our total opinion of it must find its place in our opinion of the larger whole.'

Too true. But while alcohol might excite the Yes function it also releases the No function and the Get-out-of-my-way-or-I'll-stick-you-in-the-eye function. Inhibitions that normally curdle in the belly jump out when one is drunk. It is because of this releasing action that alcohol is often called a stimulant when, physiologically, its effect is to depress the central nervous system. Disinhibition comes at low doses and most social drinking doesn't go beyond this point. In most cases the atmosphere will be all the happier for having dispensed with the leg-irons of etiquette. But in certain settings an inebriated group can perform the kind of mercilessly cruel acts that wouldn't be countenanced when sober. Its members become attracted to a certain course of action and little impressed by possible sanctions. Football hooligans are a case in point. And so is the husband and wife couple who, a court heard in February 1994[2], were inspired by drink to beat up, torment with a knife, dowse with vodka, tie with telephone cord and bundle into a cellar a South London barman – that's after the wife had had sex with the victim and the victim's girlfriend. On their way out of the pub the predatory pair grabbed £150 from the till plus a handful of pepperami sausages.

From the very first drink there will be a deterioration

41

of mental and physical performance and, as the dose is increased, these functions are progressively dulled. Death from respiratory collapse would ultimately result. On the way, memory, body co-ordination, the senses, concentration and judgment will all go.

Occasionally drivers or machine operators insist that their performance is actually enhanced by a tipple, but such claims are a product of their ailing judgment, which ails all the more as they continue drinking. The biggest boasts often come from s/he who is most hammered.

Some people exhibit more obviously drunken symptoms than others. A lot depends on social setting and the way the individual chooses to steer the experience. Someone sitting alone in a rented room is unlikely to get garrulous, witty and amorous. Similarly, a heavy drinker at work will do his/her best to conceal any signs of excess consumption. Friday night down the pub is something else. There, we are more likely to see the traditional excitement, emotion, and perhaps a little kick-fighting if the stimulation – real or imagined – is present. Men who terrorise their wives after drinking do in some respects have a pharmacologically based 'excuse' (disinhibition, lack of judgment, etc), but in reality the violence wasn't put there by the alcohol, it was simply let out. Zero Tolerance was the name of a campaign launched throughout London during January 1994. Designed to make men understand that 'domestic' violence is a crime and that women and children have the right to live free of its threat, one of the launch posters depicted a conventionally attired young man at a drinks party chatting to a woman. Above him are the words: 'He gave her flowers, chocolates and multiple bruising.'

Capacity

A person's level of drunkenness depends on the concentration of alcohol in the bloodstream. Sobriety is recovered when the alcohol is discharged. It follows, therefore, that people will get more drunk if they take in high levels quickly. It also follows that they will sooner be able to walk the white line again if they can speed the alcohol out of their bodies. In terms of alcohol absorption – which begins in the stomach and intestines and continues as blood passes from the gut through to the general circulation via the liver – we don't all start out as equals. Women show higher blood concentrations than men of the same size after drinking the same amount. That's because they have less body fluid to dilute the booze. It is also now believed[3] that women are not physically equipped, as men are, to break down a proportion of the alcohol in their stomachs before it has a chance to move on.

There are other factors that affect how drunk we get on a given amount. Food delays alcohol absorption, especially carbohydrates like bread and potatoes. But while getting drunk can be slowed or quickened, sobering up works at a steady, unvarying rate. Generally speaking, the average-sized male takes approximately one hour to reach his peak blood alcohol level after drinking a pint of beer, and another two or three hours to wipe the traces. This time-scale relates to the work-rate of the liver, the organ that metabolises 90 per cent of alcohol. The balance is peed out unchanged or excreted through the breath and in sweat. In emergency cases hospitals have been known to inject fructose – a simple fruit sugar – to speed up the metabolising, but this is risky unless done by competent trained personnel. Coffee has some merit in stunning people awake, but it won't improve co-ordination or judgment, so driving is still hazardous.

Drinking and Driving

The legally permitted amount of alcohol a driver can have in his/her bloodstream is 80 mg per 100 ml. This will usually be accumulated from about five Units of drink for a man, three for a woman; fairly smartly consumed. But since judgment and co-ordination can be impaired at much lower levels, the safest course is not to drive if you've been drinking – and that means being aware of just how long alcohol sticks around in the bloodstream, and the effect a topping-up drink can have hours after the first session.

Evidence of what happens when drivers don't heed the

43

no-drinking injunction is to be found in the journals of the Campaign Against Drink Driving (CADD). The criminal recklessness of the perpetrators is quite often matched by the trial judges who regularly hand out bafflingly low custodial sentences for multiple killers: three years and a ten-year ban for an inebriated Telford man who, it was reported in January 1994, killed three women[4]; thirty months for a twenty-year-old BMW driver who killed two little girls and, according to the *Daily Mail* (3 March 1993), was more concerned about his wrecked vehicle. 'Just look at the state of my car,' he is said to have complained, as a seven- and eight-year-old lay dying yards away after being hurled through a brick wall. The driver, who had consumed six pints of beer and was operating on a stolen, out-of-date insurance cover note, was close to his home when he took a corner at 50 mph and lost control. He hit the kerb and veered across the road into the girls. They had been skipping along the pavement.

The death toll on British roads has actually been falling during the last fifteen years, with 660 alcohol-linked fatalities registered during 1991. But while the figures compare well with other European Union countries, UK drivers are more expert than most at killing and maiming pedestrians – children especially. A third of all road fatalities are pedestrians, and two-fifths of these are youngsters. Though the deaths these pedestrian percentages represent are also down since 1970, much of the drop can be attributed to youngsters – or their parents – being too scared any longer to use the roads and pavements in the areas in which they live. In 1971, 90 per cent of junior schoolchildren made their own way to and from school. Twenty years later that figure was down to 9 per cent, many parents preferring to drive their youngsters rather than have them run over.[5]

The chairman of CADD, Derek Probart, notes in one of his *Journal* articles that we will know when road safety is being taken seriously in the UK. It will be when the government 'legislates for air-bags to open on the OUTSIDE of vehicles on impact, so as to protect the innocent pedestrian or cyclist who is mowed down by the driver's excessive speed.'

Health Effects

It need hardly be stated that the majority of people handle their drink well enough, causing no major injury to themselves or to others. This illustrates the comparatively mature attitude we have towards the drug. But when things go wrong, the implications for health can be devastating.

Hangovers

There is some debate about the part congeners play in laying on the traditional head-thumping symptoms of nausea and fragility. Some believe congeners are most of the problem, but it seems clear enough that dehydration also plays a large part. Alcohol is a powerful diuretic, prompting an increased flow of urine. As to hangover cure, the best one is to avoid further irritating the stomach with more drink. A pint of water also often helps – either cold or boiled, as though for tea.

Alcohol with other drugs

Doctors warn against taking alcohol in conjunction with most of the other central nervous system depressants such as barbiturates, tranquillisers and the opioids, since the action of one is accentuated by the other. Alcohol taken with heroin can be especially dangerous: there is the possibility of vomiting while in a coma. Alcohol also reacts adversely with the MAOI drugs (see pages 86–7), and with anti-histamines.

Body heat

Alcohol causes the blood vessels near the surface of the body to widen, leading to heat loss. For someone falling down drunk out of doors on a cold night this can prove fatal. Homeless drinkers are, of course, especially vulnerable. The elderly who drink are also more prone to hypothermia.

Long-term Heavy Drinking

In regard to longer-term effects, alcohol is associated with numerous illnesses either as the actual cause or as a complicating factor. Estimates for the number of premature deaths drinking causes vary greatly, although the government seems to favour the figure of 28,000[6] every year. This would include deaths from alcohol-related psychoses, over-dosing, heart and liver disease, cancers, suicides, and vehicle smashes.

Nutritional and digestive troubles may be the first signs of illness arising from prolonged heavy drinking. For although alcoholic drinks do contain small amounts of iron and magnesium, their principal value is as a sugar, i.e. empty calories. Alcohol can also stop the body absorbing and using vitamins – especially thiamine, other B vitamins and vitamin C. Consumed on top of normal eating, drink will deliver excess flab. Taken instead of food – which is the way with many serious drinkers – malnutrition will follow. This can be aggravated by further loss of appetite as a result of inflammation of the stomach lining (gastritis), or by poor absorption from the gut caused by irritation of the bowels. Vomiting, nausea, loss of appetite and diarrhoea are common warning signs of damage. But gastritis will invariably settle quickly if the stomach is not exposed to the irritant effects of more booze.

Ulcers. While it cannot be definitively demonstrated that ulcers of the lining of the gut (duodenal and gastric) are caused by drinking, they are certainly associated with it.[7] Ulcers may burst or bleed and require an emergency operation which the problem drinker is in poor shape to withstand. If drinking, as well as smoking, continue, the chances of an ulcer healing are greatly diminished.

Pancreatitis. The pancreas gland lies in the upper back of the abdominal cavity where it secretes enzymes necessary for digestion. Also associated with it are cells that produce insulin, the hormone that controls sugar levels in the body. Pancreatitis occurs when the gland is inflamed and, while it has many causes (infection and the use of certain drugs such as steroids and thiazide diuretics), serious alcohol consumption is heavily implicated. The main symptoms are vomiting and abdominal pains, and unless heavy drinking is stopped life expectancy is greatly curtailed.

Liver disease. The liver is the organ that probably suffers most from heavy, long-term drinking. The harm done falls into three main categories: fatty liver, alcoholic hepatitis, and cirrhosis.

The first is where the liver swells as a result of alcohol blocking its ability to metabolise fat. When drinking stops the liver usually returns to normal and, while symptoms are rarely serious (nausea, pains, bowel problems), alcoholic fatty liver does kill around forty people a year.

Alcoholic hepatitis is a more serious condition, whereby the liver becomes enlarged and tender and the sufferer experiences a range of symptoms including loss of appetite, fever, tiredness, and pain on the right side of the abdomen. The destruction of liver cells the disease causes might lead to liver failure and/or play an important part in the development of cirrhosis. However, not all heavy drinkers fall prey to the condition, even after decades of boozing, and in about 10 per cent of sufferers the condition seems to remedy itself.[8]

Cirrhosis, the best-known consequence of heavy, long-term drinking, usually takes from ten to fifteen years to develop. It is a progressive and potentially lethal condition in which changes in the fat content of the liver damage its cells, which are then replaced with scar tissue. The problem with scarring is that it obstructs blood supply to those areas responsible for producing and storing nutrients. Alcohol is not the sole cause of liver cirrhosis. Indeed, some researchers prefer to blame it on malnutrition, pointing to a high incidence among prisoners-of-war. Nonetheless, as with smoking and lung cancer, while the relationship isn't exclusive, it's a close one – best illustrated by the way in which graphs showing the ups and downs of alcohol consumption over a period of years show a broadly parallel rise and fall in the number of fatal cirrhosis cases.[9]

Women have a special problem with cirrhosis, in that they are more prone to get it in the first place and their chances of survival are, subsequently, less than men's.

The brain. Studies of living alcoholics and post mortem examinations of their brains indicate that the great organ shrinks from years of imprudent drinking.[10] The result is intellectual impairment – failing memory, sluggish thinking, and conversation that is repetitive and unresponsive to other people's input. If not gone too far, and if drink is given up, the process seems gradually to reverse itself.

Cancer. While still argued over in medical circles, evidence[11] for high alcohol intake moderately increasing the risk of certain cancers is looking fairly convincing. The parts most vulnerable are the tongue, mouth, throat and voice box (particularly when booze and tobacco are used together), the liver and breast.

Heart disease. Heavy drinking does the heart no good but moderate consumption might be better than total abstention. Regarding heavy use, it seems this weakens the heart's pumping action and may cause something known as congestive heart failure, characterised by shortness of breath, swelling of the ankles, and blueness in the fingers and toes. It may also prompt abnormal heart rhythms, although rarely of a serious nature. Evidence that moderate drinking might afford protection against coronary heart disease (CHD) – the cause of angina and heart attacks – has cheered up those who feel we are too thoroughly fussed over by 'the health lobby'. The 'lobbyists' don't deny that the data show[12] it is probably better to drink a little than nothing at all, but warn that all kinds of factors might be skewing the figures.[13] Lifelong abstainers, they point out, might well have chosen their course because their health was already compromised. Another category of abstainer – the former alcoholic – is also likely to be already damaged.

Peripheral neuritis. This is another major physical ailment resulting from heavy use, a condition that has alcoholics missing their step and crashing to the ground. Basically, it's about nerve fibres being starved of vitamins and, as a result, failing to perform properly. The condition mainly affects the toes, feet, fingers and hands. It starts with tingling and progresses to numbness. Treatment is by rest and vitamin B therapy.

Sudden deaths. As with other central nervous system depressant drugs, an extremely high dose of alcohol quickly consumed can kill. There is no amount you can point your finger at and say: this much is lethal. It depends on constitution and how much tolerance has been built up. However, anything in excess of one bottle of spirits in one bout and death is a possibility.

Alcohol and Pregnancy

Babies, being a product of their parents and everything they consume, run a risk of damage when one or both of those parents indulges in heavy drinking. So far, practically all measurements and research have been done in respect of women, but if the child can have its father's nose it can also bear the mutagenic scars of its father's alcohol habit – transmitted via the sperm.

The effects on the developing foetus of the woman continuing to drink is a heavily contested matter. Even consumption of 7 to 14 Units a week, according to a California study,[14] can double the risk of miscarriage (although this study has been challenged on the grounds that many of the women under-played the amount they drank); and work at three British hospitals seems to show that drinking more than 10 Units a week doubles the risk of having an underweight (i.e. more feeble) baby.[15]

But the most carefully examined consequence of heavy parental drinking is what is known as Fetal Alcohol Syndrome (FAS), a leading cause of 'inherited' mental retardation. The term was coined in the 1970s, although the condition has been recognised for centuries. Generally, the baby when delivered will be small and light and its facial features are also distinctive: they include a small head; broad, flat mid-face; low nasal bridge; short, upturned nose; and 'mongolian' folds at the inner corners of the eyes. Mental impairment is the most serious outcome of the full syndrome. A link with alcohol appears proven, although calculating the incidence is replete with problems, not least because the condition is not always immediately recognisable and there is not much effort, later on, put into either keeping count or finding out what happens to the children long-term. An exception was the study conducted by a team of German and Swiss doctors[16] which involved following the progress of sixty youngsters for ten years. They found that the facial malformations diminished with time but the head and the child him/herself remained small. 'Mental retardation' was the main, persisting problem, and 'environmental and educational factors do not have strong compensatory effects on the intellectual development of affected children.'

49

Emotional Impact

Apart from this catalogue of physical hazards, alcoholism also inspires a range of maladies that affect the emotional life of the user and those closest to him/her. Typically, there can be anxiety, panic, depression, guilt, paranoia, morbid jealousy, memory blackouts, agitation and, quite often, violence visited upon the spouse. It is not an exaggeration to say that the impact on the home life of a heavy drinker is the heaviest of all.

Alcoholism

Alcohol is much like any other potent mind-altering drug in that a proportion of those who use it will return to it too often and with too much relish so that a tolerance to the desired effects develops. If this attachment isn't controlled the tendency is to keep on increasing the dose, which strengthens the bond and weakens the mind and body. A point is reached where to be without the drug is to suffer deprivation. This syndrome can be called dependence or addiction, but in the case of alcohol it has more usually been called alcoholism. An equivalent term would be heroinism or benzodiazepinism. Since the 1960s alcohol dependence has often been thought of and treated as a disease – one that can be defined in medical terms.

The disease idea was a reaction against older notions that said heavy drinkers were bad or weak people, but the notion is falling from fashion. 'Disease', it is now argued, is a rigid concept that promotes rigid systems for dealing with it. It suggests some alien factor eating away at the passive victim, whereas alcoholism actually allows for a host of psychological and physical moving parts which vary from person to person and over which the 'victim' can and does have control. More contentiously, it is now being stressed that total abstinence may not be a realistic goal for some chronic drinkers; it would be better to get the dose down and steady. This coincides with the intellectual drift among workers dealing with other drugs, for whom the watchwords are *harm reduction*.

Withdrawal

Once a person becomes physically dependent on alcohol the problems incurred by suddenly withdrawing the supply are as severe as from any other drug. They are almost identical to the results of abrupt barbiturate withdrawal, including the risk of convulsions, hallucination, and delirium. The first symptoms can occur a few hours after the last drink, typically with the morning shakes. A drink will steady these. If one is not forthcoming the alcohol addict will get increasingly jumpy and agitated, unable to hold a cup or tie a lace. While in the throes of the shakes something like a quarter[17] will suffer accompanying hallucinations. They'll probably be short-lived and take the form of distorted shapes, moving shadows, snatches of music, or shouted remarks. In this state, note Kessel and Walton in their classic little volume *Alcoholism*,[18] the sufferer will be prone to reading threats into the most casual glance or remark from innocent bystanders. More awesome still is the condition known as *delirium tremens*. This, they say, 'is one of the most dramatic conditions in the whole calendar of medicine.' Kessel and Walton's own description cannot be bettered.

'The symptoms are florid. There is great restlessness and agitation. In the hospital ward the patient, weak as he is, may have to be restrained by two or more people before he can be got into bed. He is never still, tossing and turning restlessly, constantly engaged in conversation, switching from person to person, from subject to subject at the smallest stimulus and frequently shouting salutations and warnings to distant passers-by. His hands, grossly tremulous, clutch at the bed-clothes; continuously he tries to pluck from them imaginary objects, shining silver coins, burning cigarettes, playing cards or bed bugs. He is prey to ever-changing visual hallucinations and may shield his face from menacing or attacking objects, animal or man. He is completely disorientated. He may not know where he is, the time of day, the date or the month.

'No words can do justice to the picture of fully developed *delirium tremens* during the hours or days before the patient falls exhausted into a deep sleep. He generally emerges from this little worse and with his memory for the recent events mercifully blunted.'

Left to run their course, the DTs generally last three to four days, but drugs can ease the suffering. The main dangers arise from other illnesses that might be present at the same time, and from possible convulsions. They can prove fatal if unattended. Other frequently registered causes of death during the DTs are a critical drop in blood sugar, uncontrollably high temperature, and shock.

Earliest Use

To trace the history of alcohol consumption is to trace the origins of the human race itself. The natural fermentation process was probably discovered by humans in prehistoric times and would soon have been followed by the conscientious production of wines and beers from sugary and starchy plants[19]. Among the first historical accounts of wine-making is that found on an Egyptian papyrus dated 3,500 BC. Enthusiasm for the craft is also to be found in the Finnish epic, the *Kalevala*, where the 'good beer' is praised as the beverage that 'sets women to laughing, puts men in good humour, the righteous to making merry, fools to joking.' Around the world, inebriating beverages became central to every kind of religious, social and personal event – from crownings to war-making, from births to funerals. But while the socially solidifying benefits of alcohol were properly appreciated, so were its 'evils'.

The distillation of spirit is thought to be a mere 1,000 years old, although it wasn't until the late 1880s, with the introduction of improved transportation and mass production of bottles, that the first internationally famous brands emerged – Martell, Hennessy, Haig and Johnny Walker. The common folk of Britain have supped on nut-brown ale for centuries; it was as much a staple as bread and was said to be the difference between the imperial Briton

52

and the insipid continental. Between 1720 and 1750 the gin epidemic took hold, during which establishments vied to produce the cheapest and most explosive beverages, and supplied premises where the recipient could lay himself down until the faculties recovered. Artists such as Hogarth and Cruikshank presented famously dramatic evocations of the depths to which the gin-sodden lower orders had sunk, but a little research reveals that the upper classes – who preferred brandy and wine – were merely better at masking or politely ignoring their own degeneracy.[20] The worst gin-related excesses were checked by an Act of Parliament in 1751 which put a high tax on the drink and curbed its retail sale. But even after this move – which was accompanied by riotous protest – up to an eighth of all London adult deaths were said to have been caused by excessive spirit-drinking.[21]

The introduction of coffee and tea helped sober the population, but a great liquor resurgence came about during the Industrial Revolution. For the toiling, uprooted masses of the chaotically expanding cities, drink seemed the logical recourse. In the latter part of the nineteenth century the national binge inspired temperance movements, with doctors, clergy and other moral upholders imploring the public to acquire better habits. Closure of public houses between midnight on Saturday and noon on Sunday came in 1848 for England and Wales, and by 1872 there was a ban on weekday drinking between the hours, roughly, of midnight and 6a.m.

The modern system of licensing and opening hours developed through the Defence of the Realm Act(s) of the 1914–18 war. In 1921 they were consolidated under the 1921 Licensing Act which handed over powers to local magistrates. From this emerged the basic pattern of nine hours' drinking per day divided into two sessions – one from about 11a.m. to 2p.m., the other from 5.30p.m. to 10.30 or 11p.m. More modifications came in 1961 and 1964. Then in 1976 came the hotly debated Scottish reform which relaxed the whole system of opening times north of the border. Under the new measures, individual premises could apply to open earlier, close later, and trade all afternoon, Sundays included. The intention was to appease tourists and lure families in to upbeat establishments. It was also done to eliminate the afternoon chucking-out ritual in the hope that the sum total of noise and aggravation would be reduced. The Scottish experiment was scrutinised minutely. Were people getting sicker and acting more violently and recklessly as a result of the longer drinking hours? The answer depended upon the disposition of those turning over the data. Ultimately, it was officially decided that no additional harm was being done and, with the passing of the 1988 Licensing Act, broadly the same regime was introduced in England and Wales. The relaxed rules meant that some eighteen and a half extra hours were gained by drinkers and publicans – though the compulsory Sunday afternoon siesta still survived. As in Scotland, there are no obvious signs, as yet, of negative health fall-out.

Patterns of Use

It might be supposed that consumption of alcoholic drinks would have slumped in the last thirty years on account of the vastly increased use of a range of more exotic mind-bending substances, such as are described elsewhere in this book. But total booze use rose by more than 30 per cent between 1961 and 1991, with wine, spirits and cider all showing healthy gains[22]. The exception was beer. In all retail outlets, ale was performing badly. In pubs and clubs (as distinct from supermarkets and off-licences) sales, since 1979, have fallen by a full quarter.

Much of the reason is to do with price. A pub pint is expensive compared with a supermarket-purchased can of beer. But pubs are also having problems adjusting to the tastes of new generations of drinkers who have other pulls on their time, or maybe just want to stay at home and down a four-pack of export lager in front of the video. In recent years pubs have resorted to flash electronic games and flash food to supplement the primary recreational pursuit of boozing. They are offering karaoke nights, strip shows, and Belgian lagers. Many are returning to ye olde cask-conditioned traditional ales. But they are still falling away. Some 3,000 pubs closed in England and Wales between 1989 and the end of 1993, leaving around 57,000.

When it comes to regional preferences, Scotland likes its beers dark and sweet while in the West Midlands, Wales and the North-West they still go for old-fashioned mild in a big way. Everywhere, continental-style lager is supplanting the more traditional ales, although having claimed a little over half the beer market by the end of the 1980s, sales fell back a fraction in the early nineties.

Overall spending by what the statisticians call 'households' peaked in 1975 when booze represented more than 5 per cent of all outlay. It has since fallen. But we still spend much more than we did in the 1950s and twice as much on drink as on cigarettes – with the poorest, least skilled groups spending the biggest share of their income on alcohol.

Although women drink less than men (and have fewer alcohol problems) the average woman's consumption, after increasing in the 1970s, has remained constant since 1978, whereas the average male's has declined.[23]

The habits of youth are a perennial source of anxiety. *What next!* Having worked through a series of substance panics throughout the 1980s, from glue to heroin, the media discovered the 'lager lout' towards the end of the decade. It was a particularly volatile time in terms of the social climate. Yuppyism – the triumph of easy money for those who were well connected and could play the game – was at its apogee; while in the poorer, neglected parts the sense of bitter resentment overflowed. The country had been getting used to 'black' inner city riots since 1981 (the fact that whites often took part was usually ignored), but in 1987 a new phenomenon was identified: the non-urban 'white riot'. Even in the sleepy Caucasian towns and villages of the Home Counties, large-scale bust-ups were occurring, often where a licensed club or disco spilt out into an all-night fast-food joint. A chief inspector with the Thames Valley force told me that in the last eight months of 1987, a total of 1,000 youths had been involved in pitched battles with police on dozens of different occasions. Why, it was being asked, was the best of British white youth behaving so? But closer examination revealed that the participants weren't so different from their inner-city contemporaries when factors such as social class, education and career prospects were considered. Sections of youth in England's deep south and in small towns elsewhere were just as aimlessly disgruntled as the better-publicised outcasts and rebels of the big cities.

Is British youth drinking more and more recklessly? As always, it depends where and how you look. Throwing all the data into one pot the answer comes out that 'most [adolescents] drink in moderation . . . and the stability of alcohol use among this age group is emphasised by a succession of studies which indicate the normality of alcohol consumption among its members . . .'[24] This is a possibly accurate though bland account of what is taking place. Many young people now regard drink as just one item in a repertoire of mind-bending substances from which they demand a good value-for-money blast. They will judge a pint against, say, the psychoactive clout of a £2 LSD blotter. The brewers know this, or perhaps sense something of the sort, and are responding with a range of cheapish, super-potency lagers and sweet ciders; also with fruit-flavoured designer drinks (orange, strawberry, red grape) with names like 20/20, whose alcohol content exceeds 13 per cent and which are sold in hip flask-type bottles with a screw top and straw.

In studying 'cohorts' of young people in his home patch of Greater Manchester, social work professor Howard Parker deduced that 'the initiation to public drinking for contemporary youth is increasingly with alcohol-potent designer drinks. And from our younger cohort [came] almost identical reports. For example, the favourite drink for 15 year old girls is Diamond White: 8.2 per cent alcohol by volume, a sweet, sparkling cider and easy to drink. If you can only get alcohol from the off-licence then Thunderbird is another designer drink, 13 per cent by volume, targeted specifically at the teenage market in my opinion.'[25]

Parker suggested new looks at taxation, at the behaviour of the brewing industry, and the nature of health education. Overcoming the disincentive for young people to consume soft drinks in pubs might also have been usefully included on Parker's *To Do* list. A 1993 investigation by the Campaign for Real Ale found that a pint of orange juice was costing £2.77, while the same amount of mineral water might be priced at an equally unappealing £2.46.

Where drinking does spiral out of control, the seeds of the problem can often be seen, in retrospect, to have been planted surprisingly early in childhood. Philip – now twenty-two – was thirteen when, at a family celebration staged in a London hotel, he went too heavy on the sherry and wound up semi-comatose and vomit-stained in the lavatory. He was the only one of a couple of dozen invited youngsters to get in such a state.

'It was a definite intention to get drunk that evening,' he recalls, 'although I definitely didn't anticipate getting ill – just being naughty, I suppose, was the main attraction. After that, I just stood about on the streets drinking, and by the time I was fifteen I had become a regular in the pub in the part of north London where I lived, and I do mean regular – which is slightly disturbing for someone that age.'

There were run-ins with the police and scenes of extreme emotional drama with his perplexed parents. He quit school early and, in a tough labour market, bounced in and out of a series of unsatisfying jobs.

'Even though I caused havoc at home, I think my concerns were pretty selfish at the time. But when I moved out and suddenly bills were to be paid and I was still getting drunk and not paying them, that's when I saw what I was into. It's not unusual to spend £30 during a session, which in my financial situation should never happen. Even when I have earned OK money I never got round to buying myself my own hi-fi or my own TV. I'm in a squat now, which I did out really nice with a friend and turned into a home. But that's not looking too secure any more.'

Philip is an intelligent and attractive personality. Why does he drink to excess? His dad has a good thirst, although dad has never let it run away with him. And there is also the suggestion of mild dyslexia, which clouded Philip's performance in the classroom and bruised his self-esteem.

'I think basically I'm quite a negative bloke and do expect things to be handed to me on a plate, which I know is not a good thing to expect, and why I drink is because they don't get handed to me on a plate. Perhaps it's just an easy option – easier than doing all the other things you think about doing. You kid yourself you can run away from your problems, but they always appear again. They always land on you.'

Philip believes equilibrium will enter his life if two things come his way: a girlfriend and financial security. The chances of either happening, he recognises, remain less likely for as long as booze is at, or near, the centre of his existence. It's this self-awareness which offers him his best chance; that and

57

the example – all too visible these days – of what befalls a career drinker who slips down the chute.

You see them around the city centres and railway terminals up and down the country – the seriously drunk street homeless. Living by the Giro and the soup run, they bounce from police cell to magistrate's court, back on the street to be re-arrested, with none of their underlying problems ever attended to. Nor is there satisfaction for local residents, who invariably associate their *nfa* (no fixed abode) neighbours with rowdiness, aggressive begging, and mountains of discarded beer cans.

The 1971 government-commissioned Weiler committee called for a network of detoxification and recovery centres to which street drunks could be brought by the police as an alternative to being banged up in cells. But nearly twenty-five years later there are just two in the whole country – in Manchester and in Leeds – with a third planned for London's King's Cross.

The Leeds project, run by St Anne's Shelter and Housing Action, is an integrated service encompassing a first-stage detox centre, as well as a twenty-two-bed temporary-stay hostel on the same site, and a number of houses and flats that offer twenty more places for those who have gone further down the road to independence.

The first of half a dozen customers I saw arriving during a visit in the summer of 1993 initially had to be checked every thirty seconds to make sure he didn't asphyxiate. The police had delivered him from the back of a transit van, then waited while two of the three St Anne's staff on duty that evening donned rubber gloves and searched his pockets for booze, drugs, and hidden weapons. One held him as he retched up something that looked like straight Newcastle Brown into a big stainless-steel dish. (In fact, most of it went on the floor.) Then they tucked him up in bed the way Mum would have done.

Eighteen of the twenty-two hostel beds were occupied that night. Among the residents was Eric J, a forty-five-year-old former pipe layer with British Gas, who thanked St Anne's for allowing a man to be less than perfect. 'If you ever slip up twice they don't throw you out like the others do.' And there was forty-seven-year-old Tony W, a Sussex-born former keyboards player who used to work the P & O liners and the northern clubs before booze brought him down. It lost him his wife and two children and, looking back, he says he now sees that the problems started in his early teens. He had been at the St Anne's hostel nine weeks – sober the whole time and currently taking a business administration course. 'Here, they give you all the encouragement you could want, all the advice you could seek, and nothing is rammed down your neck.'

As we spoke, the police delivered new bodies to the adjacent detox unit. Some came in raging, others dropped to their beds with barely a murmur. There was a seventy-three-year-old white-haired man called Maurice who had got drunk consuming miniatures on the train up from London. He awoke in the early hours and treated the night staff to an unintelligible soliloquy about frozen pipes and prickly things outside his window. And there was Barry M, who arrived retching, coughing and demanding Librium. His reputation on the street was as an enforcer for a gang of loan sharks who preyed on homeless drinkers. Like several of the other overnight residents, Barry was off soon after first light – probably to a local grocer-cum-off-licence that sold over-priced booze from around 6.30a.m.

St Anne's recognises that there is something of a circuit-dance in operation even within their own set-up – in and out of drunken episodes and different kinds of accommodation. But at least, their social worker, Ian Harris, told me, 'we're lessening the physical and psychological damage they do themselves, as well as the problems they can cause the whole of society. The fact that the level of assaults on staff and other clients is so low here is a lot to do with the way we accord these people respect and dignity from our first contact. They might have drinking and homeless problems but it doesn't mean their value systems are wrecked.'

The Industry

They might not have the cultural or economic sure-footedness of bygone days, but the countries of the European Union are still exceptionally good at producing and consuming booze.

59

EU countries have around an eighth of the world's population yet account for half the recorded production of alcohol. The five leading world exporters of alcoholic beverages are all EU members – France, the UK, Italy, Germany and Spain – and the people of France are the world champion boozers, with an annual consumption rate equivalent to 12.4 litres per head of pure alcohol.[26]

The UK comes in at number twenty, after countries such as Hungary, Germany and Australia – but ahead of the Republic of Ireland, notwithstanding all those gormless Paddy jokes that presuppose the Irish are bigger piss artists than the British. It is also worth noting that, whereas the drinks appetite in the majority of European countries is receding – France drastically so – the UK's, in the last twenty years, has got bigger.

It seems we would consume more still if it weren't for a punitive tax regime which the brewers say penalises beer and the distillers insist hurts whisky, gin and brandy sales. Both are right, depending on how you read the figures: spirits *are* taxed almost twice as severely as wine and beer per litre of pure alcohol; but, since 1979, beer tax has risen 52 per cent in real terms and the beer market as a whole has, correspondingly, dropped 15 per cent.

The Brewers' Society, in a November 1993 pre-Budget appeal to the Chancellor, demanded a phased-in, two-thirds reduction of beer duty to bring the rate in line with the European average. If it wasn't done (which it wasn't) everyone would feel the pain, including the Exchequer, since now there were the fiscally injurious 'booze cruises' to worry about – jaunts by Britons to French ports where they were loading up caseloads of low-taxed beer and wine that were often a third of the price back home. The government's own estimate was that it was losing between £25 and £470 million a year in tax revenue, while the supermarkets claim to be down 10 per cent on their alcohol sales due to the cross-Channel competition.[27]

The health campaign group, Alcohol Concern, were unconvinced by these pleadings and produced a bundle of charts to show how drink is now more affordable in the UK than it's been for years. This, their figures show, translates into higher consumption which means more death, injury and economic loss.

Rather than reduce beer taxes, Alcohol Concern suggested 'levelling up' duties on beer and wine to match those on whisky. This would stick about eighteen pence on a pint and eighty-six pence on a bottle of wine. Even though, according to AC's calculations, the Exchequer would benefit by about £1.95 billion a year, the Chancellor resisted.

But the most avidly debated industry issue of recent years has been the 1989 Monopolies and Mergers Commission (MMC) inquiry into the brewing industry and the peculiar after-shock that has resulted.

The MMC found that the big brewers weren't playing fair. Six of them dominated production and also controlled most of the English pubs. Beer prices were rising ahead of inflation. And the brewers' own pub tenants got an uneven deal owing to their lack of bargaining power. Even landlords of 'free houses' were under the brewers' thumb since many had taken big loans from them.

In response to the MMC report the government ordered that the Big Six dispose of a total of 11,000 pubs and allow their remaining pub tenants to sell a 'guest beer'. The tenants would also get added security, as from July 1992, under the Landlord and Tenants Act.

What followed from this apparently sound set of measures? 'Beer is now more expensive,' according to Paul Vallely writing in the *Daily Telegraph* (20 November 1993) 'and sales have fallen, several [independent] breweries have stopped making beer, thousands of pubs have closed, hundreds of publicans have gone bankrupt and a number committed suicide. Instead of the big six brewers controlling 76 per cent of all beer production there is now a big five, controlling 82 per cent. Government intervention has cost the industry, according to City analysts, around £500 million with no serious benefit to the average drinker.'

Booze, fags, food and hotels look increasingly like one mega-industry, with a handful of key corporations dominant in all four sectors. Their tentacles not only reach into numerous foreign territories, they reach into each other, by virtue of a series of complex brand-sharing and property-leasing deals that make it difficult to tell where one hyphenated corporation ends and the next one begins.[28]

The three major British spirits companies together produce nearly one in three of the world's best-selling brands, with

Grand Metropolitan advancing the most powerful portfolio; it includes eleven of the world's top 100 favourites. Smirnoff vodka, J & B Rare whisky, Gilbey's gin, and Bailey's Irish Cream liqueur are all Grand Met lines. Other group interests include the Burger King chain and the Pillsbury food company.

Aside from its famous black stout, **Guinness plc** is responsible for Johnnie Walker, Dewars and Bells whiskies, Gordon's and Booths gins, and Cossack and Skol vodkas.

The third UK spirits giant is **Allied-Lyons**, whose brand portfolio takes in Teachers, Canadian Club and Ballantines whiskies, and Beefeater gin. The group also controls the international food operation, J. Lyons, Baskin Robbins ice-cream, and Dunkin donuts.

The Big Six pub-owning brewers, prior to the 1989 MMC shake-up, are now five: **Bass**, with around 23 per cent of the market; **Carlsberg–Tetley** (18.5 per cent); **Courage** (16.5 per cent); **Scottish & Newcastle** (14.5 per cent), and **Whitbread** (13.5 per cent).

All are discovering that they can garnish their profits by selling 'real' cask-conditioned ales, especially when they parade them as 'premium' products. Designer lagers are another lucrative line and there are now around 300 brands to choose from. Some are home-made, others sold in the UK on licence from continental brewers. But it is the companies' growing enthusiasm for 'branded catering' which is providing the most useful returns of recent years. The following is a *sample* of who owned what as of January 1994:

Bass – Holiday Inns (the world's largest hotel chain), 147 Toby Restaurants, five American-theme eateries, plus company catering set-ups in more than 1,000 of its Bass Taverns

Scottish & Newcastle – 1,600 Chef & Brewer houses (acquired a few months earlier from Grand Met), 50 T & J Bernard traditional ale and food houses, and 15 Home Spreads restaurants targeted at the family trade

Whitbread – the UK's second biggest restaurant chain after McDonald's, with 275 Beefeaters, 22 Pizza Huts (a joint venture with Pepsico), and 200 Brewers Fayre traditional pub grub units. Its spring 1994 stock market value was nearly £3 billion and it employs some 62,400 people

Help

Bad drinking habits derive from a dangerous spiral. They could have their roots in social ritual that got out of hand, or in pain. They can arise from biological pre-disposition or from the example of peers and parents. Good drinking habits come from understanding – understanding what alcohol is and its potential for good and for harm. Good habits also grow out of self-awareness and the determination to confront problems and overcome them in a healthy way.

Self-help

Professional help is no guarantee of success in dealing with a drink problem. Many people choose to help themselves and do very well. Here are some tips.[29]

- You may already have tried and failed to quit several times. That doesn't mean you'll fail this time. Circumstances don't remain the same, and nor do you.
- Decide if you're going to reduce or entirely eliminate drinking.
- Be clear about the reasons for the change (i.e. it will improve my health, make my friends/family happier). Perhaps jot them down on paper and take a look when you're feeling weak.
- Stay clear of – or rehearse coping with – haunts, people and situations that could trigger a relapse.
- You might need special help for the withdrawal period itself – especially if you've no one to keep a close check on you and/or if you've previously had serious

withdrawal symptoms such as fits, hallucinations, and severe shaking.

- Cut down gradually rather than stopping abruptly. The worst symptoms – restlessness, trembling, can't sleep – come in the first two days and will mostly have passed after a week. Don't miss meals, drink plenty of fruit juice and water. Take warm baths, go for walks, relax with music, keep busy around the house. Sleep will be disturbed but should return to normal after a month or so. Withdrawal is just the start of the road to recovery. See the addresses at the back of this book for help in the months and years that follow.

Professional Help

There is a range of statutory services to call upon, financed by central as well as local government. There is also an important voluntary sector which – as in the non-alcohol drug field – constantly walks a fiscal tightrope. The main plank of the government's response is the (roughly) 25 Alcohol Treatment Units (ATUs), which are usually sited in the psychiatric departments of major hospitals. All offer detoxification programmes. Some also lay on good support, counselling, therapy and follow-up. Others pitch out their patients – following a detox – ill equipped to head off a relapse and without a clue as to where to find other support. ATUs have never succeeded in serving the whole of their designated catchment areas and so other hospitals sometimes take it upon themselves to service the problem drinker either in the psychiatric or general wards.

GPs also lay on a service of sorts but, like social workers, they tend to be less able to recognise drink-related problems and/or unwilling to get involved. Probation officers are more sharp-sighted and the probation service does get involved in the running of special hostels. But it is through the voluntary sector – that part which is neither securely funded nor responsible under statute – that the major facilities are laid on. There are, for instance, about 100 alcohol advice centres providing information, advice and counselling as well as referral to special care facilities. A person may simply show up with or without a doctor's letter. The scale of these operations varies enormously and parts of the UK – including East Anglia, central Wales, and the East Midlands – are very patchily covered. There are also around 115 residential services in England and Wales, about three-quarters of which are run by the voluntary sector. All are for people with severe, long-standing habits, and they allow people to live in from six weeks to 18 months so that they can grapple with their problems. (The length of programme has generally been on the decrease in the last couple of years owing to a harsher economic reality.) The majority of 'residentials' require detoxification to have taken place before admission.

Alcoholics Anonymous is a mutual help group that is entirely self-funded and which organises around 2,000 small local gatherings than meet all over the country, usually weekly but sometimes more often. It works on the Twelve Steps to Recovery principle – employing an amount of spiritual deep-thinking and the unshakeable belief that alcoholism is a 'disease' rather than a simple indulgence and that the only cure is abstinence. AA's kith and kin are Al-Anon – for the families and friends of problem drinkers, and Al-Ateen – another mutual support fellowship for children of alcoholics.

Notes

1 Nicholas Faith, 'Gentlemen's War: A survey of the world's trade in distilled spirits', in *The Economist*, 22 December 1984.

2 'Barman gets beaten after sex threesome', in the *Hampstead and Highgate Express*, 2 February 1994.

3 This is according to research carried out at the Alcohol Research Centre, New York, and at the Trieste School of Medicine, as reported in the *Guardian*, 12 January 1990: 'Enzyme clue to alcohol inequality'.

4 'Driver who killed trio of women gets 3 years', in the *Daily Telegraph*, 8 January 1994.

5 *Private Eye*, 4 November 1994, p. 8.

6 This is Office of Population Censuses and Surveys data combined with other data contained in the *Lord President's Report: Action against Alcohol Misuse*, HMSO, 1991. A summary is available from Alcohol Concern.

7 I. Davies and D. Raistrick, *Dealing with Drink*, BBC Books, 1981, p. 51.

8 *The Medical Consequences of Alcohol Abuse: a great and growing evil*, Royal College of Physicians, 1987, p. 41.

9 See 'Taxing for Health', Alcohol Concern's Budget submission, November 1993. Its graphs are produced from data drawn from official government sources.

10 *Independent on Sunday* 'Second Opinion' health column by Tony Smith, 19 December 1993.

11 'Alcohol and cancer', in *The Lancet*, 17 March 1990, p. 634.

12 'Alcohol and Heart Disease: A review of the evidence', Alcohol Concern, 1993.

13 Ibid.

14 Harlap and Shiona, *The Lancet*, 2: 173–6, 1980.

15 *A Woman's Guide to Alcohol*, Alcohol Concern.

16 Hans-Ludwig Spohr *et al.*, 'Prenatal alcohol exposure and long-term developmental consequences', in *The Lancet*, 10 April 1993, pp. 908–11.

17 N. Kessel and H. Walton, *Alcoholism*, Penguin, 1965, p. 34.

18 Ibid.

19 Mark Keller, 'A Historical Overview of Alcohol and Alcoholism', in *Cancer Research* 39, July 1979, pp. 2822–9.

20 Ibid.

21 Kessel and Walton, op. cit., p. 54.

22 *Statistical Handbook 1992*, Brewers' Society.

23 *A Woman's Guide to Alcohol*, Alcohol Concern.

24 Carl May, 'A Burning Issue? Adolescent Alcohol Use in Britain 1970–1991', in *Alcohol & Addiction*, Vol. 27, No. 2, 1992, pp. 9109–15.

25 Howard Parker, 'Finding threads in the crime – alcohol tangle', in *Alcohol and Crime – Proceedings of a Mental Health Foundation Conference*, Mental Health Foundation, London, 1993, p. 43.

26 'Beer Facts 1993', Brewers' Society.

27 'Sainsbury's drinks to a first in France', in the *Guardian*, 27 April 1994.

28 The data for this section come from a variety of sources – trade journals, industry analyses, and national newspapers. Often the information presented conflicted, but I have done my best to summon up a reliable industry snapshot.

29 Most of these ideas are drawn from Jo Chick and Dr Jonathan Chick, *Drinking Problems*, Optima, London, 1992, pp. 85–92.

AMPHETAMINE

Intro

Amphetamine is a booster, hence the street names, *speed* and *whizz*. It boosts energy levels, confidence levels, and the powers of concentration by stimulating the central nervous system (CNS). And yet as much as any other drug it epitomises the maxim that there is no such thing as a free lunch: the additional zest is not conferred by the drug but is borrowed from the system's finite stocks. Thus, the inevitable aftermath of a 'speed trip' is exhaustion and depression.

This price might be considered worth paying. For instance, a truck driver hauling a load from Warrington to Bruges might find the sustained thrust of energy useful; similarly the writer trying to meet a deadline, or the young dance-scene adept who doesn't want to be inconvenienced by the need to sleep. If these individuals can repair their bodies with a long sleep or perhaps ghost-walk through some undemanding tasks over the next day or two they might estimate they got a good deal from their drug.

Certainly the pharmaceutical industry was at one time extreme in its advocacy of amphetamine products. A 1946 report[1] was able to list thirty-nine different disorders for which Benzedrine – one of the three main kinds of amphetamine – was *the* recommended treatment. These included night blindness, seasickness, migraine, and impotence. Even battle campaigners have made use of amphetamines. During the Spanish Civil War they were dispensed to overworked troops to provide verve and ferocity. Some 72 million tablets were issued to British forces during World War II,[2] during which conflagration German and Japanese forces were also being supplied. Hitler himself is said to have been unable to function without his daily injections of methylamphetamine (up to five a day plus tablets)[3] which would account for at least some of his paranoid ravings. The pattern continued with the Americans in Korea and Vietnam, by which time there had been two absolutely typical developments: first, after years of wanton mass production and mass prescription, the pharmaceutical/medical industry 'discovered' that amphetamine was excessively dangerous and suitable only for the most limited dispensing; and second, it had become an undislodgeable street favourite.

The wonder of speed is that it has kept out of the headlines for so many years (since the late 1960s). Cheaper and longer-lasting than cocaine and with a huge indigenous customer base, perhaps the drug isn't 'foreign' enough to excite pages of newsprint. The base materials come, not from an exotic shrub, but from commercial chemicals which (with some difficulty) can still be purchased on home soil. With a little ingenuity and O-level chemistry, anyone can go into the *whizz* business.

But perhaps an amphetamine panic is finally on the way. The convergence, in recent years, of several factors makes it more likely. Consistently low-quality street sulphate (5 per cent purity or less) is encouraging more users to inject rather than 'snort' so as to maximise the drug's impact. Once injecting starts, speed users, according to various surveys (see below), are not only more inclined than opioid users to share their works, they also have more sex with more partners without bothering with condoms. *Youth, a pump-me-up-drug, needles, sex, AIDS* – these are probably potent enough ingredients for a media feast.

What Is It

Amphetamine, popularly known as *speed, whizz,* or *sulph,* is a chemical compound that acts as a central nervous system (CNS) stimulant. That is to say it causes lots of activity in the CNS (composed of the brain and spinal cord), leading to arousal and a greater responsiveness to the external world. Structurally, amphetamine closely resembles the body's own chemical transmitter norepinephrine (NE) which plays an important role in the fight/flight response to stress and emotion. Amphetamine (and also cocaine) appears to mimic or enhance the action of NE in the brain and thus is able to charge up the central nervous system.

Amphetamine divides into three main pharmaceutical classes (their chief brand names are in brackets): laevo, or d'l-amphetamine (Benzedrine); dexamphetamine (Dexedrine); and methylamphetamine (Methedrine). The three vary greatly in their absolute potency with the strongest, weight for weight, being methylamphetamine. This delivers about twice the kick of dexamphetamine which, in turn, has double the force of laevo-amphetamine.

In addition to the original amphetamine compounds, numerous derivatives have been developed, some of which have been mixed with vitamins, others with CNS depressants. One of those in the up/down class was the 1960s princeling Drinamyl (Purple Heart) which became an enormous street favourite. In the 1970s its place was taken by Durophet M, which has also been withdrawn. There was once also a thriving home-made trade in upper-and-downer tablets of variable quality that were marketed as *Blues*. Occasionally, something of that name is still to be found (coloured white as well as blue). They can be crushed and injected but are usually swallowed.

Amphetamine Sulphate

By far the most common street speed since the mid-1970s has been amphetamine sulphate, containing equal amounts of laevo-amphetamine and dexamphetamine and recognisable as an off-white or pinky powder. Historically, it has always been heavily 'cut' (diluted). But by the early 1990s the purity rate was often 5 per cent or lower. The rest was milder stimulants such as caffeine, other drugs (e.g. paracetamol), or non-active substances, including baby milk and glucose. Sometimes flour and talcum powder were being used, causing potentially serious damage when injected because of their tendency to clot inside the veins.

Amphetamine is not particularly difficult to make, although in recent years access to the essential chemicals has been restricted throughout the European Union, with the UK coming down hardest. There are several methods of manufacture but the starting point is usually a material known as benzyl methyl ketone (BMK), which is converted into its corresponding amine via a process known as the Leuckardt route (named after the chemist who devised the method in 1931). Essential to the chemical broth are ammonium formate (or similar), a concentrated acid, an alkali, and a solvent such as ether. Some BMK is sneaked in from Holland but UK underground chemists have now become adept at making their own.

Ice

Methylamphetamine – usually cooked up from ephedrine, a less potent stimulant – is more rarely encountered in the UK. It appeals to injectors because, unlike sulphate, *meth* provides an initial 'rush' when administered. It usually comes as a white, adulterated powder, which can also be snorted, eaten or smoked.

Just as *meth* is not commonly seen in the UK, so there has been an even greater paucity of *Ice*, the heavily concentrated, crystallised form of methylamphetamine which is usually smoked but can also be injected. Ice was at one time thought to be running rampant throughout the US, following reports – in 1989 – of an unstoppable epidemic in parts of Hawaii. In fact, it met too much consumer resistance owing to its hammerblow effects. Reports of intense paranoia and debilitating comedowns became increasingly common and Ice vanished from the headlines.

But by November 1994 there were signs that Ice could be making genuine inroads into the UK club scene, with accounts of the drug turning up in places as far afield as Cambridge and Barrow.[4] Tabs, scored with the words 'Speed King', were being sold in Liverpool clubs, although their contents had yet to be confirmed. The appeal of Ice for clubgoers bedevilled with lousy-quality Ecstasy (cut with everything from battery acid to worming tablets) is that Ice is difficult to adulterate.

Initial going prices for UK Ice were around £15 a hit,

or £200 a half-gram. Some were smoking it in six-inch glass pipes or – more typically – from Coke cans and bottles.

Base

Elsewhere in the country (e.g. Exeter and Plymouth) something called amphetamine 'base' was on sale – a lumpy white crystal or paste of approximately 60 per cent purity. It was being used orally but, no doubt, injection and smoking would follow. Whether this was truly amphetamine minus its hydrochloride salts, or 'Speed King' in another guise, was yet to become clear. But the relative strength of this new variable portended problems to come. It might also have been some kind of marketing device designed to soften the punters up for the much more expensive cocaine *base* (i.e. crack).

Legal Amphetamine

Once prescribed by the million, there is little in the way of licit amphetamine tablets around any more. The main exception is Dexedrine, prescribed in 5 mg doses for people with the sleeping sickness narcolepsy, and – more contentiously – for the 'management' of hyperactive children.

Other Amphetamine-Like Stimulants

The main speed-related substances are listed below – although, at the time of writing, there seemed to be little evidence of them on the street.

Diethylproprion

A moderately less potent version of amphetamine which has been one of the most commonly prescribed slimming drugs, despite strong official warnings against issuing it in any circumstances.[5] The various branded versions have had a strong tradition of street use. Still available are:

Apisate – a 75 mg yellow sustained-release tablet with added B vitamins (riboflavine and nicotinamide).

Tenuate Dospan – also 75 mg sustained-release tablets but containing no additives.

Mazindol

Marketed in the UK as Teronac and in the US as Sanorex, it is another milder version of amphetamine which has been popularised by the slimming industry.

Pemoline

Less potent than amphetamine, its main prescribed use is to treat hyperactive children (with the risk that tics, mania, and uncontrolled jerkiness might result[6]). Less often it is used to counter the sleepiness of people being treated for severe pain with morphine and other opioids. Claimed by street users to stimulate the memory and the loins, the current branded product is called Volatil but it was once also marketed as Kethamed and Ronyl.

Filon

The trade name for a combination of phenbutrazate hydrochloride and phenmetrazine. The first is a mild stimulant. The second has the potency of amphetamine. Once prescribed as a slimming aid it is no longer issued in the UK though imported stock (branded Preludin) might sometimes become available.

Ritalin (chemical name methylphenidate)

Closely related structurally to amphetamine, Ritalin is a less potent stimulator of the CNS – a quality that made it a

74

drug preferred by doctors for treating hyperactive children. In adults it was prescribed for listless, senile behaviour, mild depression, and narcolepsy. In virtually every respect the drug produces the same adverse and positive effects as amphetamine, though of slightly lesser magnitude dose for dose. Street users have often described Ritalin as a 'cleaner high' and it was especially fashionable among serious 'polydrug' users who injected it as a companion to a downer. It was also mixed with the painkiller Diconal to make a speedball substitute. So popular did it become in unauthorised circles that in 1983 it was withdrawn and is now rarely seen in the UK.

Khat

The name of a green-leafed shrub, *Catha edulis*, that has been chewed for centuries by inhabitants of the Horn of Africa and the Arabian peninsula and is now turning up in Europe among emigré and refugee groups. Khat is legal in the UK but not so in countries such as Norway, Sweden, Canada, and the US.

The high is amphetamine-like (alertness, euphoria, appetite suppression) and the main active ingredient, cathinone, is held by those who study such things to be, in effect, a natural amphetamine.[7]

Despite its heavy usage there have been relatively few reported cases of psychosis,[8] detectable 'abstinence syndrome' involving major withdrawal symptoms,[9] and while one report found an association in Saudi Arabia with head and neck cancers, all those who fell sick had used the drug for at least twenty-five years.[10]

Nonetheless, khat has been the subject of some old-fashioned media scare pieces, not least in London's *Time Out* magazine which, in November 1993, ran a two-page item called 'Deadly Harvest' which described how a good proportion of the capital's Somalis were 'chewing non-stop for up to 15 hours at a time.'

During the last three decades, the piece reported, 'use of the drug has exploded in Somalia in particular where it is generally credited with exacerbating the civil war, crippling the economy and producing a work-shy generation of living zombies.'

Ninety per cent of London's Somalis, the piece declared, rely on state benefits, so a strong habit placed a heavy burden on finances. 'Our families are broken,' quoth a Somali community worker. 'Our men spend all their money. They chew all night and sleep all day. They are useless. Khat should be banned.'

Moreover, London had become the world's largest clearing house for illegally transporting the drug all over the world. Every morning, according to the magazine, at least half a ton of freshly harvested khat arrived at Heathrow from Nairobi. Within a few hours, leaf-wrapped bunches were on their way to distributors and to East London greengrocers who sell it alongside other vegetables. They have to be quick. The plant is psychoactive only for forty-eight hours after picking.

Blaming khat for the degraded condition of London's Somalis – most of whom are refugees – misses the point. And a Home Office ban on the drug, as the *TO* piece itself seemed to recognise, would simply drive khat fanciers on to more potent and expensive products (khat was on sale at just £4 a bunch).

Extracting cathinone, the active ingredient, is reported to be a complex matter, although it has already been accomplished in London and New York.[11] Precedent shows that if more legal pressure and media attention are forced upon this synthetic version of the drug, demand will rise, prices escalate and, in no time, synthetic khat or *Cat* could be mounting a serious marketplace challenge to cocaine and amphetamine. Such a development would probably see the advent of a new international demon-figure, more crazed than the Yardie, more ruthless than the South American coke baron: the *African Cat Fiend*.

Sensations

A standard 5 mg dexamphetamine tablet will yield results within fifteen to thirty minutes, which is fast for an oral drug. The lift from snorted amphetamine sulphate occurs quicker still. By either method the effects usually last for around six hours and produce similar sensations. It starts with a tickle in the gut and the feeling that energy is being pressed up through the body – clearing the mind and making it more powerful. The teeth start grinding. The jaws clench. There is a sensation of elation, confidence, and a desire to communicate fine new insights and witticisms. Libido might be raised and while sex might be more prolonged and athletic than usual, an orgasm could be hard to come by. Appetite is suppressed. There might be frequent weeing. If no more of the drug is administered there is unlikely to be more than a manageable level of fatigue and down-feeling when the effects wear off. The temptation on an open-ended weekend, or for someone without constants demands upon his time, is to sniff/swallow more as the comedown begins. This makes the rebound more severe when it does occur.

Regular Use

There are various patterns of amphetamine use, many of them producing no fundamental health risk. The drug has been especially popular in recent years on the dance scene as one of a repertoire of 'tonics' that includes Ecstasy, LSD, GHB, temazepam, and cocaine. Amphetamine's appetite-suppressing qualities makes it especially attractive to young women clubbers who might be keen to lose weight as well as jump all night. Inevitably, reports are coming through that some are falling into warped eating patterns, including bingeing, vomiting, and self-enforced starvation.

Someone drawn to speed initially because it overcomes feelings of powerlessness or social ineptitude may keep returning to it for a lasting 'solution'. Because amphetamine can't possibly deliver long-term euphoria, a ragged cycle of use is set up causing emotional and physical sensations that alternate between soaring and crashing. Once drawn into such a cycle the 'efficiency' of the needle often seems appealing. Similarly, the use of a downer such as heroin or temazepam might appear the only respite from the harshness of the amphetamine experience.

One victim of the up/down cycle is a former Salford nurse we can call Lynn. Aged thirty-five when I met her in 1994, she acquired her amphetamine habit twelve years earlier while working as a sister on the psychiatric ward of a large hospital in the north-west of England. She had been a bright child who went to grammar school on a direct-grant scholarship, then on to nurses' training in Manchester and further schooling at Lancaster University, where she developed speciality skills in drama therapy and psychotherapy.

'I had been working with people who had psychiatric problems as a result of drug-taking yet I was totally naive about the kind of effects they could have on me. Speed made me feel more alive, ten times more awake than without it. It's not that I lacked confidence, it was purely a social thing. But it starts creeping up on you, your use increases – subtly so that you don't realise it. Then you find you've got a habit. You get up in the morning and find you can't get through the day without it.'

For nearly seven years Lynn was injecting street sulphate, turning to heroin when amphetamine wasn't around or to 'deal with the psychosis brought on by the speed.' Her drug-taking partner throughout these years was the son of a senior figure with a pharmaceutical company. His own preference was Diconal. Together, they had three children, bought and lost two houses, and ended up flat broke.

For three years Lynn was prescribed amphetamine by a consultant working for a Community Drug Team – a rarity, given that there has always been nervousness about prescribing anything to addicts other than the heroin sub-stitute methadone. Her life stabilised, her consumption fell markedly. But then a new consultant took over and the speed prescription was withdrawn and replaced with one for – yes – methadone. There followed years of chaos while she sought to escape what she regarded as the malign influence of the father of her children, the man who got her taking drugs in the first place. When he died in 1990 there were no more excuses.

'I knew my own situation had to change, that my chil-dren needed bringing up properly and there was only me to do it.'

Today – still on methadone – she works for a support group for other dependent users in the Manchester area.

Taking It

Sniffing

The snorting method involves chopping up the crystalline powder so that it is fine enough not to scrape the nose. Chopping is done on a mirror or hard board with a razor blade. A thin 'line' two or three inches long is formed and this is drawn up through the nose either via a rolled-up banknote, a ballpoint case or – for those who don't care for any ceremony – without any accoutrement.

Swallowing

A method popular in recent years is to roll up a dose of sulphate inside a cigarette paper and swallow it, perhaps chased by a beer. Known as a *bomber*.

Smoking

The smokeable, supercharged version of regular cocaine is *crack*. The equivalent as far as amphetamine is concerned is *Ice*. But – to be technical – whereas crack is cocaine in its chemical *base* form, ice is chemically identical to methamphetamine; it has simply been concocted in a different physical form, having been allowed to 'crystallise up' during production. It is more concentrated than the sulphate and has the appearance of a dense, sparkly rock. Heating of the ice crystal is usually done in an incense burner or in a glass pipe. The resulting vapours are inhaled.

One of *Ice*'s peculiar properties is that, after being smoked, a small part remains in the pipe, returning to its solid state. This residue can then be reheated and the vapours once more inhaled – a feat repeatable three or four times, though with diminishing results.

The needle

Though crude sulphate can be injected by dissolving it in water and filtering it through a clean cigarette tip to remove the chalk, it is the more potent and difficult-to-obtain methylamphetamine (Methedrine) that is prized among the

79

cognoscenti. This is principally because of the exhilarating 'rush' the drug provides at the moment of injection. Practitioners claim the hit is like no other and compare it with an entire body orgasm (cocaine purists say exactly the same about their drug). The rush occurs immediately the liquid is injected and is gone within half a minute. In the US, methylamphetamine has developed something of a cult following, but since the epidemic year of 1967–68, illegal stocks have been hard to obtain in the UK.

The needle doesn't appeal to most snorters, even to those who use heavily. But, with speed having almost entirely escaped the negative onslaught directed since the mid-1980s at heroin junkies, the use of lots of speed – even via the needle – has yet to be flagged as a major problem. In fact, not only is speed far more popular than heroin, several surveys have shown that those who inject it tend to be younger and more sexually active than needle-using opioid consumers.[12] They probably share their needles more (because they're less likely to have dealings with drug agencies that offer free replacements), and the sex they have is more likely to be without a condom and with a wider variety of partners.

While there can be few functioning adults left in the UK who remain unaware of the rudimentary message in relation to HIV/AIDS (unprotected sex and needle-sharing increase the chances of infection), there is much less known about the equivalent risk of catching and passing on TB and the hepatitis strains B and C. The trouble with speed is that it tends to encourage feelings of omnipotence: *I am all-powerful, nothing can hurt me*.

Added to this is another consideration: while speed injectors might appreciate the risks, they might be too embarrassed to say no to an unwashed barrel of speed when it is passed their way – perhaps from a friend. Or they might feel unable, during the heat of slippery foreplay, to ask their sex partner to pull on a condom.

Disease risks aside, those who do take to injecting should take care to grind up as fine as possible (between spoons or with a bottle) their powder or pills. This is to avoid insoluble particles lodging in the small blood vessels at the periphery of the lungs and brain. Abscesses tend to be common among injectors, as is inflammation of the walls of the vein, and infections in or around the site the needle goes in. Any of these afflictions can be caused by adulterants in the street product, inept injection techniques, the use of unsterile needles, or by repeated use of the same spot.

The purity of street speed can be as low as 1 per cent. But there is always the chance that a much stronger batch could turn up and, if injectors are not forewarned, they could be putting serious strain on their heart or brain.

Runs

The phenomenon of the speed 'run' is well known in drug circles. It lasts for up to several days and is an attempt, by repeated injections, to hang on to the initial feelings of exhilaration and mastery. By the second day there is no more rush and the high feelings are replaced by agitation in body and spirit. Typically, these sensations intensify over the next three to five days, during which time the user probably won't eat or sleep and will usually inject more speed more often. The run ends when the supply or the user is spent. Sleep will follow – forty-eight hours or more. Upon waking there will be feelings of grogginess, depression, dehydration, and hunger – the last two because of the drug's appetite-suppressing qualities.

Amphetamine psychosis

Some individuals can trip into what the professionals call an 'amphetamine psychosis', so named because in most respects it is comparable to the symptoms expressed by schizophrenics. In both cases there are vivid auditory hallucinations as well as paranoid delusions. The drug-induced psychosis might start with a vague and not unpleasant curiosity; a desire to look beneath the surface of things.[13] Other people and their actions become entrancing and are scrutinised. But then those others appear as if they're scrutinising right back; watching and following. Noises, colours, and other stimuli are sharply experienced, which provokes hallucinations. Some people get into obsessional activities – ironing and scrubbing through the night, or pointlessly dismantling and reassembling gadgetry such as radios and bits of car engine.

An arresting account of speed paranoia appeared in *Journal of Drug Issues*,[14] as relayed by a San Francisco male sex worker/prostitute: 'You're walking down the street,' he said, 'or you're on a bus and you're kind of looking around and you automatically think everyone knows you are on this drug. Then you hear someone clapping their hands and you think they are motioning towards you and they may be two or three blocks away . . . You may see things like someone standing on the corner and you think they are following you or watching you . . . You think, so I've been walking up and down the street so many times and everyone is bound to know me now and so you're walking down the street and you see the bus go by and you know you may not be dressed for the day and everybody in the bus looks at you and the bus driver maybe honks the horn at somebody in the street and you don't know this and you think it's all directed towards you.'

The major difference between traditional psychosis and one that is speed-induced is that the drug user's symptoms will invariably vanish once the body is free of the substances – usually within a few days, rarely more than a week. Also, in amphetamine psychosis consciousness and memory generally stay clear and there is an acute appreciation of time, place, and self-identity. Such fundamentals can become murky in people classed as schizophrenic.

The onset of amphetamine psychosis is frequently related to heavy, long-term use. However, those in the novice class, but with a predisposition, are also vulnerable. A more serious problem is that amphetamine use could trigger an authentic schizophrenia in such persons who are latently inclined.[15]

Aggression

The stereotypical view of powerful stimulants such as amphetamine and cocaine is that they hype people up into an aggressive state. They get the nervous system over-reactive, induce sensory overload, leading to irritability, paranoia, and loss of judgment. While none of this is absolutely untrue, real life is more complex. Speed can actually give hitherto wound-up, insecure individuals the chemical elevation they need to help them relax. This works with aggressive adults,[16] as well as with some children who have been diagnosed as hyperactive/hyperkinetic. Alcohol (a CNS depressant) operates in much the same way. Some people want to fight on it, others become uncharacteristically smoochy-lovey-dovey.

What happens when alcohol and speed are mixed? Again, reports are varied. A man from north Essex told me speed obliterates any impact the alcohol might have on him. A North London woman user/dealer told me that she's OK if she drinks then takes speed but if done the other way round she gets into a foul-mouthed fighting frenzy (with no memory of her infelicities the next day). The Manchester drug agency Lifeline warns that combining alcohol with a couple of grams of amphetamine can assist a person who would normally have crashed out on a skinful of booze to 'stay awake long enough and retain the energy to act on drunken impulses. This is worrying from the point of view of both HIV prevention and public order and public safety.'[17]

Animal experiments

Inevitably, animals such as monkeys, cats, dogs, and rats have been subjected to all manner of amphetamine-related aggression experiments.[18] Multiple daily injections have been followed by electric shocks and other 'aversive stimuli'. They have been dosed up, 'brain-stimulated', and tormented to see how they might react. Parts of their brains have been scarred and/or removed. The treatment has continued until the subjects succumb to crazed repetitive motions, to self-mutilation, or to staring mindlessly into space – what the scientists involved call 'increasing behavioural disintegration'. That they have suffered to find an answer to a human indulgence (and there are surely plenty of habituated human subjects who could be studied on the basis of informed consent) is bad enough, but laboratory animals make hopeless 'models' of human beings and no usable answer is ever produced – only a cry for more of the same 'research'.

'The overall pattern of research', according to one authority, 'indicates that the effects of amphetamine on aggressive behaviour are complex and that these effects are not solely determined by the pharmacology of amphetamine but also seem to be determined by various environmental factors (e.g. social position and aggregation, previous experience with aggressive and submissive behaviours and, particularly, the dose and duration of amphetamine, to name but a few).'[19]

Physical Effects

Less serious

Most of the problems associated with amphetamine have more to do with the pattern of living and thinking it encourages rather than the toxic effects. In fact, amphetamine has a remarkably low toxicity and is rarely the chief substance in poison/overdose deaths. Unlike CNS depressants such as barbiturates and the opioids, amphetamine rarely causes vital body functions to close down. And an advantage it has over cocaine – a shorter-acting stimulant – is that, lacking coke's anaesthetic properties, high doses are less likely to cause respiratory depressions and convulsions.

Where overdose deaths do occur they are usually attributed to the collapse of blood vessels in the brain, to a sudden extreme rise in blood pressure, to heart failure, or to fever. A survey reporting in 1979 found that, after forty years of widespread street use, only seventy-nine such cases had been recorded worldwide and that all of these were associated with use of the needle.[20, 21]

None of this is to say that amphetamine is a drug without hazards. Long-term regular users experience chronic sleeping problems, bursts of ill-temper, persistent anxiety, malnourishment due to suppressed appetite, skin rashes, plus numerous other complaints associated with poor eating and sleeping.

Perhaps more worrying are reports of nerve and blood-vessel damage in and around the brain,[22] high blood pressure, irregular heart rhythms, and possible stroke if use continues.[23] Injury to the small blood vessels serving the eye is another reported outcome of, especially, grand-scale snorting, and this can lead (although rarely) to haemorrhage in the retina and loss of vision.[24]

Pregnancy

For general comments about pregnancy, women's health, and the well-being of the foetus see the cocaine chapter. This points out that poverty and smoking play at least as big a role as any drug in causing possible complications for the newborn. There is little specific research relating to amphetamine and much of what exists is contradictory. For instance, there is evidence both for and against an association with increased rates of foetal abnormality,[25] including cleft palate and heart deficiencies.[26] What was billed as the 'first report suggesting amphetamine as a direct cause of foetal death' appeared in the *British Medical Journal* in 1991.[27] The case concerned a twenty-nine-year-old pregnant 'amphetamine addict' who presented with abdominal pain and restlessness having injected 500 mg of the drug. 'Twenty-four hours after admission she gave birth to a stillborn infant. The baby's cord showed a high concentration of amphetamine and there appeared to be a clear association between maternal toxicity and sudden foetal death at 34 weeks.'

An intriguing Swedish study tried to discover whether the birth process itself affected the chances of the child, once grown, becoming drug dependent.[28] The records of 200 speed addicts born in Stockholm between 1945 and 1966 and another 200 hooked on opiates were studied to see whether the method of delivery had any impact. After allowing for the social status of the parents and various other factors, the investigating team concluded that the administration of nitrous oxide to ease delivery 'is a risk factor for adult amphetamine addiction in offspring.' Nitrous oxide also seemed to play a part, they declared, in the offspring developing a taste for heroin later in life, as did medical administration to the mother of barbiturates and opiates. How and why? By a process of *imprinting*. 'The unconscious memory of the drugged state at birth might make the individual more disposed to become addicted if exposed as an adult, or more prone to relapse after abstaining from the drug.'

Tolerance

Amphetamine is a drug against whose effects the body quickly builds a tolerance. This will necessitate an increasingly large dose to get stoned, but as with many other drugs the tolerance fades during gaps between use. Thus, someone who has worked up to a 1,000 mg daily dose would be unable to manage that quantity after a lay-off. Curiously, it has been found that children given amphetamine for hyperactivity, and in those administered it for the sleeping disease narcolepsy, tolerance does not develop, i.e. a rising dose is *not* required to keep them normalised. This could be due to the different rates at which the psyche and the body become tolerant. Yet overweight amphetamine users looking to suppress their appetite will find they can't keep a lid on their hunger unless they up the dose.

Dependence/addiction

Just as the lure of heroin for those who dabble in it has been over-dramatised, so the pulling power of amphetamine has been consistently understated. As with heroin, the attraction is a combination of the physical and psychological, with the user – if s/he is not wary – becoming dependent on the release of energy and confidence while feeling more and more uncomfortable during the correspondingly low periods between use. This can produce an escalating pattern of 'abuse'. When withdrawal is undertaken, the result will be precisely the reverse of what the drug was offering: instead of euphoria and the curbing of the need to sleep or eat, there will be excessive hunger and fatigue. While of a different nature from heroin withdrawal, there is no doubt that it can be equally or more distressing.

In association with other drugs

The interaction of one drug with another in the body is still little understood, but there are certain agents with which it is known amphetamine and its ilk react poorly. These include substances prescribed for high blood pressure and certain diuretics whose functioning is impaired when taken at the same time as speed.

Even more serious problems can arise from the simultaneous use of amphetamine with anti-depressant drugs of the type known as MAOIs (monoamine oxidase inhibitors). This is a fairly complex though important phenomenon: the body produces an enzyme called monoamine oxidase (MAO) naturally in the digestive juices. MAO is responsible for destroying potentially harmful fatty acids (amines) which occur in many common foods such as aged cheese, wine, pickled herrings, broad-bean pods, beer, beef extracts, avocado pears, bananas, and drinks containing caffeine-like alkaloids. If MAO didn't combat them, the toxic amines these foods contain would build up in the body, causing blood pressure to soar to a potentially fatal level.

Some drugs interfere with the MAO function and so allow amines to accumulate. Such drugs include certain non-stimulant anti-depressants, some obscure hallucinogens such as yohimbine, the harmaline alkaloids, and various tryptamines and blood pressure drugs. Patients being prescribed any of these should be clearly warned about which foods to leave alone. However, apart from reacting badly with numerous foodstuffs, the MAOIs also fail to coexist with many other drugs. They either distort the effects or cause them to hang around the body for long periods. Amphetamine is one such drug and the outcome can possibly be fatal. Other drugs to be avoided in the company of MAOIs are barbiturates, tranquillisers, sedatives, hypnotics, anti-histamines, insulin, narcotic analgesics, and more.

In association with medical conditions

Doctors warn about taking amphetamine when certain medical conditions are present – in particular, hypertension (high blood pressure), hyperthyroidism (over-activity in the thyroid gland), urinary retention, glaucoma (eye disease), arterio-sclerosis (hardening of the arteries), liver, kidney and brain disorders, and diseases of the heart.

History

Amphetamine is structurally related to the naturally occurring stimulant ephedrine (from plants of the *Ephedra* genus) and adrenalin (a bodily hormone). It was first synthesised in 1887, but it was in 1927 that its therapeutic potential was realised when it was discovered that the drug raises blood pressure, constricts blood vessels, and dilates (opens up) the small bronchial sacs. This last characteristic prompted the pharmaceutical manufacturing company Smith, Kline and French to go into the bronchial dilator business with their Benzedrine Inhaler[29] – an item of widespread abuse. Not only did asthmatic sufferers turn to the 'B-Bombs' for (short-lived) relief, it was soon learnt that the contraption could be invaded and the amphetamine-saturated wadding soaked in water, coffee or alcohol for a mighty beverage. The B-Bomb was jazz musician Charlie Parker's introduction to drugs. The Inhaler was but one of an ever-growing range of products using amphetamine during the 1930s and early 1940s. These were the decades of Depression and then global war, and it was little wonder that amphetamine tablets – known colloquially as *brain* or *pep* pills – looked to be the perfect pharmaceutical accompaniment to such dismal times. As early as 1935 the drug was being used to treat narcolepsy, whereby the sufferer lapses into sudden, unpredictable sleeping bouts. Amphetamines could keep them awake. By 1937 researchers had discovered the drug's paradoxical quality of being able to 'tame' hyperactive children.

Warnings about the drug's capacity to cause hypertension, dependence, psychosis, and suicidal depression had been voiced since 1939, yet the speed spree continued on an escalating scale for another twenty-five years. The Second World War was good news for the amphetamine industry. Some 72 million tablets were produced for British forces alone, the idea being to jag the young warriors into a scared-of-nothing, stay-awake mode. Amphetamine, it seemed, was the ultimate elixir and one medical text, in 1946, listed thirty-nine different medical uses for the drugs.[30] Until 1956, many of the amphetamine-based products were freely available over the counter. Then came prescription-only distribution, a signal that the government was no longer quite so rapturous about the drug. The one exception to the prescription rule was the street-celebrated Benzedrine Inhaler[31] – a curious exclusion since its wadding contained several hundred times the dose of amphetamine sulphate found in the average tablet. The Inhaler continued to be available not just in chemists but in general-purpose corner stores. The result was a surge in recreational usage, followed by a call from the Pharmaceutical Society for manufacturers either to withdraw their products, alter the formulation, or include indigestible additives. The trade complied.

The first great speed epidemic occurred in Japan when a hoard of amphetamine, often in injectable form and no longer needed to fuel the war effort, was dumped on the open market.[32] In Britain, the first speed 'freaks' were exhausted, isolated housewives; they were flab-fighters and people diagnosed as depressive or who were engaged in marathon work sessions. Prime Minister Anthony Eden reported that he was 'living on Benzedrine' during the Suez Crisis of 1952.[33] Other notable users were the frenetic US comedian and narcoleptic Lenny Bruce,[34] as well as that zesty, sexually active statesman John F. Kennedy, who is believed to have made regular use of injectable methylamphetamine.[35] [36]

The 'pep pill' fad among 1960s R & B mods centred on Dexedrine (*dexies*), Durophet (*black bombers*) and, more especially, a pill called Drinamyl. This was not actually a straight amphetamine but an exotic mixture of amphetamine and barbiturate. On the street the pills were called *Purple Hearts* due to their colour (blue) and their shape (triangular). The use of Purple Hearts by thousands of ordinarily wholesome youths of every class amounted to the country's first underground drugs craze of the modern era – and it scared their elders. Notwithstanding the previous widespread use via legitimate channels, the authorities now expressed great alarm. An exposé in the *Evening Standard* led to questions in the House of Commons and to a stately passage, with press in tow, through London's West End by the then Home Secretary, Henry Brooke. There followed, in 1964, the introduction of the Drugs (Prevention of Misuse) Act, which made unlicensed possession and importation of amphetamine an offence, but placed no restriction on the drug's manufacture, storage, or prescription. These constraints would have to come voluntarily from the trade itself and from GPs. The manufacturers responding by altering the shape of their product. (Young users simply switched its street name to *Blues* or *French Blues*.) Prescriptions began falling – from 4 million in 1966 to 2.5 million in 1967. But, like every drug that's pumped into the culture and then withdrawn, alternative sources developed. One was forgery of prescriptions, another was pharmacy thefts. Thirty theft cases were reported in Nottingham alone in 1968, while in Lancashire one young gang are said to have broken into twenty chemists in six weeks, netting some 30,000 tabs.[37]

By the mid-1960s London was seeing its first wave of needle-fixated cocaine and opioid users. Many used both drugs simultaneously to achieve a stronger initial rush and a smoother subsequent ride. Their source – prior to the advent of Chinese black-market heroin and South American street coke – was pharmaceutical stock, most of it prescribed by a handful of grasping or badly informed private practitioners.

By the latter part of the decade more doctors began issuing prescriptions for ampoules of injectable methylamphetamine. The epidemic year, according to a government report,[38] was 1967–68 – by which time the new methadone clinics were opening up and ordinary GPs had been stripped of the right to prescribe cocaine and heroin. For some of these physicians, dispensing injectable methylamphetamine seemed the perfect replacement. One GP, during a single month in 1968, is reported to have prescribed 24,000 ampoules of Methedrine to 100 patients.[39]

The speed prescribing habit began spreading from London and the Home Counties to other large towns. Numerous cases of 'amphetamine psychosis' began showing up in hospitals, and in Brixton prison during 1968, 400 intravenous *meth* users were logged.[40]

The youth underground movement of the day borrowed a phrase from San Francisco and warned, 'Speed Kills'. The trade itself reacted by withdrawing general supplies of injectable methylamphetamine and confining the product to hospitals only. The fad was efficiently curtailed. At Brixton prison in 1969, not a single intravenous *meth* user was registered.

Similar moves were being made in regard to the far larger trade in amphetamine tablets. Through a combination of self-discipline[41] and government threats, prescriptions for speed tablets and other CNS stimulants began falling – from more than 5.5 million in 1966 to 3 million-plus five years later.

But, as we keep seeing, once the taste for an intoxicant has been whipped up, no amount of curtailment or penalising will remove it. To replace those pill stocks previously derived from GPs and the ampoules of *meth* available from that small coterie of mainly London practitioners, a thriving underground market in amphetamine sulphate developed. Today it remains the undisputed market leader in the high speed stakes – probably the second most popular drug after cannabis.

Current Use

Amphetamine has been discredited as a palliative in all but two major areas of medication – narcolepsy and for hyperactive children. While there is little argument among medics as to its use for the first ailment, its use for (or 'against') children suffering what has been called Hyperkinetic Syndrome (HKS) has long been a contentious issue, especially in the US, where a number of researchers have argued that HKS doesn't actually exist and that the use of drugs on children who prove 'excessively disruptive' in school and on the streets amounts to a medical form of social control. These children also run some risk of suffering stunted physical growth.

Away from the consulting rooms, speed's unpretentious efficiency made it a big favourite with washed-out flower children in the early and mid-1970s, providing them with a physical and mental lift. From about 1975 it became popular with the dance-crazy Northern Soul crowd, and with the first and subsequent waves of punks who found they could pogo, spit, and shout more zealously on it and, of course, would no more be seen snorting that over-priced, bourgeois stimulant cocaine than wear a Paul Smith suit. (This was when coke was associated with the nobs on the hill rather than with ghetto riff-raff.)

By the early 1990s, speed had insinuated itself into a new UK-wide dance scene, a phenomenon that, starting with the 'second summer of love' in 1988, was originally known as Acid House, then Rave and, following a splintering of the original unified vibes, simply as the Dance Scene. Ecstasy had been the mind and body fuel from the start but, by the turn of the decade, the Ecstasy on offer was of such dubious quality most young clubgoers were *just saying no* to it. LSD came back, coke was also used – often smoked in crack form inside a tobacco spliff. And speed was appreciated because it was cheap, 'friendly', and powerfully energising.

While the dance scene produced its share of drug casualties – people who came to grief because they were ignorant, gauche, or plain unlucky – most of those involved have kept within intelligent limits. This was thanks largely to some avid self-policing and education. People taught each other about how much was too much. In short, while the drugs set the tone, revealed the possibilities in terms of music, art and fashion, they were not the obsessional centre of most participants' lives.

Yet amphetamine *is* one of those drugs which can command lives. Some pundits see it – to use the jargon – as the most *self-reinforcing* of all the mood-altering substances. One hit demands another, then another and, when it stops feeling good, continued use stops the user from feeling bad.

Speeding in Essex

Large parts of Essex are speed country. I travelled to Colchester in the summer of 1994 to meet a group of people, ranging in age from seventeen to nearly forty, for whom the drug was or had been a daily sacrament. Why speed in this part of the world? It could be a matter of local temperament, or a case of availability spawning a trend that became ingrained. One man I spoke to – thirty-nine-year-old 'Chris' – remembered a bountiful 'father figure' from the mid-1970s who was a main distributor. He also recalled several teams of manufacturers in the region, one of whom rented space on industrial estates for three or four months at a time, abandoning every piece of equipment when their noses told them to move on. For seven or eight years they worked their way through Essex and neighbouring Suffolk and Norfolk.

Colchester itself is the main centre of population in the north-east of Essex – a university and army garrison town that possesses one of the UK's largest post-war council housing estates, known as the Greenstead. Drugs are no longer bartered and consumed in Colchester's public places. It is done house to house in locales like the Greenstead, a furtive scene that makes traditional drop-in drug agency work almost irrelevant.

It was at the Greenstead that I met my amphetamine devotees, five out of a scene of around sixty or seventy dedicated drug consumers living on what was a fairly well-kept red-brick estate of mostly low-rise blocks.

Chris, a user for twenty years, had noted two marked

developments in the last two or three years: the rapidity with which numerous youngsters were switching from snorting to injecting amphetamine – often within eighteen months of trying the drug; and a consequent take-up by such people of heroin to ease the rawness of the speed experience – all previous taboos against dabbling with the evil *scag* effortlessly abandoned.

Was this the flipside of the government-sanctioned harm-minimisation policy? The provision of clean needles was supposed to prevent sharing of dirty works (and various surveys had shown this had been achieved, with UK HIV-infection rates looking good against those of most other European countries). But the policy also provided young snorters with the means and the 'justification' for giving the needle a try. The journey, thereafter, from speed to heroin is not only simple but 'logical'. Speed, especially when injected, is relentless. It gives the body and mind no rest. Heroin seems the perfect peace-with-the-world antidote. Seventeen-year-old Vicky crossed over from sniffing to injecting speed within the space of three weeks, and on to heroin after eighteen months.

Like so many avid drug-takers, there's turmoil to be found in her early years. Mum and Dad fought. Dad beat up Mum, then left when Vicky was twelve. School seemed pointless. By fourteen she was hanging around with an older crowd – men and women in their twenties – who transmitted to her their taste for a variety of mind-benders. Hash made Vicky paranoid. She tried speed after meeting a new boyfriend, a man who'd come to Colchester to escape drug chaos in London. He was soon back on heroin ('they spiked his tea in the homeless hostel he was staying at,' says loyal Vicky) and though he forbade that she use heroin herself, he couldn't help but let her know how *dreamy* he felt under morphine's spell. 'Beautiful, beautiful,' he'd whisper, '. . . don't ever let me catch you doing it.' And, of course, she did – as soon as he went to prison for a string of burglaries. She told his friends, who supplied her with the heroin, that it wasn't for her, it was for the boyfriend. She would be taking it to him in prison.

'He's got home leave in September,' Vicky told me. 'If he finds out I'm using he'll do his nut.'

Speed, she says, made her feel confident. But it also made her weary and lonely, up all night racing, while her manfriend and his associates were floating away on the heroin. 'Speed,' she says, 'is something you grow out of.'

How did she feel about her drug-taking career to date?

'I wish I'd never started,' she answered quietly.

The popularity of amphetamine injecting among young north-east Essex drug consumers was confirmed by a survey published in 1993.[42] Sixty-six injectors were 'sampled' in Colchester and Clacton, many of them having been reached through an innovative 'outreach' education and health-protection scheme that enlisted the services of drug users themselves.

All thirty-five respondents in the Clacton group and most of those in Colchester named speed as the drug they had injected most often in the past four weeks. And, in both towns, by far the largest number had taken to the needle before they were twenty. Clean syringes and needles were no longer difficult to obtain, and while sharing and lending of used gear had become less usual, most of the re-used works were not being properly cleaned.

More alarming, perhaps, for the non-drug-taking fraternity was the method of disposal of dirty works. Despite the provision of special 'sharps disposal' units, a fifth of those surveyed in Colchester dumped used works down a toilet, a drain, or in a regular bin. The Clacton figure was more than half.

Knowledge of HIV/AIDS and the message about how it is spread and guarded against was good. But if people's needle habits didn't always tally with what they knew to be safe practice, their performance in the sexual arena was even riskier. Most of the respondents were sexually active, more than a quarter having had 'casual partners' within the past three months. Yet only a minority used condoms – because they 'disliked' their feel. Other surveys have found that changing sexual risk behaviour among injectors is more difficult than cleaning up their needle habits.[43]

Speed, the Needle and Sex

An earlier (1988/89), though much bigger, sample of drug injectors in the north-west of England produced a whole cluster of figures that would feed nicely into a tabloid scare campaign. Even more so than in Colchester, the data indicated that speed injectors were young, sexually active, careless about disease-protection measures, more likely than heroin injectors to shoot up with several others, unlikely to contact drug services (which were for 'smackheads') – in fact unlikely to see themselves as being addicted to speed, even though they might be injecting daily.[44]

Stand by for some figures: 61 per cent of the 200 speed injectors who were surveyed for that investigation reported that the drug increased their interest in sex – in contrast to a previous sample of heroin users, 67 per cent of whom reported reduced libido. A further tickling of the data showed that speed users' sex appetite was probably twice as vigorous as their smack-taking counterparts and yet more than 70 per cent of those who (to depart from the jargon) screwed around didn't bother with condoms.

When it came to sharing injecting equipment, 55 per cent said they had used others' gear during the past six months and 68 per cent reported passing on their own. (The equivalent figures for the heroin injectors were 44 per cent and 46 per cent.)

The author wanted more attention paid to amphetamine use 'now that injecting equipment is so widely available and the dangers of HIV infection are with us.'

Speed on Prescription

All of which brings us to a so-far quietly smouldering argument about whether or not pharmaceutical amphetamine should be given to street users in the way that methadone is offered to heroin addicts. The arguments for were set out by Richard Pates, a clinical psychologist with the South Glamorgan Community Drug Team: it would help, he said, to reel in a host of young users who currently see no purpose in coming forward to a drug agency.[45] Once captured (my own, not Pates's term) they can be educated, supported, given clean works and condoms – all of which are critical resources in an age of, not just HIV, but of Hepatitis B, C, and other blood-borne diseases.

The arguments against come from the psychiatric orthodoxy and have been consistently transmitted through reports by the government's Advisory Council on the Misuse of Drugs (ACMD). The line, in summary, is that many speed users are not, so far, heavily into the drug. Prescribing might change all that and lead them into injecting. Furthermore, speed is associated with psychotic reactions, which is not something to be chanced by offering state fixes. The experience of prescribing during the 1960s '. . . is generally acknowledged to have been disastrous . . .'46

Many in the field dispute the idea that 1960s' speed prescribing was disastrous. The potential for such a service, they say, was unfairly and irrationally evaluated. Pates himself counters that street supplies in the 1960s were far purer; they were diverted pharmaceutical stocks. Today's sulphate is often of just 5 per cent purity, which means less risk of psychological problems, but more of a health risk from the adulterants. Yes, he says, many amphetamine users are not yet heavy users but many already are and find themselves 'leading unstable and chaotic lives, enmeshed in crime and prostitution.'

The problem those in the Pates camp face is how to demonstrate the worth of prescribing, given that large-scale pilot studies aren't being done – partly because not enough potential subjects are attending medical services from where they can be studied, but also because powerful figures within the psychiatric establishment put the wind up lesser colleagues who might otherwise be inclined to give it a try. The drugs treatment establishment has never faced squarely the question of stimulant addiction. Having, for historical reasons, invested its intellectual and financial stock in the study and treatment of opioid use, it finds the whole speed/cocaine issue a perplexing irritant.

Pates, meanwhile, can report on apparently promising prescribing results from places like Portsmouth, Exeter, Mid Glamorgan, the West Midlands, and his own Cardiff.

'Our first ten clients showed reduced injecting, better health, less illicit drug use, reduced prostitution and crime, and a distinct improvement in the stability of their lives.'47

He adds a warning: 'Prescribing is no panacea. It should be

96

part of a package including services such as counselling, and is not suitable for all amphetamine users, particularly those using small amounts and not injecting. That still leaves many heavy, chaotic users for whom prescribing might provide the opportunity for change.'

Tip-off Signs

You can usually recognise a keen amphetamine user by the odd hours s/he keeps – up and bouncing for long periods and then marathon sessions of sleep from which s/he'll wake ravenously hungry and dispirited. Depending on how much is being used there'll be unaccountable mood spasms: joyful and confident; anxious and irrational with outbreaks of temper. Heavy, long-term users, or those who are susceptible even at low doses, will express fears of being persecuted: *What's that noise? Why is that person staring at me?* Then the panic will pass and you'll probably see another elevation of mood.

Coming Off

Most moderate users of amphetamine, whether snorters or tablet-eaters, will face no great hardship if they decide to quit. In most cases their sleeping cycle is jarred and they'll have some depression accompanied by a sense of deprivation which soon passes. But those who have remodelled their lives to suit the pharmacological ups and downs of the drug can expect severe disruption. In the early stages there'll be a depression that has been known to lead to suicide. There could be such fatigue that much of the day will be taken up by sleep. Unlike heroin withdrawal, which goes through various fairly predictable stages, withdrawal from speed can produce unpredictable fluctuations, with paranoia, exhaustion, and restlessness waxing and waning.

A rock music writer of my acquaintance had a half-a-gram-a-week snorting habit that caused him to reprogramme each week into sleep and no-sleep portions. His habit developed over eighteen months and it took exactly that time to recover.

'I woke up one day and decided I couldn't stand it any more. The person I was living with was also a speed freak and she got hit a lot harder by the psychological factors than I did. We decided to sort of quit together, which was extremely messy. Apart from informal advice from people I knew, I went to see my GP, who said he didn't know anything about it but gave me notes to stay off work, and prescribed a lot of vitamins. When we first stopped, the day consisted of getting up at five in the afternoon, just in time to go out and buy some groceries. I'd suddenly rediscovered this appetite for food. Then we'd stay up watching TV, listening to records and smoking dope until about one o'clock and then fall over again. There was this complete lassitude and depression in the first couple of days. I don't think I've ever felt quite so low in my life. The way it was explained to me was that there was so much amphetamine in my body that it had almost packed up producing [structurally related] adrenalin, because it wasn't required. It had to adjust itself to naturally producing adrenalin again. The period was completely uncreative. I could hardly write. I could do virtually nothing, but what I would do was get up as early as possible, which effectively meant that after week two I was getting up at four instead of five, and a week after that, at noon. When I got to the point where eight hours sleep was enough and I could get up at 9 a.m. I went back to work. This took about two months, but it was eighteen months before I was restored to the kind of human being I'd been before taking the speed.'

He admits to backsliding a couple of times, tempted by the demands of work, but he got through and for some years has been amphetamine-free. His new drugs of choice are grass and hash (though less than he used to consume) and alcohol ('a little more than I'd like'). While he stays clear of speed he does have the occasional 'toot' of cocaine but is 'sufficiently indifferent to it not to seek it out.'

Help

Heavy users going through withdrawal should first settle their minds about what lies ahead, do their calculations as to whether they truly want to be rid of the drug, and then guard against succumbing to the depression that will follow. They could do with help from a friend who understands what is happening. They might want to seek help from a specialist agency which, if the habit has been entrenched for several years, might want to prescribe anti-depressants for a 'lengthy period of time'.[48] Before accepting such a prescription, it would be sensible to read up on these powerful drugs to see if you really want them.

The problems of relapse and depression were emphasised in a key document produced in the 1970s by the government's Advisory Committee on Drug Dependence.[49] It warned doctors: 'The onset of depression [during withdrawal] may bring the risk of suicide. Attention must be given to the social and psychological factors which have led to the drug abuse. Follow-up of patients is essential as relapse is the rule rather than the exception if and when supplies of amphetamine become available. Some 6 to 12 months' after-care may be required, and it seems likely that some cases will require continuous psychiatric supervision and treatment.'

The Advisory Council's warning is legitimate although exaggerated, as well as brutally mechanistic in language. It assumes practised speed users will be for the most part defeated and can only draw succour from the authorities. In fact, the best long-term 'cure' for amphetamine addiction is for the user to set about developing an improved opinion of him/herself. Friends and family can help generate this confidence by offering constructive assistance rather than by keeping a morbid watching brief. Ultimately, the process is about seeing and believing in an amphetamine-free future.

Notes

1 T. Duquesne and J. Reeves, *A Handbook of Psychoactive Medicines*, Quartet, London, 1982, p. 217.

2 M. Gossop, *Living with Drugs*, Temple Smith, London, 1982, p. 162.

3 Ibid, p. 163.

4 'Powerful new drug hits UK', in *The Big Issue*, 6 November 1994, p. 7.

5 See the standard medicines guide, the *British National Formulary* (No. 27, March 1994, p. 167), published by the British Medical Association and the Royal Pharmaceutical Society of Great Britain.

6 Ibid, p. 166.

7 O. P. Kalix *et al.*, 'Khat: A plant drug with amphetamine-like effects, in *Schweiz Med. Wochenschr*, 104 (923), 1991, pp. 1561–6.

8 C. Pantelis *et al.*, 'Use and abuse of khat *(Catha edulis)*', in *Psychological Medicine*, 19, 1989, pp. 657–69.

9 P. Nencini and A. M. Ahmed, 'Khat consumption: A pharmacological review', in *Drug and Alcohol Dependence*, 23 (1), 1989, pp. 19–29.

10 H. E. Soufi *et al.*, 'Khat and oral cancer', in the *Journal of Laryngology and Otology*, 105 (8), 1991, pp. 643–5.

11 Tony Thompson, 'Deadly Harvest', in *Time Out*, 24 November 1993.

12 See, for instance, N. V. Harris *et al.*, 'Risk factors for HIV infection among injecting drug users: Results of blinded surveys in drug treatment centres in King County Washington', in the *Journal of Acquired Immune Deficiency Syndrome*, 6(11), 1993, p. 1275. This showed that the prevalence of HIV infection among speed injectors was three to four times higher than for injectors of other drugs. Also Hilary Klee, whose articles in the *British Journal of Addiction* (Vol. 87, 1992, p. 439), *Nursing Times* (Vol. 88, No. 22, 27 May 1992, p. 36) and elsewhere point to the same dynamics.

13 G. King, 'Amphetamines and other stimulants', in *Substance Abuse, A Comprehensive Textbook*, Williams and Wilkins, Baltimore, 1992, p. 259.

14 D. Lauderback and D. Waldorf, 'Whatever happened to Ice? The latest drug scare', in the *Journal of Drug Issues*, 23(4), 1993, p. 597.

15 'The amphetamines and LSD', report by the Advisory Committee on Drug Dependence, London, 1970, p. 6.

16 King, op. cit., p. 249.

17 'Amphetamine', a pocket booklet produced by Lifeline, Manchester.

18 King, op. cit.
19 Ibid, p. 250.
20 'Drug Notes: Amphetamine', ISDD, 1993, p. 5.
21 Cox *et al.*, *Drugs and Drug Abuse*, Addiction Research Foundation, Toronto, Canada, 1983, p. 161.
22 King, op. cit., p. 255.
23 ISDD, op. cit.
24 R. T. Wallage *et al.*, 'Sudden retinal manifestations of intranasal cocaine and methamphetamine abuse', in the *American Journal of Ophthalmology*, 114 (2), 1992, pp. 158–60.
25 M. Hepburn, 'Socially related disorders: Drug addiction, maternal smoking and alcohol consumption', in *High Risk Pregnancy*, W. Dunlop and A. A. Calder (eds), Butterworth, London, 1992, p. 272.
26 *Drugs, Pregnancy and Childcare*, ISDD, 1992, p. 22.
27 J. C. Dearlove *et al.*, 'Stillbirth due to intravenous amphetamine', in the *British Medical Journal*, 304 (6826), 1992, p. 548.
28 K. Nyberg *et al.*, 'Obstetric medication versus residential area as perinatal risk factors for subsequent adult drug addiction in offspring', in *Paediatric Perinatal Epidemiology*, 7, 1993, p. 23.
29 *High Times Encyclopedia of Psychoactive Medicines*, p. 237.
30 Duquesne and Reeves, op. cit., p. 217.
31 Advisory Committee on Drug Dependence, op. cit., p. 8.
32 *High Times Encyclopedia of Psychoactive Medicines*, p. 237.
33 Duquesne and Reeves, op. cit., p. 164.
34 *High Times Encyclopedia of Psychoactive Medicines*, p. 218.
35 Duquesne and Reeves, op. cit., p. 277.
36 It would be interesting to know what drug-induced decisions are made in our own momentous times by the world's political leaders. Certainly, a rumour persists within educated drug circles that a prominent Tory Cabinet minister of the Thatcher and post-Thatcher years had a keen appetite for speed's sister stimulant, cocaine.
37 Advisory Committee on Drug Dependence, op. cit., p. 15.
38 Ibid.
39 Release, *Stimulants: A Release Guide* 1990.
40 Ibid.
41 In 1969 an Ipswich GP instigated a voluntary amphetamine ban among his local colleagues, so encouraging prescribing cut-backs nationally.
42 A. Walling, 'A descriptive evaluation of the north-east Essex volunteer drugs outreach service', Essex Rivers Healthcare Trust, Colchester, 1993.
43 M. Donoghoe, 'Sex, HIV and the injecting drug user', in the *British Journal of Addiction*, 87, 1992, pp. 405–16.

44 H. Klee, 'A deadly combination', in *Nursing Times*, Vol. 88, No. 22, 27 May 1992, p. 36.
45 R. Pates, 'Speed on prescription', in *Druglink*, ISDD, May/June 1994, pp. 16–17.
46 From the second *Aids and Drug Misuse* report of the Advisory Council on the Misuse of Drugs, as quoted in the Pates article above.
47 Pates, op. cit., p. 17.
48 'Working with stimulant users', conference report published by the Standing Conference on Drug Abuse, 1989, p. 9.
49 'The amphetamines and LSD', report by the Advisory Committee on Drug Dependence, op. cit., p. 6.

BARBITURATES

Intro

Little is seen these days of barbiturates. Yet in the late seventies to early eighties they were everywhere, and ranked by drug agency specialists as perhaps *the* most dangerous of all the street substances. If ever there was a class of drug that in actual use refuted much of what was claimed for it by the pharmaceutical industry, it is the barbiturates. Conceived as sedatives, they are capable of rousing furious and chaotic behaviour; as an aid to sleep they might bring on slumber for the first two or three weeks, but then they begin to suppress the normal sleep function, including dream sleep. They were a favourite drug of people wanting to kill themselves; they are practically the most lethal of all injected substances, and one of the most dangerous to withdraw from.

At their peak popularity in 1966, 16 million prescriptions were written out, despite their having been solid evidence as to barbs' damaging effects and their strong addiction potential for at least fifteen years, with the argument going back more than fifty. At the core of the story that unfolds in this chapter is an outrageous betrayal of the public by those to whom it has always looked for protection from the worst effects of powerful prescription drugs: doctors and the government's own regulatory authorities. The record shows that what began as a calamity for a category of GP-attended insomniacs and people with everyday anxieties ended as a major street-level catastrophe, with literally thousands maimed and killed every year.

The barb story was, in many ways, instantly repeated with the drugs that came to fill their market niche – the benzodiazepine tranquillisers. Tranks were also hyped through 'licit' channels as safe, effective, and with little 'abuse' potential – and they too landed in huge numbers on the street. We can see now that tranquillisers are the barbs of the nineties – just as barbs replaced bromides, which had earlier taken over from other once-admirable categories of hypnosedatives.

The information that follows about a drug now rarely seen on the street is offered without apology. For to understand the story of the barbiturates is to understand much about how 'monstrous youth' gets the wherewithal to mess up its brains.

It also has to be said that, while barbs are almost gone, they are still not buried. They might yet come around again.

What are they?

'Barbiturate' designates a substance derived from barbituric acid, which was discovered in 1864 following the unlikely marrying of urea, a principal component of urine, and malonic acid, a by-product of apples. Barbituric acid itself does not sedate, but many of its literally thousands of derivatives do. They are divided into three main groups according to the time they take to get absorbed by, work upon, and pass through the body. The first are called ultra-short-acting (chemical names: methohexitone and thiopentone). These get their name because, being extremely soluble in fat, they quickly penetrate the fat-laden barrier to the brain where the sedation work takes place. They also quickly evacuate the brain, after which they are redistributed to other parts of the body. It is this talent for rapid brain entry and exit which makes this category attractive for quick surgical procedures or as 'softeners' for more substantial anaesthetics. The traditional after-surgery grogginess is caused by the drug continuing to haunt the body in concentrations too low to induce sleep, but high enough to make the limbs feel leaden. Because of their fast, incursive nature, the rapid-acting type are rarely picked up by the recreational user.

At the other pole are the long-acting barbiturates (pheno-barbitone and methylphenobarbitone). These circulate in the blood primarily in water-soluble form and so take longer to penetrate the brain's fatty defence. Because they are easily picked up by muscle and body fats they carry on circulating through the blood in concentration sufficient to keep the individual sedated or sluggish for twelve to twenty-four hours – and it can be many days after that before the drug is finally excreted. The slow, unexciting nature of the long-range type again make them unappetising to pleasure-seekers. They are prescribed chiefly to control epileptic seizures.

The barbiturate group that street users have found irre-sistible are those in the intermediate range (amylobarbitone, butobarbitone, and quinalbarbitone). They fall midway between the other two groups both in terms of speed of brain pen-etration and the duration of bodily hangover. Their 'effective duration' is said to be six to eight hours. Prescription is supposed to be limited to the treatment of 'severe intractable insomnia in patients already taking barbiturates'.[1] In practice this means that they are only for people (usually the elderly) who have been using the drug for years without it solving their sleep problems – except now they can't do without their daily dose.

How they work

All barbiturates achieve their hypnosedative effects by depressing the central nervous system (CNS). But unlike the opioids, which also depress the CNS, they are not effective against pain. They might make the user sufficiently drowsy not to care, but they don't appear to lock on to the pain receptor sites deep inside the brain as do morphine and heroin. Nonetheless, when supplies were plentiful, many heroin users considered the barbs valuable weaponry to supplement their arsenals when their first-choice drug was scarce.

Identifying the products

Barbiturates come in a multiplicity of plain and coloured tablets, capsules and dry ampoules. The four leaders, as far as the diminishing number of street users are concerned, are listed below.

Tuinal: This combines two barbituric acid derivatives, amylobarbitone sodium and quinalbarbitone sodium, in equal proportions. It is made by Lilly and comes in a 100 mg orange/blue capsule. Known informally as *Tueys*, *Traffic lights*.

Seconal: Another Lilly product, featuring quinalbarbitone sodium. Produced as an orange capsule in 50 mg or 100 mg doses. Known as *Reds*, *Sekkies*.

Amytal: Also from Lilly, it comes as a white 50 mg tablet containing amylobarbitone and as 60 mg or 200 mg capsules, both blue and filled with amylobarbitone sodium.

Soneryl: From Rhône-Poulenc Rorer, it comes as a pink 100 mg butobarbitone tablet.

Sensations

In small doses (usually one tab or capsule), barbs direct themselves at mental tension, producing tranquillity without too much drowsiness. When the dose is increased, the depressant effect spreads to all parts of the central nervous system and the inclination is to sleep. If this is resisted, the results are remarkably similar to a high intake of alcohol. Inhibitions are released, thinking and speech become clumsy, the limbs go numb, emotions soar and dive, and there is a tendency to bounce into walls, fall off chairs, etc. While there can be spasms of sexual hunger, the body will be less likely to perk up as desired. Quarrelsomeness and spates of violence are common. During their 1970s peak use, of all the drug cases that fell into hospital casualty departments, the barb user was the one most feared by staff. One-fifth, according to a survey,[2] behaved aggressively. The usual duration of the barb experience is three to six hours, which is followed by sleep and a thudding, alcohol-type hangover. But the experience can be terminal if enough is consumed, for as the dose goes up the recipient will lurch into coma and death. All the sensations so far described are greatly magnified when alcohol or another

CNS depressant (heroin, temazepam, etc.) is taken at the same time.

Health

The greatest danger from barb use is the relatively minor difference between the therapeutic and lethal dose. Whereas a doctor might prescribe a 200 mg tablet for sleep, roughly ten times that amount can kill the patient – or at least send him/her into a dangerous overdose. Injecting the drug increases the risk of an OD.

Overdose

When an overdose comes it will be signalled by a weak, rapid pulse, sweaty skin, and breathing that is either very slow or rapid and shallow. In contrast to opiate poisoning there is no straight antidote to a barbiturate OD, but with quick treatment hospitals have enough in their kitbags to bring about a recovery.

Long-Term Problems

Problems of long-term use include pneumonia (because the cough reflex is suppressed), hypothermia (because the normal responses to cold are blocked), and repeated accidental overdose (due to barb-induced confusion as to how much – if any – of the drug has already been taken). There is also believed to be severe repression of dream sleep, leading to daytime emotional disturbances.

Injection

Injecting barbiturates brings all the familiar risks of septicaemia, collapsed veins, viral and bacterial infections, etc.
However, there is also a range of problems peculiar to barbs
which make them among the most dangerous of all the injected
mood-altering drugs. The main hazard comes when the needle
user has spent his/her easy-to-aim-at veins and turns to the
femoral vein in the groin. Since this corresponds closely to
the femoral artery, it is easy to hit the latter by mistake.
Should this happen, the barb will send it into spasm, causing
a drastic loss of blood to the leg below – the result of which
might require amputation of the limb. A similar outcome can
derive from hitting an artery in an arm.

Pregnancy

Massive doses of long-acting phenobarbitone in pregnancy
have been associated with distortions of facial features and
finger malformations.[3] Prolonged regular use in the later
stages of pregnancy can result in the newborn child suffering
withdrawal symptoms.[4] But pregnant women who wish to
quit the drug should seek some expert advice because of the
risk of fits.

With Other Drugs

As already noted, taking barbiturates together with other central nervous system depressants can be dangerous, since each
drug multiplies the effect of the other. Barbs should also be
avoided with 'major' tranquillisers (used to treat severe mental disorders), certain anticoagulants, corticosteroids such
as Cortisone, antidepressants, antibacterials, contraceptive
pills, and the anti-inflammatory drug phenylbutazone.

With Other Conditions

Barbiturates are not recommended for people suffering from severe liver disorders or respiratory problems, kidney disease, prostate enlargement, hyperthyroidism, diabetes, severe anaemia, heart disease, or raised pressure within the eye of the sort caused by glaucoma. They are also a problem to the elderly, increasing the risk of falls through grogginess and hypothermia.

Tolerance

There is an in-built enticement to reach a lethal level of barb use, for while tolerance to the intoxicant effects builds up quite quickly, a comparable resistance does not develop to the drug's depressant effects on the central nervous system. This means that, as the user takes more of the stuff in an effort to retrieve an ever-more elusive stoned feeling, the drug is banging down his/her respiration to, ultimately, a lethal level. The dose that finally breaks the user's back could be just one more 100 mg tab than was taken last time.

Dependence

The time it takes to get barb-dependent varies according to the constitution of the user. However, it seems very few are resilient beyond an 800 mg daily dose taken for a couple of months. The physical incentives to reach towards such levels are discussed above. The psychological factors are also considerable. Barbiturates provide an emotional lift. But while they might do this in the short term, in the medium to long term they will heighten anxiety and depression. The tendency then is to take more, which sends the user deeper into the trough from which the apparent escape is more drugs: after all, curing the blues was, for decades, the stated function of licitly prescribed barbiturates. In this way, not a few individuals have been caught in a downward spiral which has ended either in accidental overdose or suicide.

The Elixir that Failed

The development of barbituric acid derivatives, starting at the beginning of the twentieth century, is an example of science's tireless search for the immaculate elixir that will calm the human spirit. When the Bayer company's Veronal was introduced into Britain in 1903 it was advertised as 'absolutely safe and without toxic effects.[5] Within a decade, it was one of ten drugs most often implicated in fatal accidents and suicide.[6]

At that time, there was room for a promising new item. Opium, in the form of laudanum, had been discredited as an all-purpose tranquilliser, and ethyl alcohol, chloral hydrate and paradehyde were also proving problematic after initial great expectations. Yet to be unfrocked were the bromides, which, since the 1850s, had been sold in the form of inorganic salts. Like barbiturates they were prescribed for sleep and daytime sedation, but their prime function was in the management of epilepsy. It was believed then that the root cause of certain forms of epilepsy was masturbation. Since it appeared that potassium bromide reduced the sexual drive, and thus the need to manipulate the private organs, it followed that the drug would help alleviate the consequent seizures. Urged on by the suitably named Sir Charles Lowcock, physicians found that barbs did indeed reduce epileptic seizures, but not, we have to assume, because they quelled sexual fervour, rather because of their ability to depress general CNS functioning. Bromides were still considered the efficient fix until the 1950s when the phenomenon known as bromism finally received official recognition. This was caused by the body's painfully slow action in breaking down and excreting the drug. Symptoms included trembling, delirium, paranoia, hallucinations, and rashes that sometimes covered the entire body.

Just as bromides began dipping in popularity, the barbiturates were lifting off as the hypnosedatives of medical choice. By the 1960s, literally hundreds were on the market in an array of sizzling shapes, colours, and sizes. By 1966, annual prescriptions stood at 16 million, even though a minority of senior medical figures had been warning of their serious addiction potential for at least thirty years. In Lexington, Kentucky, during 1950, what looked like the definitive addiction experiment was carried out on five human volunteers.[7] But this too was ignored. For up to five months the experimental quintet were kept dosed on amounts of the drug sufficient to cause 'continuous mild to severe intoxication'. Then they were abruptly withdrawn. Their resulting agonies demonstrated for the research team that 'addiction to barbiturates is far more serious than is morphine addiction.'

Symptoms included delirium, major convulsions, hallucinations, and a feeling of such weakness that some of the subjects were unable to stand. The interpretation by the medical profession at large was perverse. The experiment, it was decided, proved that major difficulties arose only from extremely high doses; also that addiction was a problem of the patient rather than of the drug. Emotionally healthy individuals did not become entangled.

As Charles Medawar points out in his illuminating book *Power and Dependence* (Social Audit, London, 1991), barbiturate prescribing created the classic fatal spiral (subsequently repeated with the successors to the barbs, the benzodiazepine tranquillisers). Not only did the drug soon fail to have any remedial effect upon patients experiencing anxiety and depression, but the patient's suffering was reinforced by numerous, more severe symptoms caused by the barbiturates themselves. Unable to recognise the barb-induced damage, doctors carried on prescribing, perhaps increasing the dose to account for the decline in their patients' condition. If the patients, at any time, tried to quit, then the punishing withdrawal symptoms merely confirmed the need to continue as before.

Thus, wrote Guy's Hospital psychiatrist Dr Richard Hunter in a 1957 paper, 'a mild psychiatric disturbance, in all likelihood amenable to one or two sympathetic interviews, becomes converted into a serious and perhaps protracted illness.'[8]

More than a few patients followed this hopeless route all the way to multiple operations on the brain.

In 1965, the UK Department of Health was still arguing that the barbiturate menace was mostly got up by the press and that there were no more than 200–300 barb addicts in the whole land.[9] But with barbiturate-linked deaths rising to 2,000 per annum by the early 1970s, even doctors were disposed to rethink. In 1975, the Campaign on the Use and Restriction of Barbiturates (CURB) was undertaken by a group of eminently well-placed specialists who barracked members of their own profession for wanton prescribing of 'these outdated drugs . . . which are now killing far more people than heroin.' By then, they accounted for more than half of all fatal poisonings – something like 27,000 lives between 1959 and 1974.[10] At the same time as CURB was going at the loudhailer, the Committee on the Review of Medicines (CRM) was also casting its eye over the barbiturates. In 1979 came their assessment.[11] Under normal circumstances barbiturates (they then named all those being issued at the time as sleepers, anti-anxiety agents, and sedatives) should not be used in any medical treatment of the following groups: children and young adults; the elderly and debilitated; women who were breastfeeding or pregnant; patients with a history of alcohol or drug abuse. In the end, the only use the Committee could find for the drugs was in the treatment of 'intractable insomnia'. It also warned about the 'potentially fatal' withdrawal symptoms which could occur on abrupt cessation in all ages.

Prescription totals were already tumbling by the time of the CRM report – down to 9.5 million in 1974 and to 5.1 million in 1978. (The 1992 figure was 800,000.) Doctors were switching to the new benzodiazepines (Valium, Librium, etc.), and since these agents were far more expensive than barbiturates the drug companies were not exactly itching to keep the outmoded barb deployed any longer than was embarrassingly necessary. Doctors were also happy. Benzos cleared their surgeries of malingerers just as quickly as barbs had done, and the fact that benzos were already showing every sign of producing addiction problems as intractable as those of the barbs (a feature noted in 1964 by an expert committee of the World Health Organisation) was a detail that could be reflected upon at some more convenient moment.

History of Street Use

Barbs landed on the streets in a big way during the mid-sixties when they were combined with amphetamine in a famous combination called *Purple Hearts* (Drinamyl). The Purple Heart rage was essentially the beginning of the mass street drugs scene (discounting alcohol and tobacco). It was the first elephantine kick for youth, the first piece of intensive tutoring about what drugs are and how their effects call for mastery and respect. Some learnt. Some didn't. The authorities tried to come to grips with the fad, but their target was the racy amphetamine, as though the barb part of Hearts was of no consequence. Not true. The barb element was considered essential by consumers to avoid jagging out on a diet of pure speed.

New controls put a stop to the wide availability of Drinamyl, but not to the taste. Within a few years a 'licit' pill with almost identical effects was on the market, called Durophet-M. Although this too was deleted in 1981, there are today countless other ways of acquiring the up/down fix; the combination having become a permanent feature of the drugs culture.

Straight barbiturates became popular on the early eighties dance club scene in places like Manchester, into whose virtually free all-night joints recession kids poured several nights a week charged up with snorted amphetamine sulphate. On the way home they'd swallow a barb such as Tuinal, which allowed them to present themselves to Mum in a credibly worn condition – and maybe even get some sleep in what remained of the night.

Up a couple of notches, barbiturates also appealed to classic speed freaks who used the downer as a companion drug or remedy to the violence of the amphetamine experience. In fact there was a well-trodden path from speed not simply to barbs, but from there on to heroin. It worked like this: after a spell of injecting barbiturates to counteract the amphetamines, the user starts suffering collateral damage from the downer drug, including painful abscesses where the needle misses a vein. So the speed users start looking elsewhere to relieve themselves. They alight upon a downer drug that is potentially less 'filthy', but in any case brings with it (short-term) painkilling properties. Such a drug is heroin.

The speed-to-junk-via-barbs route was most easily spotted when looking at the punk fall-out of the late seventies and early eighties. British punks got lift-off in 1976, selecting no-nonsense speed as their number-one item because it gave them the chemical zest to stay the hard, sharp course. But as punk withered and its exponents either cleaned up or got more frenetic, barbs came more into their own. The peak of uptake occurred from 1981 to mid-1982 when such drugs were *the* sought-after item on the London Piccadilly scene. One support agency worker told me at the time that six of his teenaged clients died from barbs during this period, five of them girls, one of whom walked sleepily into a bus.

To meet the demands of the barb epidemic a special centre was set up in North London, called City Roads.[12] Though not exclusively for barbiturate consumers, some 85 per cent of their early traffic were registering this drug as their main problem. By 1985, in keeping with the line we are plotting, it was heroin which got the most mentions.

At the same time as barbs were hitting the West End of London, they were appearing in towns such as Bradford where in addition to punk fall-out there was already a severe recessionary frost. Prior to late 1980, £1 used to buy three or four barbs in a pub. Then suddenly, there was a rash of chemist break-ins and they were going for £1 for 100. In a letter to the music paper *New Musical Express* (to which I was a contributor at the time), a young local poet, Joolz Denby, reported 'children of 14, 15, 16 hurtling headlong to death by their pathetic ignorant use of barbiturates, especially Tuinal. In the last 18 months we have had many in hospital with colossal overdoses, three in intensive care. They seem to regard this as some kind of a test of street credibility, of how cool they can be. A hospital overdose bracelet is the latest fashion. They flirt with death as if it was nothing.' By late 1983, Bradford's young were still doing barbs, only now it was more common to inject rather than swallow them, and soon after that heroin reached town.

Though we have been examining the speed-through-barbs-to-heroin syndrome, this was only one of an incalculable number of patterns. Once a person starts loading up heavily on any sort of drug there is little incentive to remain a substance purist. A large number of people used barbs together with alcohol for an extremely ribald high, and it was thanks primarily to the unappealing spectacle of drunken barbheads that the drug achieved its gutter reputation among the great mass of conventional drug users. For drug moderates, barbiturates were for the headbanging lunatic fringe. They were about falling off chairs and squaring up to innocents.

Not until 1985 did the UK government consider barbiturates dangerous enough to control under the Misuse of Drugs Act 1971, the key piece of anti-street drugs legislation under which most other substances examined in this book had long been regulated. And even after falling within the MDA's ambit, barbiturates were placed in a class that drew moderate penalties for the punter and lax regulations for the professionals who prescribed and dispensed them.

But it wasn't the new legal controls nor even peer pressure which killed the barbiturate fad. Barbs vanished because the drug companies devoted themselves to marketing a 'superior' replacement in the form of the benzodiazepines tranquillisers. Thirty million trank prescriptions were made out in 1977 – the year the government-funded Campaign on the Use and Restriction of Barbiturates (CURB) was winding itself up, satisfied with a job well done. From then on, the volume of tranks flooding the streets increased year after year until, by the early nineties, their popularity had eclipsed most other outlawed substances, as had their capacity to blight and end lives.

Coming Off

Physical withdrawal symptoms from barbiturates can be eased considerably with special treatment (details from your local drugs advisory agency). Without it, sudden cessation of the drug will produce a range of symptoms which, again, will depend on how much has been used, for how long, and general bodily repair. Typically, symptoms start within twelve to twenty-four hours of the last dose and include shakiness, anxiety, and inability to sleep. At a more profound level there might be fluctuations in blood pressure, fever, seizures, and *delirium tremens* (DTs). The most dangerous time is between one and three days after the cut-off point. During this time it is possible for death to occur, although this is rare and usually only happens when vomit is inhaled during a seizure. Once over this peak, all physical symptoms should gradually clear. Then there comes the more lingering business of patching those parts that are in psychological/emotional disrepair.

Notes

1 *British National Formulary*, British Medical Association and Royal Pharmaceutical Society of Great Britain, London, March 1994, p. 144.

2 A. H. Ghodse, 'Drug dependent individuals dealt with by London casualty departments', in the *British Journal of Psychiatry*, Vol. 131, 1971, pp. 273–80.

3 *Drugs, Pregnancy & Childcare*, Institute for the Study of Drug Dependence (ISDD), London, 1992. p. 22.

4 *Drug Abuse Briefing: Fifth Edition*, ISDD, London, 1994, p. 11.

5 C. Medawar, *Power and Dependence: Social Audit on the safety of medicines*, Social Audit Ltd, 1992, p. 58.

6 Ibid, p. 58.

7 Ibid, p. 64.

8 Ibid, p. 68.

9 P. A. Parish, 'The prescribing of psychotropic drugs in general practice', in the *Journal of the Royal College of General Practitioners*, Vol. 21 (92), Supp. 4, November 1971.

10 'Recommendations on Barbiturate Preparations', Committee on the Review of Medicines, in the *British Medical Journal*, Vol. 2, 22 September 1979, pp. 719–20.

11 Ibid.

12 Credit is due to the casualty sister at Middlesex Hospital, Beryl Rose, who campaigned for and organised such a project, having seen a succession of damaged youths pass through her hospital department.

CAFFEINE

Intro

Now is the time to ask again a question fundamental to this whole book: what actually constitutes a drug? The answer cannot be given in terms of certain types of substances which have 'x' effect, but rather must be defined by the way in which a substance is used. The Fly Agaric mushroom with its brilliant red cap cannot realistically be described as a drug while growing in the November mist under a birch or larch. It is a fungus with its own purpose. But once plucked from the ground, taken home and infused in salt water, the resulting broth can rightly be called a drug because when consumed it will effect a psychoactive change in the consumer. The same goes for the *Cannabis sativa* plant. This can be converted into rope or bird seed, but it is only when the resin is isolated and consumed for its mind-altering effects that the plant is truly in a drug state.

The caffeine phenomenon is more subtle. Caffeine is one of a family of chemical compounds that stimulate the central nervous system (CNS), increase the flow of urine, and get the stomach churning, so accelerating digestion. While capable of being manufactured in a laboratory (it looks like baking powder) this is an expensive method. Of the sixty-odd plant species naturally containing the drug, the most commercially attractive concentrations show up in the pit of the greeny-brown fruit of the Arabian coffee shrub (*Coffea arabica*). Other important sources are the commercial tea plant (*Camellia sinsensis*), cocoa beans, kola nuts, and South American maté leaves – from which tea is made. Most of these species additionally contain one or other of two stimulant drugs closely related to caffeine, and these show up in a variety of common products: tea, cocoa, chocolate, soft drinks, as well as a large number

119

of over-the-counter painkilling pills. Caffeine's relatives are known as theophylline and theobromine. All three are generally classed as xanthines, signifying that they are methylated versions of the chemical xanthine. The most powerful of the three in terms of stimulating the CNS is caffeine. Theophylline rates second. Theobromine is virtually inactive. On the other hand, theobromine is better able to stimulate the heart and is more effective at increasing urine production. Given that each of them turns up in a diverse range of consumer products the question arises as to whether the products themselves are to be counted as drugs, and the answer surely has to be that it depends – on the quantity, frequency and manner in which the products are consumed. A pot of mocha at the end of a meal among friends cannot rightly be compared in drug terms with the imbibing habits of some early-morning coffee drinkers, who are virtually paralysed unless they get their several cups. Tea is often considered a more timid beverage than its xanthine-rich relative, coffee. But this isn't always so. An average cup of leaf or bagged tea contains very nearly as much caffeine as a cup of instant coffee and in some cases (for instance, Tetley versus Gold Blend or Maxwell House granules) a little more.[1] Tea also contains small amounts of theophylline and theobromine. Thus, someone disposing of four cups before catching the morning train is probably more taken with the stimulant effect than the impact upon the palate. Similarly, there is a syndrome, recognised in the US, called 'colalism', whereby people (usually young) are guzzling ten or more cans of cola a day and reporting sleep problems and jitteriness.

Nonetheless, when we look at the way the xanthines have been used by our society, comparing the great quantities consumed with the amount of social and physical damage that has resulted, we can conclude it might have been a good deal worse. Unlike most other drugs looked at in this book they have provoked no great political tumult, at least not in modern times. They have caused no palpable physical harm on anything approaching the scale of tobacco or alcohol. There *is* an amount of mental harm flowing from them, but this is of a comparatively slight nature.

What Is It?

Caffeine is a white crystalline powder that could have devastating effects if taken in its pure state in sufficient quantities, but it is rarely seen as such. The fact that it is invariably, and often surreptitiously, buried in among a mass of other ingredients is the secret of its success. Like the other xanthines it is everywhere and yet we scarcely see it. We even deny that xanthine consumption amounts to drug-taking. Do the xanthines actually move us? Perhaps their effects, for most people, are marginal. But then it could be argued that our whole xanthine-drenched world is suffering the clinically defined symptoms of xanthine poisoning – over-stimulation, anxiety, excitement, abnormally increased sensitivity . . .

The xanthines in nature

Here, at a glance, are the xanthines as they appear in nature and on the supermarket shelves.

Genus, species	Active principle	Used to make
Coffea arabica	caffeine	Arabian coffee
Coffea liberica	caffeine	Liberian coffee
Coffea robusta	caffeine	Congo coffee
Camellia sinsensis	caffeine, theophylline	tea
Theobroma cacao	caffeine, theobromine	chocolate, cocoa
Cola acuminata	caffeine, theobromine	soft drinks
Ilex paraguariensis	caffeine	maté

Caffeine is also included in various stimulants, painkillers, and cold cures, some available across the counter, some prescription only.

Quantities present

There seems to be no reliable breakdown on the presence of theobromine and theophylline in the various beverages and confections, and quite often the term 'caffeine' will be applied to xanthines in general. So we too must generalise and use the term 'caffeine' when perhaps other xanthines are present. The following data on average 'caffeine content' has been assembled from several sources.

Percolated/filter coffee cup	133 mg per cup (although as much as 263 mg)
Instant coffee	65 mg per cup
Decaffeinated coffee	1–6 mg per cup
Tea, bagged	55 mg per cup when brewed for 3 or 4 minutes
Loose tea	57 mg per cup
Typical chocolate bar	20 mg
Canned or bottled soft drink	10–50 mg
Chocolate drink	4 mg (plus between 50 and 90 mg of theobromine)
Standard stimulant tablet	200 mg
Over-the-counter analgesic	(up to) 50 mg per tablet

Sensations

Pure powdered caffeine has an excitory effect similar to cocaine and amphetamine and can sometimes be passed off as such. Moderate use – up to about four consecutive cups of coffee – combats drowsiness and tiredness and helps with both physical and mental performance. Larger doses start working on the lower parts of the brainstem and spinal column, affecting physical co-ordination and giving rise to jittery, anxious feelings. As with cocaine and amphetamine, the more that is consumed the more likely it is that these ill feelings will be intensified, producing the possibility of tremors and the experiencing of odd noises and flashes of light. Any dose can affect sleep, and with any dose there will be a physical and mental comedown roughly commensurate with the preceding high. This is why it is inadvisable to drink a lot of coffee or tea at the beginning of a long night-time drive and then nothing during the course of the journey. The effect of the initial dose is to plunder the body of its reserves of energy, inviting drowsiness and poor co-ordination before they would normally have been due. It is far better to pace consumption, allowing the body to deal with a dose of caffeine before loading in more.

Physiological effects can include increased heart rate, raised blood pressure, a need to pee, constriction of blood vessels in the brain (which might relieve some types of headache), and increased breathing.[2]

Medical Effects

Toxicity

Deaths from overdoses of caffeine are sometimes reported, and experts have settled on the figure of 10 grams as the kind of amount likely to lead to fatal convulsions and respiratory failure: 10 grams is about 100 cups of coffee. The lowest reported lethal dose[3] is 3,200 mg administered intravenously. Children, as always, are vulnerable at lower doses because of their less-developed defences as well as their lower body weight. One can of cola, drunk by a small child, can be equated – in terms of caffeine consumption – with an adult drinking four cups of coffee.

Stewed tea also brings with it particular dangers owing, it's believed, to the high yield of tannic acid. In what is perhaps an apocryphal story, this acid in tea was said to have been the cause of death in a group of labourers who drank from a pot constantly on the brew.[4]

Long-term use

Calculating the long-term impact of caffeine is virtually impossible because, as we've seen, people don't consume the drug straight, they take it as part of a complex mix of ingredients, some of which (sugar, dairy and artificial creamers, laboratory-made flavourings and colourants) are more physically debilitating than the caffeine itself.

Most medical research does little to untangle the confusion by its tendency – as one specialist journal admitted – 'to equate coffee with caffeine.'[5]

'It is common', according to the *Canadian Journal of Cardiology*, 'to use pure caffeine in animal experiments and to compare the results with coffee consumed by humans. If this were not confusing enough, there are additional dilemmas arising from decaffeinated coffee, caffeine in cola drinks, and differences in action of brewed versus boiled coffee . . .'

Nonetheless, we must try to distil the most plausible bits of research and leave the reader to listen to the grumblings, if any, of his/her own body.

Daily use of moderate amounts of caffeine in healthy adults is generally not considered damaging. But above the equivalent of six or eight cups of coffee (600 mg), a range of insidious effects can take hold – insidious because they are often regarded as normal symptoms of stress for which another cup would be the appropriate treatment. These include upset sleep, depression, anxiety, irritability, malfunctioning bowels, and fast, irregular heartbeat.

Internally, what seems to be happening is that a dose of caffeine is instructing the adrenal glands to release energy-giving glucose into the bloodstream as though for a fight-or-flight emergency. When this doesn't occur, rather than having the surplus sugar hang around the blood, glands in the pancreas issue insulin to prompt its uptake into the body cells. The repetition of this routine can, it is believed, lead to insulin over-reaction, causing blood sugar levels to drop too far. This leads to tiredness and the other symptoms described above.

Diabetes

The relationship between coffee and diabetes has been periodically examined, especially the possibility of whether the insulin-dependent variety of the disease can be triggered in the offspring of women who drink large amounts of the beverage while pregnant. A 1990 report in the *British Medical Journal*[6] amassed what it thought was some incriminating evidence. Finland, the authors noted, has the highest incidence of insulin-dependent (ID) diabetes in the world. Its population also drinks more coffee than any other nation. As coffee drinking has increased, so has ID diabetes. Other countries with high coffee consumption also have more ID diabetes. A breakdown of the Finnish figures showed some specific relationship between large-volume coffee drinkers and the amount of diabetes found in their offspring.

How might the damage be done? The authors blame the

caffeine which, they say, crosses the placenta into the foetus in whose liver and brain, in particular, it accumulates.

'We postulate that high concentrations of caffeine or its metabolites [by-products created during breakdown by the liver] have a toxic effect on intrauterine [within the womb] development of the pancreatic cells that produce insulin in genetically susceptible foetuses.'

They did, however, advise caution on interpreting the figures, a sensible move given that among the factors that seemed to have been left out of their calculations was sugar intake by these coffee-guzzling mothers.

Aggression

The effect of caffeine on the aggressive urges of psychiatric patients was put to the test in a 1,200-bed California state psychiatric hospital, when caffeine-containing coffee and soft drinks were banned from sale in the hospital canteen and from vending machines. (Though sales of tea, hot chocolate, and chocolate bars continued, and there was other access to caffeinated products via local stores and visitors.) Patient behaviour was analysed[7] before and after the April 1987 partial prohibition, with the following results: assaults against other patients were down 29 per cent, those against staff fell 25 per cent, and property destruction dropped 51 per cent.

Prior to the ban, it was reported that some of the patients were guzzling ten to twenty cups a day and a number were actually snorting instant coffee crystals – the tell-tale signs being their coffee-brown 'moustaches'.

But even these fairly impressive data were insufficient to convince a fellow Californian senior shrink who reported that, at another state psychiatric hospital which he had studied, aggression was substantially down without there having been a caffeine ban.[8] 'The final answer on the relationship between caffeine and aggressive behaviour', he argued, 'is not yet in.' Among his stated concerns was that any caffeine ban had 'important patient care and patients' rights implications.[9]

Asthma

Most experiments and data-crunching look for negative effects, but an Italian research team found what it believed

125

was a positive relationship between coffee consumption and the prevalence and severity of bronchial asthma.[10] The coffee, they suggested, probably worked its beneficial effects by opening up the bronchial passages. Their conclusions were based on data from the 1983 Italian National Survey. But in a subsequent issue of the same journal, a French researcher said she and her team had looked at figures from their own country's National Health survey and found no such link.[11] The Italians continued the argument by suggesting that the French study was far too small.

Heart

The effect of caffeine on blood pressure and the health of the heart has long been hotly debated in the medical literature. After a raft of dire warnings, the new consensus is that caffeine is now basically in the clear, as long as it's not taken in the form of Scandinavian-style boiled coffee – this being a fast track to a dramatic rise in blood cholesterol levels, which in turn leads to heart disease.

The all-clear was sounded by the *Canadian Journal of Cardiology*: 'It now appears that caffeine and coffee do not increase mortality from heart disease, neither do they significantly affect cholesterol or other lipid [blood fat] levels. Finally, it has been shown that their effect on cardiac rhythm in health and disease has been much exaggerated.'

One paper even suggested that four to five cups of caffeinated beverages per day is OK for heart disease and coronary thrombosis patients still in the hospital's coronary care unit.[12]

And yet ask your average doctor and s/he's likely to take exactly the opposite view: 'When questioned on their beliefs,' wrote the *Western Journal of Medicine*,[13] 'physicians will generally agree that coffee increases the heart rate, causes cardiac arrhythmias (irregular heartbeats), elevates the blood pressure, increases sympathetic nervous system activity, and is associated with a higher incidence of coronary heart disease.' None of this, said the editorial, was substantiated by the current body of research.

This, as I say, is the present state of the art. A reassessment of the data in however many years might produce a further spectacular somersault in thinking.

Pregnancy

The effect of coffee/caffeine on the developing child is another major research enterprise which has, so far, produced no credible, long-lived evidence to show that there is an increased risk of abortion, malformation, or stillbirth. However, the possible consequences of five or more cups of coffee a day are that the baby will be late to develop[14] and underweight.[15]

With other conditions

Since caffeine activates the acids in the stomach it is as well for people with peptic ulcers not to use it excessively. And the same can be said for people with heart conditions, high blood pressure, or those who suffer from anxiety – despite the uncertain state of medical knowledge regarding the drug's impact on such conditions.

With other drugs

The xanthines react badly with the prescription drugs known as monoamine oxidase inhibitors,. There are potentially dangerous side effects. See pages 86–7

Tolerance

Tolerance describes the way in which the body becomes resistant to a drug's effects and therefore requires increasingly large doses to achieve the desired psychoactive changes – that is, until a ceiling is reached beyond which no amount of the drug will achieve success and will more likely act as a poison. There seems to be some slight tolerance towards the stimulant effects of caffeine, although for many people one daily cup of coffee, particularly in the morning, will go on jolting them awake for years. Quite likely a lot of this thrust from a minimal dose is allied to expectation: the signal of aroma, steam, and so forth. But by whatever device, the body is able to remain responsive to the effects of the same unaltered dose.

Dependence

The caffeine habit is not readily acknowledged because it is so concealed in the entirely acceptable routine of swallowing cup after cup of the hot or cold brew. Not that dependence refers simply to something done every day, but rather to feelings of physical and mental torment that habitual use can lead to. Caffeine is capable of generating a host of such feelings with daily use of about half a dozen cups of tea or coffee, and so can rightly be described as a drug of dependence. Typical symptoms of excessive use are anxiety, moodiness, headaches, muscle twitches, and chronically disturbed sleep. All will usually clear once caffeine intake is reduced.

Chocolate encourages a particularly powerful dependence in some people, but this is likely to be related to factors other than its comparatively modest xanthine content. Apart from being outstandingly palatable, chocolate is the classic binge food – one invested with connotations of guilty excess. As noted earlier, xanthine-laced soft drinks (Pepsi, Coca-Cola, 7-Up, etc.) can also lead to habitual use – 'Coke after Coke after Coke . . .' in the words of a long-running US ad campaign. But, again, isolating caffeine as the vital draw might be wide of the mark. The attraction of chocolate and soft drinks is as likely to depend as much on the sugar and synthetic additives contained in them as on the xanthines.

Earliest Use

The cultivation of the evergreen cacao tree (*Theobroma cacao*) for chocolate goes back three thousands years or more, but is first reliably noted in the realm of the Aztec emperor Montezuma, who, it was believed, guzzled some fifty cups of xocoatl a day. This xocoatl was a hot beverage, not unlike our own unassuming cocoa, but instead of milk and sugar, the beverage was laced with pepper and other spices. And instead of sending the Aztecs to sleep it roused their sex drive. The Catholic Church of the occupying Spanish didn't approve.

Peppered xocoatl wasn't a tremendous hit in Europe. The Spanish mixed it with cinnamon and sugar and, by the late seventeenth century, chocolate houses were established in many of Europe's capitals where people would sup the drink and indulge in high-minded conversation.

The epoch of the chocolate bar was born in 1847 when the Bristol company, Fry & Son, combined cocoa butter with pure chocolate liquor and sugar to produce a solid block. Some thirty years later, milk was added.

Today, West Africa produces most of the world's cocoa beans, around 80 per cent of which is cultivated by smallholder farmers working from tiny plots of land. As a result of price speculation and other fluxes on the international commodity exchange market, many have been brought to the point of economic collapse in recent years.[16] The rest of the world's cocoa is grown on independently owned estates in Brazil, Malaysia, and elsewhere, many of whose underpaid workers suffer health problems including rashes, nausea, and nose bleeds induced by the toxic pesticides routinely sprayed on the crop. At least thirty chemicals are used during cocoa production, according to the UK's Women's Environmental Network.[17] WEN are trying to encourage consumers to switch to organic 'fair trade' chocolate such as Green & Black's Maya Gold.

Coffee

Coffee is a far more recent concoction than chocolate and, according to a Persian saga, one of the many miraculous bequests of Mohammed (570–632). Once, when the Prophet of Islam was suffering from a sleepiness verging on stupor, the Almighty is reported to have commanded the prophet Gabriel to appear with a deep black beverage – as black as the celestial Black Stone of the Kaa'ba, that is the holiest object in all Mecca. The name of this beverage was Kahwa or Kahveh, and it came from the pit of the fruit borne by the tree botanists now call *Coffea arabica*. Mohammed was clearly refreshed by the black drink, for not only was he able to go out and defeat a host of Arabian enemies, he also set in motion the Islamic revolution that proved so troublesome to European Christendom. One of the Prophet's strictures, as conveyed through a chapter in the Koran called 'The Table', is that wine is an evil, not to be touched. It had been the lubricant of the Classical culture, an agent of unconsciousness and darkness. Coffee, by contrast, was the great stimulator which stole wakefulness from sleep, encouraging sharp, disputatious reason which is the hallmark of traditional Islamic culture with its geometric architecture and ultra-correct procedures. Heinrich Jacob, in his 1935 book *The Saga of Coffee*,[18] suggests that there might have been no Moslem civilisation or the later empire without the special fuel of coffee.

Jacob reports that the Arabs originally got the brew from Abyssinia and Somaliland. It was shipped over the desert by camel caravan, then across the Red Sea and on to a further long land journey. This made it a commodity strictly for the wealthy, who drank it not as a beverage but medicinally – probably for migraine, since caffeine constricts the blood vessels around the brain, causing the pounding to ease.

Once the cultivation of local varieties began, prices fell, but consumption didn't increase noticeably until a prohibitionist movement got under way in the Holy City of Mecca. Like the furore that occurred two hundred years later around the London coffee houses, the movement was politically based. It was inspired by the appointment in 1551 of a new ruler of Mecca, who took exception to some local coffee-drinking satirists who were making him the butt of their lampoons. The appointee of the Sultan declared a ban on all-night establishments in which the beverage was drunk, complaining that the din from them 'wounded the night'. The ban caused a riot which was used an an excuse to outlaw coffee itself. Those who persisted in drinking it, says Jacob, were 'bound face to tail on the backs of asses and driven through the town, being flogged all the while'. But the appointee was let down in his grand prohibitory moves by the Sultan. There was nothing in the Koran, the sovereign ruled, forbidding the use of coffee. And, besides, how could he and his courtiers manage without it?

Coffee moved swiftly throughout the whole of the Islamic world, then into Christian territories where it became entangled in something of a theosophic contest with wine. Italian churchmen at first condemned the black beverage as an infidel drink, but it was 'Christianised' by Pope Clement VIII and by the mid-seventeenth century had reached most of Europe.

It was introduced to the UK initially as a medicine. Then, with great suddenness, it became a rage between the years

1670 and 1730. London became filled with coffee houses and the capital consumed more of the beverage than any city in the world. Jacob suggests it was a kind of massive sobering-up exercise after a long spell of morbid insobriety that began after the Civil War. He argues that it reshaped the native literature and political consciousness, as individuals of discrimination filled the new establishments for late-night verbal jousts. They became famous as literary resorts, with men such as Sheridan, Dryden, Swift, and Hogarth among the aficionados. They also had influence on the country's commercial life: banks, the Stock Exchange and Lloyd's all started in coffee houses. In their earliest days they enjoyed a spell as places of robust political intercourse – places to campaign, recruit, and speechify. This ended when the authorities posted a notice ordering the closure of all the capital's coffee establishments 'because in them harm has been done to the King's majesty and to the realm by spreading of malicious and shameful reports.' The powerful brewers had also been complaining of lost business and women's groups were protesting that family life was suffering thanks to the interminable tongue-flapping that the new inns encouraged. 'The Women's Petition Against Coffee', published in 1674, complained that coffee 'made men as unfruitful as deserts whence that unhappy berry is said to be brought'.

A 'compromise' – suitable to the Crown – was forced. The houses could reopen but only if the proprietors forbade the sale of all books, pamphlets, and leaflets, as well as political oratory. Notwithstanding the Crown's efforts, the coffee-house fad ended as quickly as it started. Largely it was a matter of commerce. The drive into India was under way in the early eighteenth century. The British were now landlords of a tea-bearing country.

Tea

Tea has a legend that compares very nicely with the discovery of coffee by the sleepy Mohammed. It concerns an apostle called Dharma, the Buddhist son of an Indian monarch. He is said to have travelled to China where he lived the life of an ascetic, vowing never to sleep so that his body might remain in perpetual communion with God. But he did sleep, to his chagrin, and on wakening ripped off his unfaithful eyelids and flung them to the ground.

The next day he noticed that his eyelid skins had struck roots, and from the roots a tea plant (*Thea sinensis*) had sprouted. He took two of its leaves, laid them on his eyes, and, according to the legend, two new lids grew. Then he chewed some more leaves which, as Jacob reports, 'immediately gave him a feeling of enhanced liveliness, which passed into tranquil cheerfulness and firm determination.' This seems a perfect description of a cup of 'char' when doing its best.

The Chinese were using tea as a substitute for strong drink from as early as the third century AD, and five hundred years later it was being harvested commercially. The Dutch East India Company were the first to import it into Europe in around 1600, and England got hers about sixty years later, with the import monopoly being held by the British East India Company until 1834.

Decaffeinated Coffee

Caffeine was first extracted from coffee by a German chemist, Ferdinand Runge. The year was 1820, and Runge had apparently obtained his boxful of beans from his friend, the poet/dramatist Goethe, who was seeking an explanation for the cause of his insomnia. Runge's work meant that the drug was now available in high-street apothecaries. But it also brought an awareness of just how potent an experience heavy consumption of coffee was liable to be. A clamour grew about the possible deleterious effects. There were condemnations – now extremely familiar – of the speeding-up of modern life for which coffee was held to be partly culpable. A breakthrough was needed. It came from a young German-based merchant called Ludwig Roselius, whose own father was a coffee taster and had died from what Ludwig believed to be coffee poisoning (modern tasters spit out their samples).

Roselius's feat, following on from Runge, was to extract the caffeine, or at least the greater proportion of it, while retaining the essential flavour and aroma. This was done by exposing the raw beans first to steam treatment, then to a wash in solvents that worked only upon the caffeine. The resulting product was well received throughout Europe, although whether the customers of Roselius's Kaffee HAG company were better off with the caffeine intact or the solvent-streaked alternative is debatable. Decaffeinated brands caused worry some years ago in the US when it was learned that the chemical solvent employed – trichlorethylene (also found in cleaning agents) – was a suspected cancer-forming agent. It was banned.

British decaffeinated brands do not use trichlorethylene but they do use other solvents such as methylene chloride (used in some paint strippers and cleaning solutions), ethyl acetate and dichloromethane. As in the Roselius method, the unroasted bean is fattened with steam, solvents are flushed though, taking the caffeine with them, and then the bean is washed or steam-flushed to remove, it is claimed, around 97 per cent of the remaining chemicals.

Newer methods avoid the use of such solvents, calling instead for 'supercritical gases' such as carbon dioxide, or plain water and 'activated carbon' – as in the so-called Swiss water process. It is not always possible to tell which decaffeinated brand has been made using which method because of the lack of labelling information by some manufacturers, who prefer to remain shy on the detail.

Consumption Rates

Daily individual caffeine consumption in the UK has been variously estimated at between 360 and 440 mg, with the most voracious age category being sixty to eighty-year-olds whose prime source is tea.[19] Smokers drink more caffeinated drinks than non-smokers and men more than women. Children, inevitably, get much of their caffeine from fizzy soft drinks and chocolate. Each week they consume, on average, seven bars (or other sweets) and six cans of drink.[20] This is in contrast to a weekly consumption of three small apples and four small carrots, with a quarter of children eating no vegetables whatsoever.[21] For the population as a whole chocolate-eating, after decades of steady growth, has stabilised at about four bars each a week.

Notes

1 Figures from Nigel Scott *et al.*, 'Caffeine consumption in the United Kingdom: A retrospective survey', in *Food Sciences and Nutrition*, 42F, 1989, p. 185.

2 *Drug Abuse Briefing: Fifth edition*, ISDD, 1994, p. 43.

3 Cox *et al.*, *Drugs and Drug Abuse*, Addiction Research Foundation, Toronto, Canada, 1983, p. 209.

4 S. Linn *et al.*, 'No association between coffee consumption and adverse effects in pregnancy', New England Journal of Medicine, 1992, Vol. 306, issue 3, p. 141–5.

5 Robert Beamish, 'Coffee, caffeine, cholesterol, cardiologists and confusion', in the *Canadian Journal of Cardiology*, Vol. 6, No. 3, April 1990, p. 93.

6 Jaakko Tuomilehto *et al.*, 'Coffee consumption as trigger for insulin dependent diabetes mellitus in childhood', in the *British Medical Journal*, Vol. 300, 10 March 1990, p. 642.

7 Marshall Zaslove *et al.*, 'Changes in behaviours of inpatients after a ban on the sale of caffeinated drinks', in *Hospital and Community Psychiatry*, Vol. 42 (1), January 1991, pp. 84–5.

8 Harold Carmel, 'Caffeine and aggression', in *Hospital and Community Psychiatry*, Vol. 42 (6), June 1991, p. 638.

9 Letter from Harold Carmel, by then superintendent at the Colorado State Hospital, to Marshall Zaslove, Napa State Hospital, California, 5 July 1991 (copy in ISSD library).

10 R. Pagano *et al.*, 'Coffee drinking and prevalence of bronchial asthma', in *Chest*, 94, 1988, pp. 386–9.

11 Isabella Annesi *et al.*, 'Coffee drinking and prevalence of bronchial asthma', in *Chest*, 97, 1990, p. 1269.

12 A. Lynn and J. F. Kissinger, 'Coronary Precautions: Should caffeine be restricted in patients after myocardial infarction', in *Heart Lung*, 21 (4), 1992, pp. 365–71.

13 Martin Myers, 'Caffeine under examination – a passing grade', in the *Western Journal of Medicine*, 157 (5), November 1992, p. 587.

14 L. Feinster *et al.*, 'Caffeine consumption during pregnancy and fetal growth', in the *American Journal of Public Health*, 81 (4), 1991, pp. 458–61.

15 S. Narod *et al.*, 'Coffee during pregnancy: A reproductive hazard', in the *American Journal of Obstetrics and Gynecology*, 164 (4), 1991, pp. 1109–14.

16 Tess Swithinbank and Rebecca Downham, 'Choc Horror This Easter', in *The Big Issue*, 29 March 1994, p. 8.

17 Ibid.

18 Heinrich Jacob, *The Saga of Coffee*, Unwin Ltd, London, 1935.

19 Nigel Scott *et al.*, 'Caffeine consumption in the United Kingdom: A retrospective survey', in *Food Sciences and Nutrition*, 42F, 1989, p. 187.
20 'Bitter water hits the big time', in the *Guardian* (Education Section), 29 March 1994, p. 10.
21 Source: National Forum for Coronary Heart Disease Prevention.

CANNABIS

Intro

Cannabis is by far the most dangerous of all the illicit drugs in its effects upon the authorities. By continuing to penalise it as an innately dangerous substance, despite a lack of supporting evidence, they find themselves at odds with literally millions of citizens, more than 40,000 of whom are fined, imprisoned, or cautioned every year.

Policing cannabis not only undermines social cohesion, it is financially expensive, both in terms of the costs of processing such large numbers through the 'justice system' and in the potential tax revenue lost to the Exchequer.

Calculating the size of an illicit trade is, in the end, a matter of guesswork. But as useful a guess as any came from the European Community in a 1991 report which judged the total cannabis trade throughout member states to be worth $7.5 billion a year.[1] This was three times the size of the heroin market and nearly $1 billion more than the value of cocaine.

Even when 2,200 tonnes of cannabis are taken out of circulation, as European enforcement authorities managed to do in 1990, they still found there was 'no appreciable effect on availability or price on the market.'[2]

The argument for resisting the immense cannabis tide is the same as that used when insisting that thieving and violence (unless state-sanctioned) must be opposed, even though many people take pleasure or profit from these activities. Furthermore, goes the argument, loosening up the cannabis laws would send out the wrong 'soft-on-drugs' signals, especially to the young, who might be catapulted from reefer-smoking into heroin and cocaine addiction.

You can spin the data any way you choose – although it is statistically simpler to prove a causal link between early alcohol use and 'hard' drugs than to join together hash and heroin junkiedom. And there is even some reasonably plausible evidence to suggest that those who have never experimented with any drug during adolescence are 'relatively anxious, emotionally constricted, and lacking in social skills', compared with youngsters who went in for a little drug use (primarily cannabis). The total abstainers, according to this American survey[3] – which followed 101 subjects between the ages of five and eighteen – fell into the same uptight, 'maladjusted' category as heavy users. Imagine, if you will, how popular these findings were in *Just Say No* Reagan's America.

Can cannabis cause physical and emotional harm? While no cannabis-linked fatality has ever been reliably recorded, any drug is potentially damaging; it depends how and by whom it is used. Conversely, even the most excoriated substances can be 'self-administered' benignly. This is why categorising substances as 'hard' and 'soft' (usually to score points on behalf of cannabis at the expense of other drugs) is a bogus exercise, one that's bound to lead to constant revisionism as different drugs fall in and out of style and modes of ingestion change. (Note the way the sleeping pill temazepam has, in recent years, raced from the bottom to the top of the hazard league.)

While all the evidence indicates that there is no real medical case any more against moderate use of cannabis by adults, many people reading this chapter will be able to bring to mind friends or family members whose senses have been made mushy by dope. Invariably it's a temporary condition, one that rights itself when smoking stops. But how many people do we know who seem unable to curb their intake, despite firm resolutions. The trend favouring home-grown sledgehammer-type weeds, such as skunk and Northern Lights, makes it all the more important to talk straightforwardly about what cannabis is and what it is not.

But the essential point to remember, as the centuries-old legalisation/decriminalisation debate creaks along, is that millions of people in this country now choose to consume this adaptable, rapid-growing plant. They find it nourishing and relaxing. It makes them giggle and eat a lot. It extends their sensory range and often causes them to perform a double-take on 'reality'. This last characteristic is probably the most dangerous of all and is the reason why making war on the plant and on its champions merely confirms the always-fashionable theory among alert youth that the first duty of the state is to safeguard orthodox brands of thinking and acting rather than preserve the freedom of all its citizens.

If this analysis is right, then cannabis presents a first-class challenge. For it is a drug, according to *Food of the Gods* (Bantam) author Terence McKenna, that 'has a mitigating effect on competition, causes one to question authority, and reinforces the notion of the merely relative importance of social values.'

The government's present pseudo-strategy in relation to cannabis is a failure. It is expensive, unworkable, and breeds alienation and cynicism on both sides of the penal divide. We now have several alternative models to consider – everything from free market access, to rationing, to control within a medical context or within a licensed premises context (much like alcohol). And there is also Harvard Medical School psychiatry professor Lester Grinspoon's suggestion of a 'harmfulness tax', which would oblige users to buy a kind of insurance against the harm their drug use might cause society. Such a scheme would be guaranteed to prick national self-righteousness on the subject of drugs, given that cannabis is responsible for zero deaths every year, compared with around 110,000 caused by tobacco.

The calls for change are now coming from top policemen and from politicians across the spectrum. In a discussion paper on the subject,[4] the legal advice agency Release worked through the various options and suggested a 'step by step' approach designed to draw along neighbouring countries while avoiding turning the UK into an easy touch for those who want to smuggle out our (inevitably) moderately priced, state-authorised dope to countries where there remained a prohibitionist regime.

The Release proposals, and those like them, are anything but cast-iron. No scheme can ever be devised that will accommodate human beings' propensity for greed and stupidity. 'What is required,' Release pleads, is 'a degree of vision and the courage to make a "leap of faith".'

The alternative is to maintain the status quo. But with the political and social costs rising every year, that won't remain an option for much longer.

139

What is it?

Cannabis is the name the international regulatory agencies give to the group of intoxicating products derived from a green and bushy plant with saw-toothed leaves, fluted stalks, ranging in height from three to twenty feet. It is the male which produces the tough fibres from which hemp cloth and rope is made, the female which generates the sticky aromatic resins. Most of the resin is exuded from the flowering tops, but some is also found in the leaves. The traditional view has been that all cannabis plants are members of the same genus, *Cannabis sativa*. But botanists have also argued that *sativa* is but one species of the genus and that there are two others – one they call *Cannabis indica* and the other *Cannabis ruderalis*.

Of the three sorts, *sativa* is the lankiest and requires the most light for the flowers to mature adequately. It flourishes in equatorial regions, with Thailand, Colombia, and Nigeria among the major source countries. *Indica* is the finely formed, extremely resinous plant originating in India. Shorter than *sativa*, it requires a shorter flowering period and lower light levels. *Ruderalis* is the tough, stocky type that has traditionally grown wild by the roadside in central Asia and whose seeds are capable of surviving icy Russian winters.

From the raw material of these basic types, the plant engineers have been at work producing strains to fit the modern market. Skunk is the most celebrated – a noxious-smelling product that is both famously intoxicating and sturdy enough to do nicely outside a greenhouse in temperate climates such as that offered by Holland, the country in which it was first bred. Sales of the seeds from these new potent strains have encouraged a home-grown market throughout Europe and, by 1993, some twenty UK skunk 'farms' were discovered by the authorities, many of them in rural Wales.[5]

Home-grown

More significantly, a new breed of city-based dope growers began flourishing around this time, serviced by new-wave seed companies (asking anything from £5 to £15 per seed for top-quality material) and equipment suppliers who could lay on a start-up kit (lights, timer, fan or CO_2 spray, nutrient broth, and pumping system) for maybe £800 to £1,000. This was a lot of money for a dole kid living/squatting in a council flat to find. But with one ounce of weed fetching £150 to £200, and with some growers producing 200 to 300 plants at a time inside their lofts, the profits soon rolled in.

As I write this (October 1994) experienced drug-watchers were expecting a major assault on what had so far been a lightly policed phenomenon.

Hashish and herbal

While the home-grown herbal market was booming by the mid-1990s, the cannabis product still most often found in the UK is the caked resin of North African plants which comes in slabs, chunks, sticky balls, or powdery flakes and is called *hashish*. Here, it is smoked, but in its home regions it is often eaten in a spiced, fruity confection called *majoon*. In India hash is known by its Hindi word – *charas*. The other domestically consumed cannabis product is made up of the dried and chopped leafy parts of the plant. It is home-grown or imported from as far afield as the West Indies, Africa, Thailand, and South America. Many are its names: *ghanja, ganga, marijuana, draw, blow, weed, grass, dope, bush, puff* . . . Most people know it as an unpredictable mix of sticks, seeds, leaves, and flowering tops, but some fine distinctions are made. For instance, *ghanja* and marijuana are apparently not the same thing at all. Marijuana should be devoid of seeds and twigs, whereas *ghanja* can have everything thrown in.

Exotica

There are several more cannabis variables, but these are rarely found on the streets of the UK. There is *bhang*, which is the leaves of the plant pounded into a fine powder, spiced and brewed into a beverage. *Bhang*, confusingly, also refers to a smoking mixture of leaves plus stems and twigs. Other kinds of exotica include: *Tibetan Temple Balls* – dark, soft, resinous nuggets from the Chinese-occupied realm of the Dalai Lama; *sinsemilla* (the word is Spanish for 'without seeds'), a high-potency herbal speciality made from the unpollinated flowers of the female plant; and *Thai sticks*, another super-strong variety in which the dried herb is tied by hemp fibres to a stick. The stick formula is now used for other grasses in order to kid consumers that they are getting a quality product.

Other rarities include the high-powered Colombian grasses, *Chiba* and *Gold*; *Oaxacan Red* from Mexico; and some famous blasts from Hawaii, including *Maui*, *Oahu* and *Maui Wowee*. Then there are *Surfboards* from Afghanistan, *Moon Discs* from Kanhairi, *Finger Clusters* from the Himalayas, and *Pellet Rubbings* from Nepal.

But, as with street pills and powders, the name under which a cannabis product is marketed more often reflects the fad of the moment than the real nature of what is on offer. Any dried herb can be tied to a stick. And if the customer prefers *sensi* to African then it is a simple matter to sift out the seeds and throw in a little parsley. UK cannabis *cognoscenti* will be best served by the coffee bars of Holland, in which arcane varieties of hash and grass are legally served. Aside from the more traditional concoctions, the best-stocked bars will also have on offer the new intensively reared hybrids of which skunk is the best known but which also include items known as Northern Lights, Hash Plant, and Haze.

Oil

For those who prefer a more concentrated experience there is *hash oil*, also known as *honey oil*, five times more potent weight for weight than resin. It is made by boiling finely powdered hash in a solvent such as alcohol and straining out the cellulose solids. The solvent then evaporates, leaving behind a sticky greeny/brown oil. This can be further refined down to colourless, tasteless tetrahydrocannabinoil (THC) which is the plant's main psychotropic ingredient.

First isolated in the 1940s, it was not until 1966 that THC was first reproduced synthetically. Since then is has yielded up more than eighty derivatives, many of which are being used experimentally in the treatment of ailments such as glaucoma, multiple sclerosis, epilepsy, and to ease the nausea and vomiting caused by chemotherapy given to cancer patients.

Medical Dope

It is not generally realised that until 1973 one of the most potent products of the plant was available on general prescription in the UK, chiefly for 'exploring psychiatric states.'[6] Known – like the plant species – as *Cannabis indica*, it came as a green tincture or as a green extract. Both comprised the flowering tops of the best Indian cannabis, pounded, sifted, and treated with alcohol. One London man tells me his doctor prescribed it for him 'to relieve the paranoia that overcame me' at the thought of being busted for possession of illegal dope.' In fact the prescription of medical cannabis goes back to the mid-nineteenth century, when it was considered the standard treatment for migraine.

Source Countries

Assumptions about how much cannabis is coming into Europe and from where are generally made on the basis of Customs and police seizure data. Such figures more accurately reflect politically driven enforcement priorities than genuine trafficking patterns. Even so, it's a fair assumption that Morocco, Pakistan, the Lebanon, and Afghanistan are the principal suppliers of hash; while Jamaica (especially for the UK), Thailand, Colombia, and western and southern Africa provide the bulk of herbal cannabis.

Lebanese hash, grown in that country's Bekaa valley, was once the UK market leader, but the Moroccan product now seems to dominate. Some estimates[7] suggest that Morocco grows one-third of all cannabis consumed in Europe and that it has some 31,000 hectares of land, in the essentially 'lawless', sparsely populated Rif mountain area, under cannabis cultivation. In an effort to divert local farmers into growing more wholesome products, the European Community agreed in September 1993 to a £1.5 billion five-year subsidy programme. Without the Euro cash, claimed Moroccan government officials, it would take a century to cure their indigenous farmers of their hash dependence.

As it is, experienced consumers often talk testily these

days of Moroccan and other 'bog standard' resins. They complain that the modern product is bland and homogenised – a feature, they say, of new production methods, whereby different-quality resins, from wherever in the world, are combined and reprocessed after arriving in Europe. In this way, 'Moroccan' and 'Paki' become terms denoting a type of hash rather than the country of origin. And just as the blending of variable-quality whiskies results in an inferior nip compared with the pure malt, so the authentic hash experience is increasingly hard to come by.

Hash, for other reasons, was going out of style in the mid-1990s – losing ground to weed, which is generally considered a lighter, less stupefying experience.

Getting it here

The chief gateways into Europe are judged to be Holland, Spain, and France – because they are geographically convenient and/or have useful ethnic ties with the source countries which provide cover for those involved.

There are ten thousand schemes for avoiding apprehension, calling for a high order of acting, persuasion, bribery, practical mechanics, force, and the manipulation of the innocent. Small amounts are smuggled in through commercial airports. Large volumes come by truck and ship. Cargo vessels are specially leased or purchased, with the contraband taken on board, perhaps, just outside the territorial waters of the country of origin.[8] Busy shipping lanes are avoided where possible. Vessels carrying consignments to the UK, for instance, will dodge sailing the Channel and aim, instead, for more remote coastal waters.

Most official reports declare that the cannabis trade is increasingly organised and violent, with some of the prime players now also caught up in illegal arms trafficking, contract killings, and the promotion of 'subversive' political groups. The European cannabis trade, after all, is said to be worth in excess of $7.5 billion.[9]

Without doubt, it is a more desperately bloody business than in the hippy 1960s. But the menace can be exaggerated. The enforcement authorities, with their perpetual concerns for future funding, have an interest in painting the bleakest picture possible. And, being large, cumbersome bureaucracies, they tend, instinctively, to see their most potent foes in the same light: as ruthless international gangs, governed by hierarchies and by a common method. They find it difficult to acknowledge the often small-scale, ad hoc dimension that is at work in international trafficking of all outlawed drugs, heroin and cocaine included. Drug markets, argues Nicholas Dorn of the London-based Institute for the Study of Drug Dependence, are actually dominated by medium to small players. He sees Europol, the drugs intelligence unit of the European Union, which was established in February 1994, as 'a giraffe on a virtually tree-less plain'.[10]

Methods of Ingestion

Every conceivable route has been used for getting cannabis into the body. It can be eaten in a sweet or savoury concoction, or drunk in tea or other beverages, but smoking is the method employed by those wanting to partake of the intoxicant effects most efficiently. In the UK this usually involves rolling a *joint* or *spliff* from several cigarette papers stuck together. It will contain tobacco sprinkled with heat-softened resin or a quantity of grass. The ratio of grass to tobacco is usually two to one in favour of the tobacco. For a hash joint, a pellet the size of a grain of corn will suffice. Joints are often completed with a half-inch-long rolled cardboard filter.

Both hash and grass are also smoked in pipes. The types include clay *chillums*, brass *grill tops*, and the venerable *hookah* which cools and softens the smoke by passing it through a channel of water. Blobs of hash can also be balanced on the hot end of a cigarette and the snake of smoke inhaled straight through the mouth or via a ballpoint casing. These pellets can also be heated on a sheet of foil and the smoke sucked up, or they can be clamped between hot knives, the smoke trapped in a milk bottle and sucked up in an enormous gust.

Unlike cigarette fumes, cannabis smoke is not carelessly blown around the room. It is inhaled deeply into the lungs and held there for several seconds. This often causes the novice to erupt in a fit of violent coughing, but the lungs eventually learn how to cope with the experience and veteran smokers are even able to talk, though in a faintly silly voice, while holding the fumes deep inside them.

Sensations

The specifics of the cannabis experience can't easily be set down. This is not simply because of the great range of resins and grasses, or because of each person's varied response, but because, as much as any other drug, cannabis is supremely responsive to the flickering of human emotions, more so even than the Big Gun hallucinogens such as LSD and Liberty Cap. For while this so-called 'soft' drug does not create LSD's big psycho bang, it does create changes in feelings and perceptions that can be profound. Even so, cannabis's *soft* reputation means that it is inadmissible in certain 'experienced' circles to show any outward sign of being affected. This kind of bottling-up doesn't make for the happiest experience, especially where the new, purpose-bred, high-potency super-weeds, such as skunk, are being sampled.

Smoking

Smoking a couple of grains of medium-quality hash mixed with tobacco will have a less forceful effect on the brain than gulping a lungful of the same via the hot knives method. But however it is inhaled, no smoker will have to wait more than about ten minutes if the resin or grass has anything to offer. The initial feelings depend on the quality of the cannabis. Hash is often more immobilising, grass lighter and speedier – although there are certain grasses that are capable of pinning the user to the floor after just a couple of 'tokes'. More usually there will be feelings of uninhibitedness, dreaminess, heightened awareness of sound, colour, textures. Music will probably sound more magnificent than usual. Hidden layers

146

and meanings can be revealed and there'll be an impulse to utter profundities, to giggle and eat a great deal.

Younger, less repressed smokers can close their eyes and witness, for instance, vivid cartoon hallucinations. Skunk and other powerful weeds can generate sub-LSD mind-warping effects even with the eyes open. They can also make the ground shift and, on occasion, lead to vomiting.

The communion between fellow smokers is often powerful. Intimacies, both sexual and mental, might be shared. Higher doses and/or heavier blends ultimately lead to a paralysis of the imagination and a reluctance to move a single limb.

A description of the cannabis experience from 1854, by the American writer and lecturer Bayard Taylor, still stands the test of time. He was on a visit to Egypt when, in 'a spirit of inquiry', he tried the drug.

'The sensations it then produced were . . . physically of exquisite lightness and airiness – mentally of a wonderfully keen perception of the ludicrous in the most simple and familiar objects. During the half-hour in which it lasted, I was at no time so far under its control that I could not, with the clearest perception, study the changes through which I had passed. I noted with careful attention the fine sensations which spread throughout the whole tissue of my nervous fibres, each thrill helping to divest my frame of its earthly and material nature, till my substance appeared to me no grosser than the vapours of the atmosphere, and while sitting in the calm of the Egyptian twilight I expected to be lifted up and carried away by the first breeze that should ruffle the Nile. While this process was going on, the objects by which I was surrounded assumed a strange whimsical expression . . . I was provoked into a long fit of laughter . . . [the effect] died away as gradually as it came, leaving me overcome with a soft and pleasant drowsiness, from which I sank into a deep and refreshing sleep.'[11]

Eating

While smoking provides almost instantaneous effects, those delivered by eating hash or grass can take ninety minutes to become noticeable. The results come on stealthily, sometimes deepening beyond what the user desires. A hash smoker who has had too much simply stops toking. A hash eater might already have eaten too much without knowing it yet continues to fill up on the cake, pudding, or whatever the means of delivery. The edible high is often described as more of a 'body experience'. There will more likely be sub-LSD-type hallucinations, with objects swelling and shrinking.

But the idea that leaves and sticks can be steeped in water and the resulting solution washed down for the kind of effects described above is unequivocally put down by the cannabis gourmand Adam Gottlieb in his pocket-book *Cooking with Cannabis*.[12] 'If the plant is good quality,' says Gottlieb, 'strenuous boiling might encourage some resin to float off into the water, but this is wildly inefficient.' He maintains that THC, the main active ingredient in cannabis, is not soluble in water, only in oils and alcohol. So it's in these that it should first be soaked or sautéed before combining with whatever other ingredients are to be used.

Paranoia

This crops up fairly regularly among dope smokers and is typically caused by an inability to relax. It is often said mainly to affect novice users and will, therefore, vanish after a few sessions. But older dopeheads – though, perhaps, reluctant to admit it – can also get into an anxious state from their first inhalation. Apart from the mental state of the user, bad adulterants are thought to cause paranoia. It is believed that camel dung is sometimes mixed in with Moroccan resin, while South African grass has been known to contain *datura* – a less marketable psychoactive plant that is renowned as a stupefying agent and poison. *Datura* is one likely cause of what drug professionals call Cannabis Psychosis (see below).

No Effects

In a percentage of resistant individuals cannabis has no psychoactive effect at all. For some it produces nausea. One young woman reports that it did nothing at all for her except 'made me lose control of my bladder so that I weed myself.'

Regular, Heavy Use

A sizeable proportion of cannabis users consume it on a regular, even daily, basis, and as a consequence tend to live in a fog. In especially heavy users the fog becomes so thick as to cut off a sharp appreciation of 'reality'. Lethargy sets in. They can become dull and ponderous in conversation, with thoughts tailing away mid-stream. A case history is Colin, a thirty-five-year-old former charity worker, now doing freelance research work.

'Definitely, you get into this fog and there are certain things you can't do like learning to drive a car or learning a new piece of software. I find that when I'm writing something I can do the first draft better stoned but not the final one. There's always a tendency to start and not finish stuff. When it comes to long-term memory you can recall visual images but lose a lot of numbers. You lose specific words and have to grope for alternatives, which is frustrating because I think of myself as good with words.'

Colin says it generally takes three days of abstinence to clear his head and another couple to purge his whole system. During such times he finds himself drinking more.

'Is cannabis a *soft* drug, as it's usually portrayed? It depends how and how often it's used. Certain personalities will destroy themselves on whatever is available.'

Paul, from Camden in North London, is eleven years Colin's junior, an athletic, upper-middle-class individual whose mother designs house interiors, while his father is 'in property'.

Paul had his first joint aged fourteen but used only sporadically for the next five years. Rugby absorbed him more and he was good enough to be signed up by the Wasps. He quit sport after starting at his Midlands university – fed up with the bruises, the five-times-a-week practice and playing sessions, and the infantile low jinks – 'the willy-dipping in the beer', as he calls it. Instead of studying, he succumbed to indiscipline and idleness. He dealt cannabis to his fellow students and organised music promotions.

'I rapidly became the most successful cannabis dealer in the place and managed to completely fund my university days with it, whizzing down the M40 and back to pick up more stuff.'

Upon re-entering civic society, he took a dive. 'I would find myself getting badly stressed because I couldn't get the kind of job I felt I deserved. So rather than be pissed off all day I'd smoke a joint. But then you don't get anything done though you half don't realise the state you're in because everything seems a bit easier and you don't mind so much. Then, of course, you do mind after a while. Mentally, it's slowed me down a lot, slowed down my brain. And I'm now short of breath.'

He describes a typical night in with one of his mates. 'Whatever happens I'll have been smoking a few joints after getting back from work, or if I haven't been at work I'll probably be completely stoned already. Pete will arrive with a few beers. He'll smoke a few joints as well which will completely whack him out and he'll be just talking shit for a while with me grunting. Then we'll get it together a little bit when it's almost time for him to go home, and it's all very unsatisfying. That's when you end up being annoyed with yourself and that's when you realise it's a real day-to-day thing because you don't get anything out of it.'

He says it's not unhappiness or any kind of personality disorder which drives his cannabis appetite: 'I just happen to have the flavour for it and a certain addiction does build up. There's no doubt about that.'

But he says he's fed up with not working, with the barren days, and has recently managed to curtail substantially his intake. 'It's easier to stay in the doldrums than get off your arse, and it takes a certain amount of time before you realise you've got to. That's where I am now.'

Impact on Health
[The World Health Organisation Report]

In the past twenty-five years there have been numerous substantive reviews of cannabis and its general impact on human health. As consequential as anything yet issued was the report that arose out of a meeting in Toronto during the winter of 1981.[13] Chaired by the Canadian Addiction Research Foundation and the World Health Organisation, the resulting document doesn't exactly clear up all the loose ends (the *realpolitik* of drugs research requires ambiguity and calls for further research) but it does have something to say about how cannabis is received and conducted through every imaginable part of the body. Its main findings are as follows:

General toxicity

Intermittent use of low-potency material doesn't generally produce obvious symptoms of toxicity. Daily or more frequent use, especially of the high-potent preparations, can produce 'chronic intoxication' taking weeks to clear after drug use is discontinued.

Respiratory system

Cannabis smoke appears more injurious to the lungs than cigarette smoke, and hashish smoke is worse than herbal. Possible consequences are bronchitis and, 'after sufficient exposure', lung cancer.

Heart

Little evidence of toxic effect on the heart muscles, but users with pre-existing heart disease risk compromising that organ further.

Growth and body weight

No reliable data.

Gastro-intestinal

May produce vomiting, diarrhoea, and 'abdominal distress'. Chronic use could make the intestine more susceptible to infection.

Chromosomal damage

Studies to date show no cell abnormality or mutagenic effects attributable to cannabis.

Cancer

'Analysis of cannabis smoke, animal studies and one clinical report suggest that cannabis may have significant carcinogenic potential.' Cannabis tar (the dark, sticky substance which forms as the smoke cools and condenses) is considered the chief culprit, and while no evidence of cannabis-induced cancer in humans exists, it could show up in the future.

Immune system

The body's natural defence systems play a major role in defending it against infection and preventing the growth and spread of malignant cells. There is 'suggestive, but not conclusive' evidence that consumption of cannabis or THC may produce immune dysfunction.

Allergic potential

It has some, although it appears 'uncommon'.

The male reproductive system

Animal tests indicate 'prolonged intake' leads to decreased sperm production and other disruptions of male reproductive capacity. But these effects are apparently reversible, and in any case tests have been confined largely to immature rats. In humans nothing conclusive emerges.

The female reproductive system

There was one report of disrupted menstrual cycles among cannabis-smoking women – otherwise the subject is virtually unexplored in human females.

Fertility

No consistent evidence of decreased or increased fertility.

Driving ability

It can and often does impair driving-ability and actual performance – even in small doses – but whether this translates into vehicle accidents and how often hasn't been satisfactorily demonstrated.

Intellectual function

'A host of studies have demonstrated impaired functioning on a variety of cognitive and performance tasks during marijuana intoxication.' The faculties to suffer include memory, sense of time, reaction time, motor co-ordination, attention, and signal detection. In most laboratory studies 'memory alterations' last just a few hours, but for some there may be 'more lasting problems with transfers of new information into long-term memory storage.' For the most part, cognitive task impairment is 'dose-related', but there are apt to be 'multiple marijuana effects' depending on the exact demands of the task. 'Performance on some cognitive tasks might even improve when low doses are used.'

Amotivational syndrome

A term used by researchers to encompass apathy, loss of ambition, impaired ability to carry out difficult tasks, neglect of personal appearance, etc. The syndrome cannot be tied plausibly to cannabis use – 'better to discard it and adopt *chronic cannabis intoxication*'.

Psychiatric effects

The existence of short-lasting panic and paranoid states arising from cannabis use 'are no longer questioned'. They could be due mainly to the user's lack of experience or 'adverse social conditions'.

Problems of chronic use

Most important among them is the cannabis-related psychosis whose symptoms, lasting up to four weeks, include mental confusion and impulsive behaviour. In Western societies the incidence is 'quite low'. It seems mainly to affect very heavy users who already have a disturbed personality. The higher frequency in, for instance, North Africa and India 'may soon disappear as the validity of this diagnosis is being questioned and the use of this term is being abandoned in that region'. However, the West will likely show a rising incidence as the number of heavy users in the population increases.

Tolerance

Tolerance to most of the effects of THC (the main mood-altering ingredient) develops in much the same pattern as that for opioids, nicotine, and alcohol. So-called 'reverse tolerance' (the effects of the drug coming on more easily for the practised users instead of needing an increased dose), 'if it occurs at all, is likely to be due to conditioned responses linked to familiar cues'. (Namely, the user responds not pharmacologically, but to the setting and ritual.)

Dependence

Although scientific opinion is divided, there is now 'substantial evidence' that at least mild degrees of both psychological and physical dependence can occur.

Withdrawal

Some reports note elements of withdrawal similar to those caused by opioids, alcohol and sedatives, with reports of sweating, nausea, and muscle spasms. Other studies have found only 'post-drug irritability'.

Vulnerable groups

Fast-growing adolescents and older people who metabolise drugs more slowly may be more sensitive to the drug's effects, while a variety of conditions in the general population can be exacerbated. These include mental illness, heart disease, and epilepsy.

WHO summarised and evaluated

The use of moderate doses of cannabis produces intoxication associated with dose-related impairment of driving and machine-operating ability. The desired state is euphoria, although in some situations the user experiences short-lived reactions ranging from mild anxiety to an acute psychosis. Daily or more frequent use, especially of potent material, can produce chronic intoxication taking several weeks to clear after use is discontinued. Respiratory toxicity is observed in heavy users and may depend on smoking techniques and the combustion properties of particular material. Effects on the hormonal, reproductive and immunological states of heavy users is unclear. Chronic administration can lead to the development of tolerance to a wide variety of the drug's effects, although opinion is divided on dependence. To a mild degree, at least, physical and psychological dependence are believed to occur.

Certain groups such as the young and old are 'susceptible to the effects of cannabis', but in general a low prevalence of adverse effects has been observed even among heavy users. 'Given that millions of individuals are now using the drug, even relatively infrequent but serious adverse consequences could be of public health significance.'

Many users of cannabis, as well as experienced workers in the drugs and medical field would consider the ARF/WHO vision of cannabis as obsessively strict. No human fatalities have as yet been reported as a result of cannabis use, which makes it safer than virtually any other mood-altering drug – licit or illicit – now available. The report, and others like it, also omits from its brief an analysis of the drug's therapeutic potential (see below). It also omits an analysis of the wounding effect its illegal status has on relations between smokers and the authorities. Research into adverse medical consequences nonetheless carries on apace with the focus of concern settling, at the time of writing, on the impact on pregnancy, 'cannabis psychosis', and intellectual performance.

Pregnancy

The effects of cannabis on reproduction remain a complicated and disputed issue. In men, a single dose of THC lowers sperm count, as well as the level of the sex hormone testosterone.[14] But there seems to be no evidence – other than from animal experiments – that these changes affect sexual performance or fertility.

THC has also been shown to reduce the level of female hormones in various laboratory animals, and when pregnant monkeys, rats and mice are exposed to the equivalent of a heavy human THC dose, stillbirths and decreased birth weight are sometimes found in their offspring.[15] Elsewhere in this book I argue about the invalidity of animal experiments, pointing out that non-human animals continually respond to drugs differently from ourselves – being unaffected by substances that would kill us, and vice versa.

Nonetheless, there are reports of low birth weight, prematurity, and even a condition resembling the foetal alcohol syndrome (see alcohol chapter) in some children whose mothers smoke a lot of cannabis during pregnancy.[16] Like the animal-based data, this kind of research is also far from wholly trustworthy. The main problem facing the data-gatherers is how to extract non-cannabis factors that potentially have a powerful impact on pregnancy: for instance, the use of other drugs such as alcohol, tobacco, and caffeine; and the general condition of the parents. It is well established that virtually every kind of human malady – from TB to cancer to sickly babies – is most commonly found among the poor.

Lester Grinspoon, associate professor of psychiatry at Harvard Medical School and a leading campaigner for relaxing the cannabis laws, offers this advice: 'To be safe, pregnant and nursing women should follow the standard conservative recommendation to avoid all drugs, including cannabis, that are not absolutely necessary.'

Cannabis psychosis

This is an ornate term for what used to be called 'madness', or at least for one branch of madness. History shows that insanity has always been an affliction disproportionately affecting the 'unproductive poor'. In British Imperial India the lunatic asylums were filled with people for whom the authorities could find no other good purpose.[17] And where no reason could be found for incarcerating them, 'ghanja insanity' was as convenient a diagnosis as any. Those running such establishments have admitted as much.[18]

Today, the principal group under investigation are young West Indian males, a category for whom there is no obvious economic or social niche within modern Britain. That many of them use ghanja and, while under the influence and even when straight, act in a way that baffles and/or disturbs upright, middle-class white psychiatrists, is reason enough to bracket them as cannabis psychotic. That various medics have made something of a career out of researching this field (seeing how many black male ghanja smoking schizophrenics they can find) signals that it is time the areas of race, madness, prejudice, and the political/medical power élite were better scrutinised. I remember a few years ago visiting the secure unit of a psychiatric hospital that served a large London catchment area and being dismayed to see that virtually every face – made long and vacant by licitly prescribed sedating drugs – was a black one.

While there is no convincing evidence for the existence of a 'cannabis psychosis' – that is to say, a long-lasting state of mental derangement for which the drug is responsible – cannabis can precipitate short-lived mental disturbances, probably as a result of the toxins in the drug interfering with brain function. The condition is more likely to be caused by eating large quantities than by smoking, with symptoms including restlessness, confusion, bewilderment, disorientation, dream-like thinking, fear, illusions, and hallucinations.[19] Sobriety invariably brings an end to the misery. Being coldly examined and questioned by a man in a white coat is likely to make matters worse.

157

Intellectual performance

This has already been touched on in this chapter. Aside from what the WHO had to say, we have heard from two heavy users – Paul and Colin – who were convinced that they were functioning less well as a result of their cannabis intake. They could be right. But broad-based human studies fail to confirm that prolonged heavy use leads to lasting loss of intellectual performance or to neurological damage. Perhaps the salient point here is that compulsive drug users are often bored, listless, alienated, and otherwise troubled personalities whose problems pre-date the substance use. Yet the drugs are often identified as the damage factor. Cannabis can, in some circumstances, precipitate or quicken a decline, but its use can also be a form of self-medication; without it, the descent might be that much steeper.

Therapeutic value

Oddly enough, the most compelling argument to date as to the value of cannabis therapeutics has come from that scourge of drug pedlars, the US's Drug Enforcement Agency. Between 1986 and 1988 it heard evidence from doctors and patients and studied thousands of pages of documentation. The conclusions reached by administrative law judge Francis J. Young, on 6 September 1988, caused a major political tremor.[20]

'Nearly all medicines have toxic, potentially lethal effects,' declared Young, 'but marijuana is not such a substance. Marijuana in its natural form is one of the safest active substances known to man. By any measure of rational analysis marijuana can be safely used within a supervised routine of medical care.'

In the last century, the therapeutic value of cannabis was widely recognised, but then it was found to be politically and commercially profitable to ditch the drug. Today, substances such as cocaine, morphine, barbiturates, and temazepam are all available as legal medicines, but not cannabis – despite the latter being the only one on that list which has never been reliably linked with any human fatality.

Informal (illegal) as well as Home Office-licensed testing of the drug and its chemical derivatives does continue, with promising developments in the area of multiple sclerosis, glaucoma, epilepsy, appetite stimulation, asthma, pain relief, and as a remedy for the nausea and vomiting caused by standard anti-cancer chemotherapy drugs. The evidence of countless patients speaks of the sometimes spectacular benefits of the weed. MS sufferers swear that it relieves muscles spasms and other symptoms to the point where they can leave their wheelchairs; people with glaucoma (a disease in which fluid pressure within the eyeball increases until it damages the optic nerve) say that cannabis can restore dwindling eyesight by reducing such pressure.

Lester Grinspoon reports on one young man whose severe muscle spasms throughout his paralysed body – caused by an accidental gunshot wound – were relieved within minutes of smoking a joint.[21] The man also found he could achieve an erection when smoking, whereas this was only possible before by injecting prostaglandin E (a manufactured hormone with potentially severe side effects) directly into his penis.

Grinspoon saw at first hand the beneficial effects of cannabis when his own son, Danny, contracted an ultimately fatal case of leukaemia. After being given a powerful new drug for his illness, Danny – then aged fourteen – suffered prolonged vomiting and nausea. When he began self-administering marijuana joints, the puking stopped and he was able to eat normally.

The major problem with cannabis therapy, as perceived by the political authorities, is the 'high' the drug provides. That many other-products in the national formulary also alter consciousness (not least morphine and benzodiazepines) is considered an irrelevancy.

The main objection voiced by the drug companies is that, in its plant form, it is difficult to deliver a precise amount of drug to the patient, given that all plants vary in potency. (Tobacco companies – officially restricted in the amount of nicotine each cigarette may contain – seem to hit the mark regularly enough.) The pharmaceutical companies' unspoken objection is that whole cannabis would be difficult and unprofitable to market. It is a weed for which a moderate pricing policy would be expected. Nabilone, on the other hand, the only synthetic cannabinoid legally prescribable in the UK, costs the NHS (in 1993) £39.70 for just twenty capsules. Apart from its punitive cost, Nabilone is also physically more dangerous than the whole plant. In the US, testing of it was discontinued after the death of laboratory animals and after adverse reactions were found in human beings.[22]

Extracting the 'active ingredients' from a mind-altering plant inevitably produces products of greater potency and, thus, potentially greater harm. The process also kills stone dead, say the 'free cannabis' advocates, the magic of the weed.

More than eighty chemicals have already been identified in cannabis and it is their combined effects – their synergy – which is held responsible for its healing qualities. Pharmaceutical companies, as a matter of credos and economic logic, are devoted to the man-made. They are hooked on synthesis and antipathetic to the marketing of anything that springs naturally from the soil.

If the potential therapeutic benefits cannabis holds are to be made generally available, it will be as a result of winning the legalisation argument and not through any drug company initiative.

History

Like the coca shrub and the opium poppy, *Cannabis sativa* has been recognised as a plant of great utility for thousands of years. There is no part of it that has not been co-opted, most often for hemp and medicine, but even for the production of fibrous wands used to drive out demons. The wild version is believed to have originated in Central Asia. Further abroad it was carried and planted by nomads. The ancient Chinese are believed to have been especially adept at its cultivation, understanding from the earliest that, when sown close together, tall, thick-stemmed plants result – ideal for hemp fibres. From these twines came textiles, fishing nets, ropes, and mats. The seeds of the plant were extracted to make oil for cooking as well as herbal therapies for fever and menstrual cramps. It is in a compendium of medicines compiled for the Chinese emperor Shen Nung (circa 2727 BC) that the earliest record of cannabis use is to be found.[23]

Aryan nomads are credited with taking the plant into India

during the second millennium BC.[24] Here it was especially appreciated for its therapeutic properties. It also formed the basis of spicy beverages which were consumed by both mortals and gods. Knowledge of the plant is then believed to have spread to the Near East, Africa, Europe, and the New World.

The Ancient Greeks used juice from the seeds to cure after-dinner flatulence. The Romans took a more utilitarian approach, using the fibrous stems to make sailcloth and rope. It was they who brought hemp to Britain, but it was the Anglo–Saxons who inspired widespread husbanding.

While there have been no arguments about using the cannabis plant to produce rope, there have always been rumblings about making use of the plant's psychoactive properties. Any substance that can alter mood and perception is potentially injurious to the orthodoxy. Some saw it as the road to moral ruin. The Arab historian, Al Magrii, blamed the decline of Egyptian society on its use[25] (it was impassioned pleading by Egyptian delegates in international forums which led subsequently to the panoply of modern prohibitions).

With the sudden proliferation of sea traffic during the sixteenth century, *Cannabis sativa* in all its forms began travelling to those parts of the world where it hadn't yet been seeded – notably South America. The Europeans were chiefly interested in cultivation to make hemp for rigging on ships, and encouraged their own populations as well as those they colonised to grow it. Cultivation began in the American settlement of Jamestown, Virginia by 1611 and, before long, money, charts, maps, canvasses for oil paintings (the word 'canvas' is said to be the Dutch pronunciation of the Greek word *kannabis*[26]), and even the first draft of the American Declaration of Independence used hemp fibre. George Washington grew the plant at his Mount Vernon home; and some have concluded 'after careful study of his diaries' that the first president separated the potent female plants for his personal 'medicinal' use.[27]

It was the revival of classical learning which inspired the new appreciation of cannabis's therapeutic properties. The noted medieval herbalist Nicholas Culpepper (1616–54) listed a variety of ailments for which the common European hemp (*C. sativa*) could be useful, including inflammation, parasites, and aches and pains. Culpepper's work, according

161

to researchers Sean Blanchard and Matthew Atha,[28] probably owed much to the folk herbalism of British witches who, until the Christian persecutions, provided most of the health care to the rural populations. By Victorian times, traditional plant medicines had been all but expunged and in their place came tinctures, tonics, and other extracts. After the British physician W. B. O'Shaughnessy reported, in 1839, on what he'd learnt in Calcutta of cannabis's analgesic, anti-convulsant and muscle-relaxant properties, the modern history of the drug began. The research literature began stacking up as pharmacologists worked harder and more hazardously to obtain the best possible extracts from what were often inferior crops. Some died in the attempt – blowing themselves to pieces. By the end of the nineteenth century, cannabis preparations were seen as the answer to coughing, fatigue, rheumatism, asthma, delirium tremens, migraine headache, and painful menstruation. Queen Victoria's personal doctor, John Reynolds, a leading advocate of what came to be marketed as *Cannabis indica*, described the drug as 'one of the most valuable therapeutic agents we possess.'

Of all the Europeans it was the sybaritic French who took most joyfully to the metaphysical dimensions of cannabis. While Napoleon was cutting a swathe through the hashlands of North Africa, the people back home were immersing themselves in all that was Arabian, bowing to the style and the artefacts.

A man who travelled to those new Arab outposts and had witnessed for himself the effects of hashish was the physician Jacques Joseph Moreau de Tours. So convinced was Moreau of the similarity between hash intoxication and mental derangement that he felt certain the study of the first would help the treatment of the second. He turned to his friend, the novelist Theophile Gautier, who was so enthralled by the idea that he helped to establish – in the 1850s – a club dedicated to thorough immersion in the hash experience. It was called Club des Haschischins, a weightier forerunner to Tim Leary's acid-based League for Spiritual Discovery, and had a membership that included Dumas, Balzac, Baudelaire, and Flaubert. They gathered in the Hotel Pimodan, Paris, where their hash experiments were observed by Moreau and gave rise to descriptions such as this lushly melodramatic one from Gautier:

'My body seemed to dissolve and I became transparent. Within my breast I perceived the hashish I had eaten in the form of an emerald scintillating with a million points of fire. My eyelashes elongated indefinitely, unrolling themselves like threads of gold on ivory spindles which spun of their own accord with dazzling rapidity. Around me poured streams of gems in every colour, in ever-changing patterns like the play within a kaleidoscope. My comrades appeared to me to be disfigured, part men, part plants, wearing the pensive air of Ibises.'

Baudelaire dedicated *Les Fleurs du Mal* to his good host and penned an essay called 'On Hashish and Wine as a means of expanding individuality' by way of explaining the club's creed. The art produced by this magic circle was oddball and sensuous. It was 'foreign' and scandalous, and when Baudelaire succumbed to psychosis and an early death, hashish, inevitably, took the rap; unfairly, according to the latest thinking. The poet had relatively little experience of the resin, being far more familiar with laudanum and booze (he is said to have been an alcoholic). He also suffered from tertiary syphilis.[29]

The British tended to be more earthbound in their approach to cannabis. Romantic youths such as Coleridge and De Quincey weren't above sampling a pellet of hashish, but mostly it was important as the base for sailcloth, tinctures, and tonics. Though the British didn't take to cannabis as an intoxicant in the manner of the smart French, they were responsible for introducing the habit to the Caribbean. It was an indirect introduction, affected by indentured Hindu workers the British were shipping out to the West Indies from about 1840 to work on the sugar plantations. The black people of the Caribbean, who perhaps dimly remembered the plant from their African homeland, welcomed its introduction both for its varied medical properties and to smoke the laborious day away under the British.

But while the descendants of those former black slaves brought *ghanja* with them to the UK, they consumed it very much in a private way. The cannabis rage among young British whites, starting from the early 1960s, was learnt from their Caucasian counterparts in the US, from the hipsters, beats, and their flower-children spin-offs. But where did the American whites learn it?

163

They learnt it from their black fellow countrymen, who probably got it from Africa. The circle was joined.

The American scene

Like France, America also seems to have experienced cannabis fever in the mid-nineteenth century. There were the usual medicinal therapies made from *C. Indica*, but in addition there grew a fashion for chewing quids of ground betel nuts mixed with cannabis's flowering tops. Straight hash-smoking through a hookah was also in vogue in the most fashionably dissolute circles.

A sharp downturn in the reputation of cannabis came as a reaction to the political/racial exigencies of the day. There was no serious problem while smart New York ladies were smoking *bhang* in their uptown apartments, but Mexicans and dope was another matter.

Mexicans had been flowing into the south-west states of the Union from the turn of the twentieth century and were welcomed as a source of cheap farm labour. They brought with them their smoking pleasures, and although there were local statutes outlawing the weed, these were not seriously enforced until the Depression years of the 1930s when the migrants and their habits were suddenly surplus to national requirements. The chase for jobs between whites and Mexicans generated grave tensions, and just as cocaine had earlier been blamed for the poor humour of American blacks, marijuana (a Spanish word meaning Mary Jane) was now identified, half cynically, half in earnest, as the cause of the dispiritedness of the Mexicans; thousands were deported.

Black Americans, particularly young jazzers, were also turning themselves on in the first two decades of the century, as an alternative to the prohibited alcohol. In New York, hundreds of 'tea pads' opened up in which cannabis was sold, either for consumption on the spot or for carry-out. The city authorities did a double-take but they seemed to tolerate these parlours fairly well, again until the onset of the Depression. By this time a new commissioner of the Federal Bureau of Narcotics was in place, one Harry J. Anslinger. In dope, Anslinger saw an opportunity to raise some big congressional dollars for his bureau during what was, at the time, a fiscally tight period. Suddenly, he was a man reefer-obsessed, someone who saw marijuana-induced crime waves everywhere. His portrayal of the drug as one that immediately led to homicidal insanity did much to facilitate some extraordinarily harsh criminal sanctions, such as in Georgia, where selling dope to a minor could result in life imprisonment or death.

Squalls were coming in from abroad too. Turkey and Egypt had come before the League of Nations to beg assistance in beating the cannabis menace that was doing so much to destroy the fabric of their nations. Then, in 1937 – urged on by Anslinger – the US federal government passed its decisive Marijuana Tax Act. From now on the drug was banned except for 'licit' traders such as doctors, druggists, and birdseed sellers, and these would have to register, pay a tax, and keep such cumbersome records that the whole enterprise was considered pointless. Cannabis was dropped from the US National Pharmacopoeia and National Formulary. And though the American Medical Association initially protested about the passing of what it considered a useful therapeutic, it soon fell into line.[30]

Viewed from the UK, America was in a curiously repressed mood by the post-war 1950s period. She seemed fearful of perversions – ideological and sexual – in all places. But then beneath the writhing exterior there was indeed something outlandish taking root. Mescaline and LSD had been discovered. Intrepid beats were penetrating the Upper Amazon to explore native hallucinogenic cults, and figures like the poet Allen Ginsberg and the radical academic Timothy Leary were doing their utmost to cleave a bloody hole in the body of US society. By the time the 1960s arrived, a sizeable proportion of young Americans believed they knew exactly how to articulate their complaints, and to an important degree this involved the use of the medium of drugs. Theirs was a reaction against soulless materialism. American youth dressed up rough and steeped their senses in 'organic' pleasures. The important drugs were LSD and cannabis. But whereas the first was considered a spiritual emetic, cannabis was the dependable companion. It was warm and giggly and, moreover, a badge of affiliation. Smoking 'dope' in 1960s America earned instant access to a sub-nation of 'heads'.

Cannabis reviled

But hippies get old and the political weathervane blows one way and then the other. By the mid-1970s, cannabis-smoking was back in the closet. To the new youth, the 1960s generation were dopes and cop-outs, their revolution of the mind having achieved precisely nothing; America was still America. Nancy and Ronald Reagan proved the point with a War Against Pot that out-Anslingered anything the great man himself could have dreamt up.

The Reagan administration introduced America to such legal innovations as helicopter surveillance of private homes and gardens, pre-trial forfeiture of land and houses belonging to alleged growers, police surveillance of garbage cans, and mandatory random sampling of body fluids in the workplace.

One man who fell foul of the Reagan initiatives was Donald Scott, wealthy heir to his family's chemicals business, a gadfly and ranch-owner, who was gunned down at his California estate one bright morning in October 1992 by a small army of thirty-two individuals from the Los Angeles Sheriff's Department, the Drug Enforcement Administration, the California Bureau of Narcotic Enforcement, the National Guard, the US Forest Service, and even two officials from a jet propulsion laboratory owned by the space agency NASA, who were apparently invited along to test the air for marijuana pollen.[31]

Scott was supposed to have been a major cannabis cultivator but nothing was found except – at a late stage – a few fragments of marijuana in a cigar box.

An investigation by the local district attorney was scathing of the way the raid was prepared. The millions of dollars to be gained from forfeiture of the land was a motivating factor behind the enterprise, he decided. Under Reagan's 1984 forfeiture statute the authorities can seize any property that is the fruit of a crime or was used in committing one. This can be done without securing a conviction but on the basis of a less than punishing standard of proof known as probable cause. It is for the property-owner to prove his innocence.

Of even greater consequence for the health of America at large was the war waged on the basically peaceful counterculture communities in the back country of California, Hawaii, and Oregon, where much of the country's marijuana was grown. In the early 1980s, an influx of profiteers and thieves led to sporadic outbreaks of violence.[32] The government response was an invasion by helicopters, paramilitary eradication teams, and liberal use of the new land forfeiture laws. Most of the 'mom and pop' growers were forced out of business with consequent damage to the local economy estimated to be in excess of $1 billion. A serious cannabis drought followed, which was reflected in escalating street prices. Simultaneously, prices for cocaine (a much simpler and more profitable drug to deal in) were plummeting and, by the late 1980s, crack had displaced marijuana as the most widely available street drug in America.[33] These were the fruits of Reagan's Drug Wars.

Cannabis revived

But by the early 1990s the wind had once more changed direction. Even as the US authorities were moving to outlaw the limited medical prescribing of marijuana that still existed – leaving some well-publicised AIDS and cancer patients to go to their end without their chosen comfort – dopey old cannabis was back in fashion among the young. Cannabis motifs began turning up on T-shirts and record sleeves. Smart magazines wrote about how smart it was to shift into THC orbit, and there was even a new mode of taking it (emptying a cheap cigar and packing the shell with grass; known as a *blunt*). The world had moved on. Acres of American cities were rotting, giving way to tin and plywood shantytowns, TB, AIDS, killer girl gangs, rioting citizenry, rioting police. Much of the flavour was communicated through the new, hardest-yet strain of hip hop, called 'gangsta rap'. But even within this unstintingly aggressive milieu, hitherto the preserve of crack cocaine, cannabis suddenly became the hip thing to do. Tracks like *Pack the Pipe*, *Fellowship Mary Jane*, *Yo Yo Pass It On We Got the Last Joint* and *Blunted* spoke of the new mode.

At the head of this trend was Cypress Hill, who told *i-D* magazine (September 1993) that by altering the nature of hip hop they were hooking into 'unfinished business' – namely the 'politics of consciousness' left over from the 1960s and 1970s. In the 1960s, group member B Real told the magazine, 'smoking pot was considered part of freedom of expression, the right to freedom of consciousness which Timothy Leary called "the fifth freedom".'

Sen Dog added: 'When you get high and relax, and just chill, notice the way your mind plays tricks. Take advantage of that, 'cos your mind has been opened up. You can see things for what they really are. You can look right through the government and see the devil. The government doesn't want your mind to be expanded.'

Much of the responsibility for cannabis's revised reputation as an instrument of revolution rather than as a brain-deadening hippy weed falls to author Jack Herer, whose 1990 underground best-seller, *The Emperor Wears No Clothes* (Hemp Publishing, Van Nuys, California), reads, in outline, like the ultimate stoned conspiracy theory.

If cannabis is such a powerful medical therapy, Herer asks, why was it criminalised in America with the 1937 Marijuana Tax? His answer is that prohibition was only marginally to do with medicine, much more to do with the plant's utility as a fibre and fuel. By the 1930s, paints, varnishes, paper fabrics, and thousands of other commercial products were all made from this sturdy, fast-growing weed. The success of hemp, claims Herer, threatened to bankrupt the paper industry, stifle an emerging synthetic fabrics industry, challenge the dominance of petrol and oil – and, yes, cause problems for the pharmaceutical trade, which, at that time, didn't know how to convert the plant into an easily marketable chemical product. It was these forces, Herer argues, which conspired against cannabis, helping to stigmatise it as an irredeemably dangerous narcotic. Herer's imaginative thesis has since been amply garnished by various Hemp protagonists and utopian dreamers who are convinced that pot can save the world. *Hemp for Fuel . . . Burn Pot Not Oil* was the cry that was going up on American college campuses in 1991, according to the *Wall Street Journal*.

'Ultimately, the structure of society would be completely different if hemp were legal,' a UK Green Party spokesman noted in 1993.[34] 'If there was a society based on cannabis or hemp it would allow the raw material for paper, clothing, plastics and oil to be grown almost anywhere locally. This would lessen the need for trade movement, CO_2 emissions, competition, inequality and all the pitfalls capitalism has to offer, so its possibilities are endless.'

If that sounds like something someone dreamt up while stoned, the hemp visionaries would say that's the beauty of it.

The British scene

Given that the UK has long been infatuated with American youth culture – a compliment that is periodically reciprocated – the US movements of the 1940s, 1950s and 1960s inevitably had their counterparts among British youth. From the 1950s there was a semi-flourishing jazz scene in the clubs of Soho where 'pot' was ingested along with cool blues and bebop music. Another strong pro-ghanja faction was found among the new young West Indian immigrants – lured into the big UK cities to do the menial jobs the whites wouldn't do. Just how much ghanja was smoked by those Caribbean imports in the early days is difficult to gauge, but there are reports of young black men freely walking the streets of West London's Notting Hill pulling on spliffs. The young smokers would not have found favour among their more proper church-going elders, but local police, in common with the rest of white society, would scarcely have known of the drug's existence.

One of the first serious attempts to provoke a cannabis scare came from the barrister Donald Johnson in his 1952 opus *Indian Hemp, a Social Menace*. I am indebted to the author Peter Laurie[35] for uncovering this work, which included extracts from a series of articles in the *Sunday Graphic*.

'After several weeks I have just completed exhaustive enquiries into the most insidious vice Scotland Yard has ever been called on to tackle – dope peddling.

'Detectives on this assignment are agreed that never have they had experience of a crime so vicious, so ruthless, so unpitying and so well organised. Hemp, marijuana and hashish represent a throughly unsavoury trade.

'One of the detectives told me: "We are dealing with the most evil men who have ever taken to the vice business." The victims are teenage girls and, to a lesser extent, teenage youths . . .

'The racketeers are 90 per cent coloured men from the West Indies and West Coast of Africa. How serious the situation is, how great the danger to our social structure,

169

may be gathered from the fact that despite increasing police attention, despite several raids, there are more than a dozen clubs in the West End at which drugs are peddled.

'As a result of my enquiries, I share the fear of the detectives now on the job that there is the greatest danger of the reefer craze becoming the greatest social menace this country has known . . .'

He goes on to describe entering a 'tawdry' West End club where he and his contact were among just six white men.

'I counted 28 coloured men and some 30 white girls. None of the girls looked more than 25. In a corner five coloured musicians with their brows perspiring played bebop music with extraordinary fervour. Girls and coloured partners danced with an abandon – a savagery almost – which was both fascinating and embarrassing. From a doorway came a coloured man, flinging away the end of a strange cigarette. He danced peculiar convulsions of his own, then bounced on to a table and held out shimmering arms to a girl. My contact indicated photographs on the wall. They were of girls in the flimsiest drapings. I had seen my first bebop club, its coloured pedlars, its half-crazed, uncaring girls.'

Writings such as these, though not particularly plentiful, gnawed away at national policy-makers during the 1950s, cementing the reputation of cannabis as a dangerous narcotic that imperilled the integrity of the race. Such panics can be seen as echoes of other panics from others parts of the world in different ages: the Spanish encountering the coca-chewing Incas; Napoleon when his troops first discovered the hash-eaters of Egypt (the Emperor tried to ban the drug); the Americans and their black coke-sniffers; and the English in response to the numerically insignificant opium smokers of Limehouse, East London, who were simultaneously regarded as inert and physically menacing.

No matter the dimensions of the 1950s dope scare, cannabis continued to be confined to a fairly small, outré crowd right through the decade, with rarely more than a dozen prosecutions each year under the Dangerous Drugs Act. Aside from hip Jamaicans, there was the odd Nigerian sailor passing through London or Liverpool, and there were the US-influenced white jazzers and shaggy-sweatered beats who perhaps dug CND. Sources were informal – a parcel from Jamaica, a little 'personal' picked up in an African port.

The rapid rise of the drug in the 1960s was in one sense part of the sensual awakening of Western youth following the drubbings of the Second World War. It was also linked to what might be called the 'proletarian renaissance'. This was a movement spurred by cheap travel which saw the hitherto hidebound masses pour into the Mediterranean where they discovered that foreigners also have some good ideas. They brought back pasta, retsina, mosaics, Cuban heels, halva, incense and, a little later, hashish. In the early part of the decade such items signalled cosmopolitan modism. They went with the little PVC skirts and funny sculpted haircuts. The prime desire then was to be dynamically on the go. Drinamyl (a mixture of amphetamine and barbiturate) became the preferred fillip both through licit channels and on the street where the pills were known as Purple Hearts. But by the middle of the decade the mood changed again. Manic fabbism was displaced by something more contemplative. The *Commissar* (to use the late Arthur Koestler's phraseology) was ousted by the *Yogi*, and as the trails to the Eastern hashlands became more and more comprehensively trod, cannabis started to infiltrate the art schools, the colleges, and then sixth forms – places where speed had previously been the essential mode.

The swell began in 1966. In 1967 the first wave had rolled in, and by 1968 the whole culture was drenched.

Servicing the new cannabis consumer was still very much an ad hoc business until the early 1970s. Hash was being brought back in VW vans from Eastern source countries, like Afghanistan and the Lebanon, and divided among friends. A small portion would perhaps be sold on the street to provide for future liquidity. Black dealers would score hash from white dealers, while white youths who wanted a bag of herb could go to certain pubs and clubs where it would be cut up on the back table. (The specialisation of whites in hash and blacks in herb still survives.) But, gradually, cannabis-dealing became less of an amateur game. With more planning and resources required to escape detection, many of those involved calculated that it was better to lose their liberty for a useful amount rather than a kilo or two. The easy profits attracted traditional criminal firms who found cannabis-dealing less stressful than robbing banks; and – according to all the specialist international enforcement agencies – the major crime syndicates, such

171

as the Sicilian and Neopolitan Mafias, the Corsican gangs of France and the Turkish Clans, also staked their claim.

The scene, according to this scenario, has become violent and rapacious; the antipathy of the union of elevated souls that marijuana was supposed to have represented.

But the official version is disputed by those who argue that much cannabis trafficking, from source country to consumer, remains small-to-medium scale. Invariably, they say, it is plain business (albeit a legally risky one) free of any overt drama.

In the UK, as in America, the drug fell out of style for several years from the mid-1970s. Punks were the ascendant youth tribe and, because punks hated hippies, they hated the number-one hippy drug. They said it made users moronic and witless, and preferred speed and glue.

But, of course, the wheel turned again. Too much stimulation, whether political, financial, or biological, sooner or later requires a dose of sedation. It was probably the horrors of crack (or, at least, the images of violent paranoia associated with it) which restored cannabis's credibility. By 1993, it was the smartest drug around. Magazines like *The Face*, *i-D*, *NME* and *Mixmag* devoted pages to it: the cultural history, Herer's immaculate conspiracy, the new super-hybrids, even the beauty (presented life-size in good-enough-to-eat colour) of the serrated leaf. Cannabis (it was smart now to call it *hemp*) appealed to clubbers done in on too much Ecstasy and to coke/crack habitués whose lives were spiralling out of control.

Non-intoxicating hemp, which the Home Office were permitting to be grown on trial plots, was also the vogue fabric among some top fashion designers. And even the legalisation/decriminalisation argument – moribund for years – was energetically revived. Top cops, politicians from both Houses, and periodicals of every persuasion (e.g., *The Economist*, the *New Statesman*, the *Independent*) all argued for a let-up in the law. The legal advice agency Release set the debate in context: the status quo was criminalising 40,000 mostly young people a year and undermining the country's moral and legal fabric.

'Prohibition of cannabis subverts the acquisition of civic values for a large number of young people at precisely the time that their view of themselves as citizens is being shaped. They are criminalised by a law they widely believe to be unjustified, their respect for which is further undermined by the impossibility of its effective enforcement.'[36]

Policy

'Straight' society in the late 1960s was quick to see the symbolic importance of cannabis-smoking and launched many attacks upon it. There was still an idea, lingering from the 1920s and 1930s, that it was a morally perilous drug, and if masses of British youngsters were going through their weird metamorphosis, challenging every last conceit of society, then the drug that was so central to them had to be in some large measure culpable. A great disappointment to the Labour government of the day was the 1968 report on cannabis prepared by the Hallucinogenic Sub-committee of the Advisory Committee on Drug Dependency. Chaired by Baroness Wootton, it was the first attempt by any British government to investigate the drug properly since 1894. It came at a time when controls had been in existence for some forty years. Home Secretary Jim Callaghan no doubt anticipated a reinforcement of standard policy. Yet Wootton and her panel delivered a political grenade.

There was no evidence, said her report, that the drug, which was widely used by young people of all classes, caused violent crime or aggressive, anti-social behaviour, or produced dependence or psychosis requiring medical treatment in people who were otherwise normal. It pointed to a 'body of opinion that criticises the present legislative treatment of cannabis on the grounds that it exaggerates the dangers of the drug and needlessly interferes with civil liberty.' And yet despite the penalties there were no signs that consumption of the drug was diminishing. Among the recommendations were that:

1. The association in legislation on cannabis and heroin be ended and a new law to deal specifically and separately with cannabis and its derivatives be quickly introduced.
2. Possession of small amounts should no longer be considered a serious crime to be punished by imprisonment.

3. Preparations of the drug should continue to be available on prescription for research and medical treatment.

The popular press fumed, subjecting Wootton's panel to what the Institute for the Study of Drug Dependence described as the 'most explosive campaign of vilification ever visited upon an official drugs advisory body.' Hundreds of items were generated. George Gale, writing in the *Daily Mirror*, suggested the Committee was part of the 'conspiracy of the drugged.' The 1967 *Times* advert calling for liberalisation and signed by many notables was once more fulminated against.

It was the 'escalation' syndrome – the possibility of cannabis leading to heroin – which worried most people. It worried particularly those who participated in the Commons debate on Wootton during which both government and opposition were at one on the need for holding the line against what Callaghan called 'this so-called permissiveness . . .'

The level of discernment among certain government ministers can perhaps best be judged from a note in the late Richard Crossman's diary: 'Thursday, August 14, 1968: Barbara Wootton had come to talk to us about the drug problem. She got into trouble with Callaghan for recommending that oh, what's it called, not heroin but one of the other drugs, should be categorised as a harmless drug, although many people regard it as leading to addiction.'

Home Secretary Callaghan rejected most of Wootton's advice, of course, and five years later, in June 1973, the Misuse of Drugs Act came into force, placing cannabis possession, trafficking and manufacture in the Class B category, along with amphetamine. The maximum penalty for possession was now to be five years and/or an unlimited fine. Cannabinol and cannabinol derivatives, such as synthetic THC, were placed in the more serious Class A category, along with heroin and cocaine. These carried seven years for possession as well as the unlimited fine. (See Appendix I for the current position.)

History of Controls

The Legalise Cannabis Campaign traces the origins of British control back to 1912 when an international conference was held in The Hague to discuss controlling opium traffic. The conference also decided to investigate the cannabis question. There was a lull until 1923 when the South African government proposed to the League of Nations that cannabis be treated as a habit-forming drug and internationally regulated. (The Durban government was apparently concerned that the weed was causing African labourers to slacken off in the mines.)

Britain wanted the matter fully investigated and a decision on international controls to be considered when the League's advisory committee met in 1925. But some couldn't wait. At the second Opium Conference in 1924, Egyptian and Turkish delegates begged and won support for more urgent action. 'The illicit use of hashish', the Egyptian delegate intoned, 'is the principal cause of insanity in Egypt.' Proposals were drafted which controlled unlicensed consumption, import and export. Britain signed, giving effect to her undertakings. She signed because it was the course of least resistance, there being no domestic medical or non-medical use of the drug to speak of. She signed even though she believed the drafting committee's analysis lacked credibility, and even though Britain herself had produced a more solid analysis of cannabis some twenty years before which argued *against* prohibition. That investigation was carried out by the Indian Hemp Drugs Commission (IHDC) which, in studying the drug's use in India, spent two years interviewing 800 witnesses, reporting in a 3,000-page, seven-volume work, with an additional confidential volume on hemp drug use in the Army.

In support of its recommendation not to prohibit in India, the IHDC noted: 'Moderate use of these drugs is the rule and excessive use is comparatively exceptional. Moderate use produces practically no ill effects. In all but the most exceptional cases the injury from habitual, moderate use is not appreciable. Excessive use may certainly be accepted as very injurious, though it must be admitted that in many excessive consumers the injury is not clearly marked. The

175

injury done by excessive use is, however, confined almost exclusively to the consumer himself.'

In India, the recommendations of the IHDC report for control by taxes rather than by prohibition went into force quietly – the laws and tariffs on cannabis being standardised in all provinces.[37] But not in England, where cannabis use was not an issue and where it was inconvenient to have either a debate or a new set of laws.

Until the Wootton Committee was charged in the 1960s with looking at the drug again, the Indian Hemp Commission's report was the only substantial analysis of cannabis in existence anywhere in the world. And yet this did not prevent the League of Nations and its successor, the United Nations, from further turning up the heat so that signatories became obliged to restrict, not just lay consumption and trading, but use in medical circles too. In Britain for many years the drug was in the same legal category as heroin and, still today, its hazard rating under the Misuse of Drugs Act (the main penal instrument) is equal to that of barbiturates (both being Class B drugs) and in excess of the Class C benzodiazepines, such as temazepam.

Research Booms

Since the rejection of Wootton, the cannabis investigation market has boomed. There have been perhaps 20,000 scientific papers as well as cartloads of government-commissioned reports subjecting the drug to the kind of scrutiny that wouldn't pass a runner bean fit. Where a consensus on physical/mental impact does suggest itself, it is that there is no clear and significant damage to be found in adult humans resulting from moderate use of the drug – something the Indian Hemp Drug Commission stated more than one hundred years ago. And where there is a social policy recommendation, it is that locking people up or fining them heavily for simple possession cannot be justified; the drug should be demoted in the penal league table. This suggestion has been made in the US, Australia, Holland, and in the UK (post-Wootton). In each case it has been rebuffed by a central government too fearful of the political consequences. But, informally at least, there has been elasticity on the part of the police and judges who recognise that there would be no room in the jails for anyone else if cannabis smokers were stalked too actively.

The two key UK reports since Wootton were both produced by the Advisory Council on the Misuse of Drugs – the first in 1979 by a technical sub-committee and a follow-up three years later by an 'expert group', saying much the same thing but more elaborately. The 1979 team found 'no compelling evidence that occasional moderate use of cannabis was likely to have detrimental effects' and recommended that magistrates should not imprison for possession. They could either impose a fine or submit the offender to crown court. Since most possession offences are dealt with by magistrates, the proposal would 'reduce cannabis possession to the level of possessing an unlicensed TV – a status that in practice it has already achieved in some parts of the country.'[38] No government action was taken. The 1982 team supported the idea of reducing the penalties, and though the format of their report was changed to allow the eight professors, four doctors and one retail pharmacist their independent heads of steam, the gesticulations were familiar '. . . insufficient evidence to enable us to reach any incontestable conclusions . . . research undertaken has so far failed to demonstrate positive and significant effects in man attributable solely to the use of cannabis.'

A decade later, the debate was that much more intense. The illicit drugs trade, according to estimates in the 'quality press', was now worth somewhere between £1.8 and £3 billion a year; and not a penny of it was reaching the government by way of tax revenues. On the contrary, the authorities were annually forking out around £500 million on 'overall responses to drugs (international and national)'.[39]

Cannabis convictions and cautions in 1992 topped 41,000 – representing some 90 per cent of the total for all drugs. Ten years earlier the figure had been 'just' 17,447.

Not that all was gloom. The Drugs War, as purveyed on our TV screens and in sections of the press, had become a major prime-time entertainment. With the cameras invited along, we could be there at the dawn police raid on the sink estate; eavesdrop while yet another secretly miked-up bad guy incriminated himself at the prompting of an informer. We could watch Mr Nasty, his face 'pixilated' on our screens so as to avoid impeding the course of justice, being ordered flat-out on the ground prior to being cuffed and body-searched. Those who were remote from such things could be convinced that this was a winning game. Good was licking evil. But the bad feeling such policing engendered was immense. Cannabis smokers could see no crime in what they were doing, and even a 'telling-off' or a moderate fine was resented. Moreover, many in the black population believed that the drug laws were being used by the police as an excuse to exert undue control – a perspective apparently borne out by research in Notting Hill, West London.[40]

In the 1980s, the street disturbances in Brixton, Bristol, Birmingham, and Broadwater Farm, North London were all, at least partly, triggered by drugs policing. Subsequently, the ill-will (felt by many white youths as well as blacks) simmered rather than boiled over, only making the news when, for instance, a patrolling cop was brained by a brick through his windscreen, or a WPC had a screwdriver driven through her heart by a drug-using suspect. Many officers failed to see the hopelessness of the situation they were caught up in; some showed every sign of enjoying the undercover intrigue and the beating-down of doors. But various significant seniors – Commander John Grieve of the Metropolitan Police; Raymond Kendall, head of Interpol and a former Scotland Yard superintendent; Brian Hilliard, editor of *Police Review* and another ex-London cop – were calling for the controls on cannabis to be loosened.

Informally, things had already slackened by the 1990s. Several police forces were cautioning first offenders found with small amounts of cannabis rather than taking them to court. Customs, too, had a scheme whereby those found with a 'small' amount could negotiate an instant cash penalty. But inconsistencies remained. In rural courts, and those not used to dealing with drug cases, the sentences were usually more severe than in urban ones. And there were varying interpretations as to what constituted dealing as opposed to simple possession.

'The popular myth', I was told by Mike Goodman, director of Release, 'is that people just tend to get cautioned for cannabis possession, or get what's called an informal disposal where they just throw it away and tell you not to do it again.'

178

But, he says, whereas more people *are* getting cautioned, more people are also going to court to face a fine or imprisonment. And in the newly commercialised state schools, young people were being expelled at the first whiff of a cannabis scandal, thereby imperilling their education.

'The truth is, a cannabis possession bust can ruin a life. There are people still losing their liberty, losing their careers, suffering a great deal because of simple cases of possession.'

Given the widespread dissemination of cannabis throughout the whole of society – at least among the under-45s – the continued prickliness on the part of the authorities is badly judged. Aside from nourishing a sense of grievance among the main target groups, notably black and 'suspect' white youth, it also alienates literally millions of normally conformist individuals well past their adolescence, on whom governments depend for their mandate.

Notes

1. Committee of enquiry into the spread of organised crime linked to drugs trafficking in the member states of the European Community, draft report, 28 October 1991, p. 43.

2. Ibid, p. 11.

3. Shedler and Block, 'Adolescent Drug Use and Psychological Health: A longitudinal inquiry', in *American Psychologist*, 45, May 1990, pp. 612–30.

4. *A Release White Paper on Reform of the Drug Laws*, Release, London, 1992, p. 17.

5. Provisional figures compiled by the National Criminal Intelligence Service from Customs and Home Office data.

6. A. H. Douthwaite, *Hale–White's Materia Medica Pharmacology and Therapeutics*, J. & A. Churchill, London, 1963, p. 178.

7. 'EC cash for Moroccan "pot farms"', in the *Daily Telegraph*, 9 September 1993; 'Hash bonanza in Morocco', in the *European*, 18 March 1993.

8. Jan van Doorn, 'Drug trafficking networks in Europe', in the *European Journal on Criminal Policy and Research*, Vol. 1, No. 2, p. 103.

9. Committee of enquiry into the spread of organised crime linked to drugs trafficking in the member states of the European Community, op. cit., p. 43.

10. 'Drugs intelligence unit sweeps into action', in the *Independent*, 3 March 1994.

11. L. Grinspoon, 'Marijuana', in *Substance Abuse, A Comprehensive Textbook*, ed. Lowinson *et al.*, Williams & Wilkins, Baltimore, 1992, p. 237.

12. A. Gottlieb, *Cooking with Cannabis*, Greenham & Gotto, London, 1981.

13. 'Cannabis Use', World Health Organisation, Addiction Research Foundation, Toronto, 1981.

14. Grinspoon, op. cit., p. 242.

15. Ibid.

16. Ibid.

17. A. Sherdan, *Michel Foucault: The Will to Truth*, Routledge, London, pp. 13–14, 23–4.

18. See Amit Basu's 'A brief, critical look at cannabis psychosis', in the *International Journal on Drug Policy*, Vol. 3, No. 3, pp. 126–9.

19. Grinspoon, op. cit., p. 241.

20. *i-D*, September 1993, p. 16.

21. L. Grinspoon, in *Searching for Alternatives: Drug control policy in the United States*, ed. M. Kruass and E. Lazear, Hoover Institution Press, Stanford University, California, 1991, p. 383.

22 Grinspoon, 1992, p. 244.
23 *Comprehensive Handbook on Drug and Alcohol Addiction*, ed. Norman Miller, Marcel Dekker, New York, 1991, p. 355.
24 *High Times Encyclopedia of Recreational Drugs*, Stonehill Press, New York, 1978, p. 118.
25 Miller, op. cit., p. 355.
26 *The Face*, October 1993, p. 96.
27 Miller, op. cit., p. 356.
28 'Indian hemp and the dope fiends of Old England', unpublished essay, spring 1993, p. 6.
29 Grinspoon, 1992, p. 237.
30 Grinspoon, 1991, p. 382.
31 P. Reeves, 'Forfeit: Your money and your life', in the *Independent*, 3 July 1993.
32 D. Gieringer, in the *International Journal on Drug Policy*, Vol. 1, No. 6.
33 Ibid.
34 *i-D*, September 1993, p. 16.
35 See Peter Laurie's *Drugs*, Pelican, London, 1969, p. 88.
36 Release, op. cit., p. 14.
37 'Indian hemp and the dope fiends of Old England', op. cit., p. 1.
38 'The Cannabis Cover Up', Legalise Cannabis Campaign, London, 1978.
39 A. Kershaw, 'Medicine, man', in the *Guardian*, 'Weekend' section, 18 September 1993, p. 21.
40 Release, op. cit., p. 14.

COCAINE

Intro

Cocaine is one of the great bogey drugs of the West, periodically rousing waves of great terror. It derives from the pulped leaf of the South American coca plant and in its unadulterated form is of great utility, particularly for the undernourished Indians who occupy the high Andean plains where the air is thin and the labour hard. Aside from providing mild physical stimulation, a daily dose of two ounces of leaves – the average for 90 per cent of the Indians – is said to yield virtually all the vitamins needed. The greenery is particularly rich in thiamine, riboflavin, and vitamin C, and is believed to tone the muscles of the gastro-intestinal tract, aid breathing during physical exertion, act as an aphrodisiac, and relieve fatigue of the larynx; hence the popularity of the old coca wines with singers and orators. In fact, the coca plant much resembles the opium poppy which carpets great tracts of South-East and South-West Asia. Both can offer many blessings and both are easily over-indulged in once the active ingredient is extracted and used in concentrated form.

At the time of the first edition of this book (1986) the drug was rated, not just by social commentators but also by some medical authorities, as a comparatively harmless fillip, low in its toxic effects compared with the likes of heroin and barbiturates and presenting only a remote chance of lethal overdose.

It was used by the chic and glamorous in what were better economic times. They could handle it; it focused their creative energies, made them more potent in every sphere. Then came, as it always does, the period of revision, prompted as much by a new delivery mode (smokeable crack) as by the unravelling of social and economic confidence following the sham boom of the middle eighties.

Crack became the explanation for much of what was wrong in the black American ghettos: it caused crime, violence, disease, poverty, and social disintegration. And, while it's true that such phenomena were already eating away at the crumbling urban centres, cocaine did nothing to help.

Were we in the UK going to get a 'crack epidemic'? By the turn of the decade, the headlines, the police and politicians were all saying, 'Yes . . . it's happening now.' But experienced drug agency workers resisted the idea. History had taught them that when the authorities identified a new drug menace, what inevitably followed was a frenzy of (usually racist) scapegoating from which flowed a series of idiotic policy initiatives.

Yet in those same black communities – which the white, liberal-minded drug workers were seeking to 'protect' from the crack backlash – people were saying crack *is* tearing us apart, and it is racist to *deny* that fact, or to treat crack solely as a crime problem.

All of which goes to show that understanding drugs is about more than understanding pharmacology or the physiology of the human organism. It is about recognising competing versions of reality, as well as in which direction politics and money flow.

The best that can be said is that the future of cocaine in the UK is unclear. Amphetamine – cheaper, longer-lasting, but also increasingly adulterated – has been the traditional stimulant of mass consumption since the early 1960s. And so those who market cocaine in this country face the continuing problem of to whom and how to pitch their product: at the unstable, self-destructive *gangsta* market, or at the more elevated social echelons. Both scenes, in the States at least, have taken a knock in recent times. That's thanks to the plethora of crazed crack-fiend stories. But while casual use of all forms of the drug is down in the US, there remains a larger-than-ever repository of daily 'problem users'.[1]

Here, by 1993, coke was returning to the dance clubs (especially the 'jungle' variety) as an accompaniment to immobilising strains of hash and grass. Before dope it had been Ecstasy in the clubs, but E lost much of its market share because quality became unreliable.

A feature to watch was the appearance of crack itself in these settings[2] – crushed up and smoked inside a tobacco or from this mild beginning, the freebase phenomenon took root. The first legitimate freebase was produced through a four or five-step process that involved heating up hydrochloride with water and a volatile liquid such as ether. A famous casualty of that method was US comedian Richard Pryor who, in June 1980, while brewing up freebase at his home, nearly blew himself apart.

Today, non-explosive reagents such as ammonia and baking powder are used to produce what is now called 'crack'. The name probably comes from the sound of sodium chloride (table salt) residues burning as the crack is smoked.

Other Routes of Admission

It is possible, though not very usual, to smoke cocaine hydrochloride inside or on the tip of a cigarette; not usual because of its comparative inefficiency in terms of intoxicant effect per given amount. Other rare ingestion methods are to eat or dissolve the crystal in a drink. Again, these methods are considered inefficient.

Though crack is usually smoked, it is also increasingly injected. Thirteen of 149 users identified for a 1990 survey were administering it via the needle. A year later, 31 of 147 users were going the needle route.[5] There are various ways of breaking down what is normally an indissoluble product.[6] Usually it's done by the addition of an acid such as vitamin C, but also, and more dangerously, by heating the crack in water or alcohol. This forms a viscous substance that blocks the small-gauge needles normally available from drug agencies. Large-bore veterinary needles have been used – items that are more likely to be shared because of their scarcity.

The rarely seen pasta is too 'dirty' to inject and impossible to freebase because of its non-solubility. Cocaine hydrochloride, however, is extremely soluble in water, making it possible to inject large amounts for rapid gratification. It is not unusual – because of the short duration of the hit – for cocaine to be injected fifteen times daily. It might be injected straight, with a synthetic opioid such as methadone, or with heroin itself. This latter combination is called a *speedball*.

188

cannabis joint. If all this seemed a long way from the grimy, watch-your-back street scene, another lesson from history is that memories are short, and as with any other product – from hairsprays to AK47s – there will always be something good to be said about it.

What is it?

Cocaine is a powerful though short-lasting central nervous system stimulant and local anaesthetic. In terms of sustained wallop it pales beside amphetamine, whose effects last six to eight times longer.

The source of much of the West's recreational coke is the plant *Erythroxylum coca*, found in the moist tropical forests on the eastern slopes of the Andes throughout Bolivia, Peru, and Ecuador. A second cocaine-rich species is *E. novagranatense*, which is husbanded in the dry mountainous regions of Colombia, along the Caribbean coast, and in certain parched areas of Peru. The coca leaf, or its derivatives, can be consumed for intoxication in four basic ways.

The leaf

This is the ancient method employed by some 90 per cent of the Andean Indians. A wad of leaf is moistened with saliva and spiced with a lime-rich material such as burnt seashell or a cereal. The lime facilitates the separation of the leaf's active alkaloid. The wad is placed between the gum and cheek and gently sucked.

Pasta

Also known as *paste, base, basa, pitillo* and *basuco*. Chemists recognise it as cocaine sulphate. A brownish, sometimes damp material containing numerous impurities, it is all the rage in urban Peru and neighbouring countries where it is usually mixed with tobacco or marijuana and smoked. The fast, intense high it produces often leads to compulsive use with a range of attendant problems.

This sulphate is the intermediate stage between the leaf and finished hydrochloride cocaine crystal. There seem to be various methods of production but all involve dowsing and brewing up the leaves in a strong chemical broth. A typical method is as follows[3]: the leaves are stripped and dunked in a plastic pit with a solution of water and sulphuric acid. Three or four times daily a barefooted man will climb in and step on them and shove them around with his hands. When the leaves turn greyish the fluid is drawn off and is mixed and stirred in plastic buckets with lime water, petrol, more acid, potassium permanganate, and ammonia. A liquid is filtered off, dried, and wrung out in a cloth such as a bed sheet. The resultant granules are the cocaine base – still laced with some of the chemicals that went into its production. The yield per acre of shrub is not high – perhaps 400 grams. Low-grade, brown pasta is the stuff that reaches the South American urban slums. The rest goes to the labs for conversion into cocaine hydrochloride.

Cocaine hydrochloride

This is an odourless, white crystalline powder with a bitter numbing taste, known informally as *charlie, toot, blow, candy, dust* and *snow*.

Snorters chop it up finely with a razor blade, draw it into two-inch-long lines and sniff it up one nostril at a time using a variety of implements. A plain straw might be used. The conspicuous rich will employ a rolled-up £50 note or specially made jewelled and gold implements.

The hydrochloride is made by subjecting the pasta to further refinement. It is first washed several times in kerosene, then chilled and the kerosene removed so that 'gas crystals' of crude cocaine are left at the bottom of the tank. The next stage will probably be to dissolve the crystals in methyl alcohol, recrystallise them and dissolve them once more in sulphuric acid. They go through a further complex procedure of washing, oxidation and separation calling for such mouth-watering materials as potassium permanganate, benzole, and sodium carbonate. The result is cocaine at the mid-90 per cent purity level.

While the capacity of cocaine to blight the lives of some individuals and communities has been endlessly documented, little attention has been paid to the environmental impact of the production process. According to a Peruvian trade ministry official,[4] 'it has devastating effects on the soil, encouraging deforestation and desertification . . . the intensification of erosion, the extinction of plant and animal species and the pollution of air and water' – the latter through the lavish application of highly toxic agrochemicals for increasing the harvest or for killing weeds.

By the time the hydrochloride reaches the street, the purity will have been substantially compromised by a chain of dealers, each of whom 'cuts' the product in order to maximise his/her own profit. Some of these cuts are inert (glucose, the baby laxative Mannitol), some are psychoactive in their own right (amphetamine, the local anaesthetics lidocaine, novocaine), others might provide no 'charge' but, when injected, prove highly dangerous (cornstarch, talcum powder, flour). Other cuts are plain pernicious whatever the route of administration (quinine, strychnine, glass). In the UK, so far, there is no tradition of dangerous cuts. Most often glucose is used to thin out coke.

Crack/Freebase

Freebase is cocaine hydrochloride that has been chemically treated to 'free' the potent 'base' material from the salt. Crack is merely a modern version of the original freebase – made more simply and with less risk of the chemicals involved blowing up in the producer's face.

Because of its indissolubility in water, freebase/crack cannot be sniffed or satisfactorily injected (unless further treated). It is smoked from 'pipes' – often made from soft-drink cans and the like – mixed with tobacco/cannabis in a 'joint', or burnt on a piece of tin foil.

Freebase is a form said to have been invented by the *Yanqui* traffickers of the early 1970s as a means of testing the purity of their South American-purchased hydrochloride. Originally, it meant burning a sample of the merchandise on a strip of tin foil, then sniffing the vapours and examining the ashes to establish its quality. The vapours were enjoyed and, from this mild beginning, the freebase phenomenon took root. The first legitimate freebase was produced through a four or five-step process that involved heating up hydrochloride with water and a volatile liquid such as ether. A famous casualty of that method was US comedian Richard Pryor who, in June 1980, while brewing up freebase at his home, nearly blew himself apart.

Today, non-explosive reagents such as ammonia and baking powder are used to produce what is now called 'crack'. The name probably comes from the sound of sodium chloride (table salt) residues burning as the crack is smoked.

Other Routes of Admission

It is possible, though not very usual, to smoke cocaine hydrochloride inside or on the tip of a cigarette; not usual because of its comparative inefficiency in terms of intoxicant effect per given amount. Other rare ingestion methods are to eat or dissolve the crystal in a drink. Again, these methods are considered inefficient.

Though crack is usually smoked, it is also increasingly injected. Thirteen of 149 users identified for a 1990 survey were administering it via the needle. A year later, 31 of 147 users were going the needle route.[5] There are various ways of breaking down what is normally an indissoluble product.[6] Usually it's done by the addition of an acid such as vitamin C, but also, and more dangerously, by heating the crack in water or alcohol. This forms a viscous substance that blocks the small-gauge needles normally available from drug agencies. Large-bore veterinary needles have been used – items that are more likely to be shared because of their scarcity.

The rarely seen pasta is too 'dirty' to inject and impossible to freebase because of its non-solubility. Cocaine hydrochloride, however, is extremely soluble in water, making it possible to inject large amounts for rapid gratification. It is not unusual – because of the short duration of the hit – for cocaine to be injected fifteen times daily. It might be injected straight, with a synthetic opioid such as methadone, or with heroin itself. This latter combination is called a *speedball*.

Known in medical circles as a Brompton Cocktail, it is given orally to 'terminal' patients suffering pain. It is said to impart a euphoria greatly surpassing that achieved by either drug taken alone. The American comedian John Belushi is reputed to have been killed by this combination.[7]

Sensations

As usual, there is a tremendous subjective element involved here. Crack is supposed to be the version of the drug that induces a demented craving for additional doses, thus producing instant, irresistible addiction. This has been said of other drugs that, in earlier times, have been the subject of intense public anxiety. It hasn't proved true in the past. Nor is it true of crack. For instance, a systematic survey conducted among 308 Miami adolescent drug users[8] found that, while 90 per cent of them had tried crack, only 29 per cent were using it daily, and even then not more than one or two hits at a time. The findings are supported by at least two other US surveys.[9] And the authors of a 1991 South London research project reported that, among 150 cocaine users they surveyed, the severity of dependence experienced by the crack smokers in the group fell midway between the coke sniffers and coke injectors. Two-thirds of those who used crack 'reported only minor signs of dependence during the year prior to interview'.[10]

The crack experience is essentially a compressed version of what befalls snorters of hydrochloride powder. Most snorters say that it gives them a feeling of exhilaration that comes on within about three minutes and tapers off within fifteen to forty. The crack rush happens almost instantly, starts diminishing within a couple of minutes, and is over after about twelve. As with amphetamine, there is the sense of confidence and potency – mental, sexual, and physical – as well as a suspension of appetite and fatigue. But, in comparison with common speed, it is rated a smoother, more aristocratic ride. Typical users snort repeatedly through a session of fun or work, especially through tasks requiring stamina, concentration, and imagination. The problem with the drug, again like speed, is that nerves become jangled as more is administered in one session, and at high doses – or if the user happens to be susceptible – a 'toxic psychosis' can develop. The effects may include paranoia, confusion, hypersensitivity, and the sensation of bugs crawling under the skin.

The cocaine injection 'rush' affects people differently. Some are made nauseous and distressed, while adepts often talk in sexual terms – 'of total body orgasm' or of 'body electrification'; precisely the same language used by crack smokers.

The higher and longer a person trips on cocaine, the bumpier the landing. But after virtually any dose there are degrees of melancholy, tiredness, and hunger.

The subjectiveness of the cocaine experience was demonstrated by a team of researchers at the Yale University School of Medicine. In administering doses of various substances to experienced cocaine users they found none 'could distinguish a single dose of cocaine taken intranasally [through the nose] from the same quantity of a synthetic local anaesthetic, lidocaine.'[11] Investigators at the University of Chicago School of Medicine, moreover, found that their subjects 'could not distinguish the immediate effects of intravenous [injected] cocaine from those of amphetamine, although at later times the differences between the drugs were apparent.'[12] Such results, they were satisfied, debunked 'the overwhelming mythology' about cocaine being an exquisitely inimitable experience.

The Crack 'Mission'

Otherwise known as a binge or run, the crack mission can last twenty-four hours or more and one person might consume in excess of half an ounce. 'It starts with a massive rush,' says 'Lewis', a twenty-eight-year-old West London man. 'Your heart beats harder and your thinking's going faster and faster in ever-decreasing circles. You want more because it leaves you so quickly. It's like being cheated of this great feeling. But the first rock's always the best and you'll never get that feeling back even though you'll spend the rest of the evening chasing it. After eight or ten rocks you start getting paranoid, you're hearing things, you're panicking with these feelings of imminent doom. But you still carry on if you've got any left.

'I know of someone who had half an ounce and couldn't get out of a room in Shepherd's Bush until his lung literally collapsed. He got through 800 quid's worth. Three years ago I personally blew a whole load of social fund money that was supposed to go on furniture for a new flat. I thought, *Ooh, I'll just treat myself to one*, and before you know it you've spent 1300 quid. It took a weekend.'

Where a group get together in a so-called 'crack house' and pool resources, the mood after a few pellets can quickly become unhinged. Lewis remembers being in a flat on the Mozart estate in West London where, after a pipeload, one of those present, in a spirit of exaltation, took out a gun and fired it through the ceiling. 'People are coming in and out,' says Lewis, 'begging and hassling, scratching around on the floor for dropped crumbs, moving in on other people's weaknesses. Many times the mood gets violent, especially when you're running out of gear. As usually the biggest one there, I've often taken what's going if I've wanted more. It's done with threats.'

Physical Effects

Less serious

Most commonly, the mouth goes dry, there is sweating, increased heart and pulse rate. Sniffers might get cold-like symptoms – e.g. runny nose and general nasal irritation.

Regular users are prone to diarrhoea, buzzing in the ears, chest pains, twitches and tremors, and – among smokers – various respiratory problems such as chronic coughing, racked, wheezy breathing, loss of voice, and damage to the membranes lining the nostrils and to the tissue separating them.

Other potential consequences of a big, long-term habit are a range of problems associated with loss of appetite, including decreased weight and dehydration. There might also be irregular or abnormally rapid heart beats.

When injected or smoked the drug can produce a sponta
neous ejaculation, without any handling of the organs. But
ultimately, the sex act can be made more difficult if no
impossible. Men find it hard to mount an erection and womer
have problems reaching orgasm.

More serious

This is a highly subjective, even political area, where hos
pital data and information gleaned from scientifically dubiou:
laboratory experiments on animals are mobilised to make
the case for or against the drug. Some American medica
textbooks, just a decade ago, talked benignly of cocaine
detecting few if any major complications from its use. Today
it is held responsible for everything from heart failure and
stroke to epilepsy, hyperthyroidism, asthma, spontaneous
internal bleeding, and horribly malformed babies.

'The medical and psychiatric complications associated with
cocaine use are so numerous and severe that it would take an
entire book to describe them completely,' said one American
authority.[13]

In fact, cocaine is a drug of low toxicity compared with
barbiturates, alcohol and heroin, with deaths from overdose
being fairly rare. The fatal dose is often put at around one
gram, but there are reports that more than twenty grams of
pure coke have been survived.

But cocaine, particularly at higher doses, does present a
toxicity problem not offered by the stimulant with which it
is usually compared: amphetamine. This is due to coke's
local anaesthetic properties and, especially, its depressant
effect on the lower brain centres which control respiration.
US drugs expert George Gay[14] has noted that, while it
is primarily the higher centres which are stimulated by
low to moderate doses, when more is ingested (or in
susceptible people) the low brain centres begin triggering
tremors and convulsions. Confusion, dry throat, and dizziness may set in, with breathing fluctuating wildly between
rapid large gulps and shallow breaths. Erratic heart beat
develops quickly, and the individual could die either from
cardiac arrest or respiratory failure. The episode has been
called the 'Casey Jones Reaction' – after the puffing loco-
motive driver. While it is usually set off by injection or

freebasing, a sniffer also runs some (much more remote) risk.

Another concern to be taken seriously is so-called 'crack-lung', a condition involving chest pains, breathing problems, and high temperature. There is also some, so far circumstantial, evidence of crack-induced stroke.

Injection of the drug carries the familiar risks of abscesses, blood clots, and – where works are shared – an increased chance of receiving and passing on HIV/AIDS and the various forms of hepatitis.

Psychiatric Problems

Unlike amphetamine, which demands hours of wakefulness and, consequently, might force adjustments to daily routine, it is quite usual for cocaine to be sniffed long-term without the dose escalating or the needle/freebasing being taken up. At the same time, there is a significant proportion of coke habitués who do develop problems. These may include mood swings, poor sleep patterns, agitation, bouts of paranoia, aggression, confusion, hypersensitivity, auditory hallucinations, and the like. All these symptoms generally clear up once use is discontinued, although the healing process can take months.

People with pre-existing psychiatric problems might turn to cocaine and other stimulants in the expectation that the drug will relieve whatever feelings of depression, anxiety and hopelessness they might be suffering. But while initial relief might be forthcoming, problems are ultimately likely to deepen.

Medical Complications

Cocaine presents some risk for people suffering from hypertension (high blood pressure), severe cardiac disease, abnormal activity of the thyroid gland, epilepsy, liver damage, respiratory ailments, and muscular disease.

In Association with Other Drugs

Cocaine is one of many drugs and common foods that react badly with a class of antidepressant called Monoamine oxidase inhibitors (MAOIs) (see pages 86–7). There is also a problem with hypertensive drugs.

Cocaine and heroin (or a kindred depressant) mixed together in a syringe for a speedball combination can be more than normally hazardous because of the unpredictable effect each drug has on the other. The presence of coke can cause an overdose when taken on top of the amount of heroin the user is accustomed to handling. Similarly, the heroin might tend to provoke a dangerous reaction to what in the past has been a manageable amount of cocaine.

Pregnancy

Because of cocaine's tendency to induce high blood pressure and irregular heart beats, taking it during late pregnancy could bring extra risks to the mother of a possible heart attack. Any danger is exacerbated by the anaesthetics that might be used during labour.[15]

As to the baby, the consumption of any drug during pregnancy (illicit or medical) increases the risk of damage to the foetus and the subsequent normal development of the child. S/he might be born early and small, and, therefore, be prone to potentially serious complications such as feeding problems and infections.[16] There will be a higher than normal risk of what's called 'perinatal mortality' – that's death before birth or within the first week of life.

The risk of congenital abnormalities from drug use in general is also increased, especially where they are used in the first three months of pregnancy. After that, any problems are likely to relate to delayed growth.

But attributing specific problems to specific drugs is complicated, given that potential 'insults' to the developing child come from all directions – not least from traffic, factory and water pollution, and from what might be the poor eating habits of the mother.

In fact, poverty and smoking play at least as big a role as drugs in causing possible complications for the newborn; and the fact that damaging drug consumption is closely correlated with economic and social deprivation[17] indicates the kind of statistical tangle medical experts can get into and, as a result, just how imprecise the art of substance-blaming really is.

At the time of writing, crack was the product traumatising the US (from where most drugs-and-pregnancy research is generated) and the medical evidence has reflected that anxiety. Certain common strands have emerged but there is also much contradiction.

Where cocaine-specific problems have been identified they relate to the drug's powerful capacity to constrict the blood vessels and, as a result, the flow of blood to and from the mother and her foetus. This is said to lead to more spontaneous abortions, maternal high blood pressure, and separation of the placenta – the last being a virtual death sentence for the child since it is then starved of oxygen, blood, and nutrients. The evidence for all these damaging vascular effects is convincing, according to a leading UK authority, Dr Mary Hepburn, consultant obstetrician at Glasgow's Royal Maternity Hospital.

Crack babies

That some babies of opioid-using mothers go through a withdrawal syndrome when born is undeniable. Symptoms range from mild to severe (see chapter on heroin). The issue of so-called 'crack babies' is more contentious. Panic stories in the American media during the early nineties claimed that some of these newborn perished, having 'lost the will to live'. However, there is now less certainty about this issue in medical circles, with some of those working in the field asserting that babies of crack-using mothers do not suffer any kind of withdrawal syndrome.

We should not be amazed if expert thinking undergoes another bout of revisionism.

Tolerance

Tolerance can be defined as the need to use more of the drug in question to maintain the same effects. The consensus view in recent years has been that the high from cocaine can be achieved each time on a stable dose. But because such matters are essentially subjective (how can one 'high' be measured against another?), this assumption was bound to be revised. In the era of crack it is now assumed that tolerance may indeed develop to what is a short-lived intense experience, and that this leads users to keep on escalating their intake. The word from users themselves suggests that some do and some don't. 'The craving is with you for an hour,' a Liverpool man told me. 'Whether you take it again depends if you're in that culture and whether you're that type of person. If I'm trying to resist, I, like, hold on to a chair and wait to land.'

While more coke might be needed to get the same old high, there is a reverse tolerance syndrome whereby the body seems to build increased sensitivity to the drug's convulsant and anaesthetic properties – i.e. less ends up doing more.

Dependence/Withdrawal

Users do not build a classic physical addiction to the drug whereby they suffer convulsions and other serious bodily traumas when separated from it, but an intense psychological entanglement is possible, particularly where the drug has been injected or freebased.

Abrupt withdrawal from a heavy habit will produce the kind of long-term fatigue, depression, anxiety, feelings of isolation and agitation known to quitters of amphetamine. These could last for months, depending on the individual's constitution and the amount of emotional energy invested in the habit. Danger of relapse lies in meeting with old drug-taking cronies, or getting reinstalled in or even simply revisiting former drug-taking haunts.

Earliest Use

Andean Indians have been chewing on coca leaves for five thousand years or more. During the Inca period the habit was a prerogative of the ruling classes, but in later and current times some 90 per cent of the population took to it. Known as a *coquero*, a leaf-chewer moistens a wad with spit and places it between cheek and gums in much the way quids of tobacco are pulped in the southern US. Claimed to be rich in protein, vitamins, calcium, iron and fibre, the immediate benefits include increased energy, nourishment, and easier breathing while labouring in the thin Andean atmosphere. The leaf is also said to improve contact with the spirit world.

The invading Spanish *Conquistadores* believed that coca chewing symbolised the Indian people's pact with the Devil and that it encouraged unworthy sexual practices such as sodomy and bestiality, representations of which the Moche people of northern Peru were carving into their sculptures and pottery at least a thousand years before the Spanish landed. Because of these tendencies the Spanish initially prohibited coca use. They later relented when it was found that more gold could be extracted from the Inca mines if the natives were under coca's invigorating influence. Still today, impoverished miners will resort to coca, as a substitute for food, to get them through the day.

European History

Specimens of coca leaves were despatched to Europe soon after Spain's 'discovery' of South America, and yet despite favourable reviews the chewing practice failed to take off. This was perhaps partly a matter of aesthetics but largely due to the leaves' inability to retain their potency once dried and put on the long boat-ride across the Atlantic. Had they travelled as well as tobacco, tea, opium, or coffee beans, our view of the drug might have been markedly different. Even when the German chemist Friedrich Gaedcke isolated alkaloid of cocaine in 1855, and fellow countryman Albert Niemann further refined the process some four years later, the drug failed to implant itself into the medical mainstream. Not for twenty years were cocaine's principal benefits recognised by medical academics. In 1880 the Russian nobleman and physician Vasili von Anrep noted that there was no pain from a pinprick when cocaine was administered under the skin. In 1883 the physician Theodor Aschenbrant reported on marvellous feats of endurance and energy by cocaine-high Bavarian soldiers. And in the US, physicians were noting the drug's ability to excite the central nervous system, and studying it as a possible antidote to morphine and alcohol addiction.

All these possibilities were pondered by the young Sigmund Freud, at that time a house physician at a Viennese hospital. It is said of Freud that he latched on to cocaine as a means of promoting his name and fortune, and yet his subsequent 1884 treatise on the subject – *On Coca* – is far from wholly laudatory in regard to cocaine's effects. He warned that moderate use was reported to cause 'physical and intellectual decadence' together with weakness, emaciation, and 'moral depravity'. But to this he added: 'All other observers affirm the view that the use of coca in moderation is more likely to promote health than impair it.'

Specifically, Freud listed the following major therapeutic applications: as a central nervous system stimulant, for digestive disorders of the stomach, for the wasting disease cachexia, for alcohol and morphine addiction, for asthma, as a local anaesthetic, and as an aphrodisiac.

It remained for Freud's friend and associate, Carl Koller, to demonstrate the drug's full potential as a local anaesthetic by applying it to the eye during surgery. The medical community was astounded and until recent years the drug was still widely employed for such procedures. In the UK its use is now mainly confined to the treatment of certain conditions of the ear and larynx.

Freud's attempts to show that cocaine cured morphine addiction were less than wholly successful. One of his earliest subjects, his friend and colleague Ernst von Fleischl, simply switched from morphine dependence to cocaine dependence and within a year was using up to one gram a day. Recorded as Europe's first cocaine addict, he went into serious psychological decline. Freud also came unstuck in his claim that 'there seemed to be no lethal dose'. One of his own patients apparently died from a quantity of the drug he had himself prescribed. Reports of cocaine 'intoxication' and cocaine addiction soon began showing up in the medical journals and things reached such a pass that in 1886 Europe's leading addiction specialist, Albrecht Erlenmeyer, accused Freud of unleashing the 'third scourge of mankind' (to go with morphine and alcohol). Erlenmeyer was apparently alarmed at the by-now widespread touting of cocaine as a cure for morphine addiction – as if the simple switch of drugs promised a cure.

Freud made some grudging concessions to his critics.[18] In an 1887 paper he agreed that some people did seem to get addicted but only because they had previously been hooked on morphine. He also claimed that the apparent addiction was activated by use of the hypodermic syringe – a mode of administration he had himself commended. Finally, any addiction 'was not, as was commonly believed, the direct result of imbibing a noxious drug, but to some peculiarity in the patient.'

Freud had his own drug-linked peculiarities.[19] He smoked heavily for most of his life and acknowledged that the habit probably caused the cancer of his jaw and mouth for which he underwent thirty-three operations during the last sixteen years of his life. For forty-five years he tried, on and off, to quit. But right up until the end in 1939, he admitted to smoking 'an endless series of cigars'.

The touting of one drug as a cure for dependence on another is a recurring theme in pharmacological history. For those hooked on opium, the far stronger morphine was once advanced. For morphine addicts, cocaine, and then heroin, were pushed. For overcoming heroin addiction, methadone (another potent, addictive drug with more protracted withdrawal symptoms) is currently being dispensed by the state. A similar line can be drawn through the hypnotic/sedatives, starting with chloral hydrate, on through bromide, the barbiturates, and the benzodiazepines – none of which have stood the test of intelligent scrutiny. But even as I write these words, new categories of 'entirely safe, non-addictive' replacements are up and running, with more in the works.

What is true about all these categories of drugs is that problems rapidly accumulate when the leap is made from the comparatively mild substance found in nature to the synthesised, streamlined compound product of the laboratory. The problems are further aggravated by claims made by manufacturers, regulatory agencies and doctors who seem incapable, or perhaps unwilling, to learn the lessons of the past.

American History

Whatever the cocaine backlash of the 1880s, numerous patent remedies containing coca leaf extract proliferated. They were set against everything from nasal congestion to syphilis. This was particularly true of the US where the choice was between nose powders, suppositories, throat lozenges, and cigarettes. One of the most successful promoters of the drug was the Corsican chemist Angelo Mariani whose tonic wine – bearing his name – became a favourite with the great figures of the day. They included the Czar of Russia, the commanding general of the British army, the Prince of Wales, and the kings of Norway and Sweden. Pope Leo XIII called Mariani's wine 'a benefactor of humanity' and presented him with a gold medal.

Coca-Cola was among numerous drinks of the late nineteenth/early twentieth century infused with the leaf's psychoactive ingredient. The king of colas, developed by Atlanta druggist John Pemberton, was originally sold as a 'valuable brain tonic and cure for all nervous afflictions' when introduced in 1886. It was also touted as a 'temperance drink' because it contained not a drop alcohol – although it was boosted by a double helping of chemical stimulants: caffeine as well as cocaine. By 1903 the manufacturers were forced by public pressure to abandon use of the cocaine-laced syrup (but not the caffeine) and, instead, employed a flavouring derived from the 'decocainised' coca leaves. The same unstimulating leaf extract is still used, the source being a dry valley in north-eastern Peru.

The pressure against Coca-Cola was worked up by the American media – the low and high ends of it – in which cocaine was being identified repeatedly with crime-crazy

Southern blacks. There were reports of superhuman strength and guile, such as a story of 'black rapists' in the *New York Times*, in which it was claimed that 'bullets fired into vital parts that would drop a sane man in his tracks failed to check the "fiend".' The same *NYT* story branded the drug a 'potent incentive in driving the humbler negroes all over the country to abnormal crimes' and indicated that 'most attacks upon white women of the South . . . are the direct result of the coke-crazed negro brain.' There was, of course, a political dimension to this panic. As *High Times* magazine puts it, 'the optimism of the [post-slavery] Reconstruction era had been replaced by legal segregation and lynchings', and while bullet-proof blacks weren't all that seriously fretted over, there was the more worrying prospect of the drug providing the stimulus to a more organised and energetic resistance.

As important as the social/political pressures was the intensifying commercial struggle as to who was to exert decisive control over the supply of the new, booming drug products market – pharmacists, the drugs' manufacturers, or doctors – the latter increasingly well organised under the aegis of the American Medical Association (AMA).

The AMA's aim was to restrict virtually all drugs to prescription-only use and, thereby, seal their own status and commercial hegemony. With regard to cocaine, the AMA's battle was virtually won by 1914, when the Harrison Narcotic Act (which erroneously listed cocaine as a 'narcotic') banned the drug's use in 'patent' medicines and restricted the manufacture and distribution of all coca products.[20]

At the same time, the US federal government was spearheading international moves to curb not just the production and trading of coke, but of a range of opiates too. America was, by this time, experiencing its first great wave of street use of several substances and it aimed to do something about it on a grand scale.

British history

Britain also went through a series of cocaine tremors. The roots lie in the nineteenth century when various coca-based medicines and tonics were promoted as the solution to a broad range of maladies. 'Party' use was still comparatively rare at that time, even amongst the aristocratic-boho set, whose preference was for the more dreamy indulgences of opium and hash.[21]. Arthur Conan Doyle had his fictional detective, Sherlock Holmes, using the drug 'recreationally' for the first time in *A Scandal in Bohemia* (1886). In *The Sign of the Four*, published two years later, Holmes explained the drug's lure. 'I suppose its influence is physically a bad one. I find it, however, so transcendingly stimulating and clarifying to the mind that its secondary action is a matter of small moment.'

Conan Doyle and his mainlining alter ego have been psychoanalysed into the ground these past couple of decades. The emerging wisdom – enunciated[22] by the likes of Dr David Musto, psychiatrist and medical historian at Yale University – is that the detective's later obsession with Professor Moriarty, the evil master criminal Holmes believes is persecuting him, was probably an evocation of cocaine-induced paranoia. In fact, the author himself was dropping hints to this effect by the time of *The Missing Three Quarters* (1896).

The first real-life jolt to the general public occurred in 1901 when two young actresses suffered overdose deaths. A greater shudder came during the 1914–18 war when an ex-convict and a prostitute were convicted of selling cocaine to Canadian troops stationed at Folkestone. That troops charged with the Empire's defence should be using 'narcotic' drugs was serious enough. That the likely source was Germany herself – at that time the world's largest pharmacological cocaine producer – gave the episode an even more rank odour. There quickly grew the idea, false as it turned out,[23] that an epidemic of cocaine sniffing was raging amongst British troops. To counter it, and to comply with the obligations incumbent upon Britain under the US-led international control initiatives, a new regulation was passed which, in effect, established the hardline reaction to drugs which exists to this day.

Regulation 40B under the Defence of the Realm Act (DORA) reserved most of its detailed restrictions for cocaine. For the first time, simple possession was banned, except by medical persons, pharmacists, and vets. Cocaine, in future, could be supplied only on prescription, and these could be dispensed once only.

DORA 40B became defunct after 1918, but it lived on in the apparel of the Dangerous Drugs Act 1920. This was DORA 40B extended to conform to the guidelines set down by the 1912 International Opium Convention.

Though Britain didn't have bullet-proof blacks to contend with, it did have the spectre of the degenerate Chinaman living in East London's dock area and peddling drugs and vice to tender young white things. The novels and yellow press of the day were replete with stories spelling out this theme. The Chinese of Limehouse were seen principally to be involved in the opium trade, while the roots of the cocaine menace were often attributed to a shadowy Vice Trust centred in London which used female 'drug fiends' as its missionaries. They could be found in certain teashops in the fashionable areas of the West End, notes Terry Parssinen in his excellent book on the subject,[24] and were apparently recruited to their mischief by wealthy Bohemian types, behind whom was a Mr Big, often a businessman or aristocrat.

The real-life model for such lurid tales was the case of Billie Carleton, a beautiful young actress who, after attending a 1918 Victory Ball at the Albert Hall, was found dead in her flat, supposedly killed by an overdose of cocaine – although depressants such as opium and sleeping pills have since been implicated.[25] The Carleton case combined a delicious cast of characters for the press. At the coroner's inquest it was revealed that Billie had begun smoking opium in fashionable West End haunts and had moved on to sniffing cocaine and heroin. There was apparently a Chinese source in Limehouse, while her immediate supplier was a slippery dress designer called Reginald de Veulle with whom Billie was said to be having an illicit affair. The Carleton case triggered off not just a lava-flow of newspaper stories, books, and films, but created the new 'junkie' archetype. It also made the new laws both possible and essential.

The reality of recreational cocaine use throughout the early decades of the century is meticulously traced from court records and other sources by Parssinen. He finds that while a recreational subculture similar to that existing today was visible in American cities by the 1890s, the British scene didn't really fruit until about 1916, and even then it was comparatively tiny – confined to a few areas of London and centred on cocaine rather than morphine and heroin. But, as in the States, the London street users were, typically, young working-class or criminally inclined males and prostitutes. The origin of most stock was probably Germany. These, however, were the cases that came before the courts. There was also a certain amount of smart use by the Bohemian/theatrical crowd. Billie Carleton made that clear, while Aleister Crowley's *Diary of a Drug Fiend* gives a good indication of use in aristocratic circles. Such smart folk usually had the sophistication and connections to give the judiciary a wide berth. They might also have preferred morphine to coke as their habitual indulgence since it could be obtained from private practitioners. Cocaine and heroin were scarcely ever prescribed.

Given the size and fragility of the English cocaine scene in the early decades it was possible to harass it almost to extinction by 1930. Most users decided it was too troublesome a habit, notes Parssinen, and 'while the odd opium smoker popped up and a few elderly morphine addicts lingered on into the next decade, Britain's drug problem was essentially solved by 1930.'

By 'drug problem' Parssinen is no doubt referring to the illicit scene. But the trafficking of toxic and habit-forming substances was probably increasing thanks to the pharmaceutical industry's aggressive marketing of barbiturates and, by the late thirties, of amphetamines. This last was the stimulant that, in terms of efficiency, easily outstripped cocaine. It worked longer, jerked the user higher gram for gram, was available in pills, powders, and injectable form, and, though the ride was reputedly more ragged, it was at least legal. Yet by the 1950s cocaine began showing up again. It was traded in one or two Soho jazz clubs and used almost exclusively as an accompaniment to heroin – taken through a hypodermic syringe in a 'speedball' combination. The model was the American cool jazz scene. The practitioners here were musicians, a few Nigerians, and some early beatsters. Supplies came from hospital pharmacy thefts, so the stock was guaranteed pure. Then some doctors began prescribing and the scene grew moderately, though it rarely strayed beyond the usual Soho haunts. The circle was subsequently swelled by the arrival of a couple of planeloads of Canadian heroin and cocaine addicts who had been told by a visiting British doctor that both drugs were being lawfully prescribed in the UK.

Then, in 1967, came another turnaround with the establishment of the government's new drugs policy: special clinics for addicts were opened; ordinary doctors were squeezed out of the picture; security on pharmacy and hospital stocks was tightened; and the number of addicts provided with cocaine on prescription reduced down to half a dozen or fewer. (For the background to this policy change, see heroin chapter.) Many switched to Methedrine – there being a glut for a year – but when this source was also stepped on the injectors had to look elsewhere for their stimulation.

Current Use

The association of cocaine with heroin-injecting 'junkies' had by now taken the drug down a step in terms of public image. It was equally unfashionable among the new wave of Sixties experimental drug users who largely confined themselves to marijuana and LSD. Dealers trading in those drugs often considered it a matter of principle not to handle cocaine, and for the same reason avoided heroin and injectable methylamphetamine.

Then in the mid-1970s – by which time the Sixties 'youth culture' had fractured, and with it the old drug rules and rituals – cocaine re-entered the scene. This time it was as a chic tonic for musicians. It travelled from there to other glossy circles, some of which were entirely unused to drugs other than alcohol and cigarettes. The key to its rehabilitation was the return to a method of ingestion popular in the early decades of the century – snorting. Snorting made the drug seem safer and less sordid (snorting subsequently allowed heroin to get a toehold), and because cocaine still had its dangerous past it could impart glamour to establishment sniffers such as lawyers and City of London brokers, or to the nearly-chic like advertisers and press officers. It said of them, 'I am a rebel. I live (a little) dangerously.' They would have known that, taken in moderation, intranasally, the drug not only allowed them to function at their work, it was as safe or more so than many stimulants and depressants available through the health service. Such factors caused cocaine's appeal to

205

widen. It became *de rigueur* wherever smart and successful people worked and played; a feature of black circles as much as white. And because it was now associated with success the lower social ranks began coveting it. (Either that or they came to detest it as a frothy bourgeois thing – particularly true of English punks.)

Boom Times in the USA

In the US, consumption boomed to 'epidemic' levels, with an estimated 12 million users by 1985. Between 1976 and 1986, cocaine was said to have prompted a fifteen-fold increase in the number of admissions to public treatment programmes, as well as a corresponding rise in the number of emergency room visits.[26] Such data need to be digested with care, given that somebody dying from gunshot wounds but with cocaine in them could be logged under 'cocaine-related'; while inside the body of emergency admissions there will often have been other drugs working in tandem.

Nonetheless, there was clearly a quantum leap in US consumption and this spawned the familiar crop of horror stories and morality tales, with little in the way of analysis as to the structural problems facing – especially – the run-down black urban communities. Much simpler was to pathologise those without jobs, without homes, to treat their situations as a product of personal deviancy.

Better still were the stories of the mighty fallen. In June 1986 cocaine poisoning was reported to have taken the life of football star Don Rogers. That same month came news that All-America basketballer Len Bias, just drafted by the Boston Celtics, had celebrated with so much cocaine that he died of cardiac arrest.[27] There followed a stream of such stories before attention returned to the ghettos and the new cocaine mode of crack: crack houses for buying and selling the drug, dealers with submachine-guns infesting low-income housing projects, gangsters dripping with gold and cruising around in BMWs, kids shot on the way to school, children – barely past toddling age – used as runners, muggings, AIDS, TB, prostitution . . .

In the Bohemian 'fifties and hippie 'sixties the appetite was for 'amotivational' dope, plus a range of psychedelics that posed the big, awkward Question about what any of it meant: life and all that. Then there was a kind of polymorphism before heroin emerged as the fix for the years of disappointed ideals, until it too was eclipsed by the substance that delivered to the user feelings of drama and personal potency – this in an age when the power/money quotient appeared to be the ultimate measurement of worth. This was the message reaching the street. It was reaching emasculated black and Hispanic youth who, with crack, had the perfect economic stimulant with which to buy their piece of the American dream.

But how interesting that crack should have dug its deepest roots in the cities of Los Angeles, New York, and Washington – the first the celebrity capital of America, the second the centre of money, the third the base of political power.

Urban Ruin

In LA the story was about the gang war between, on the one hand, the Crips and the Bloods and their camp followers and, on the other, the LA police force led by chief Daryl Gate who, in 1988, likened his foe to the Viet Cong. 'This is Vietnam here,' Gate declared,[28] while leading 1,000-cop blitzkriegs and rounding up literally thousands of young blacks at a time. The explanation for the violence that came from most quarters – older blacks and whites of whatever political persuasion – was the traditional one of the failure of family values in the ghetto, abetted by welfare dependency and the decline of paternal role models.

But there were other changes going on in the Los Angeles industrial landscape, charted by an article in *New Left Review*,[29] which couldn't be easily discounted.

For working-class blacks, relentless economic decline had been occurring for fifteen years; professional blacks had left for better areas, and city resources were being absorbed in financing the corporate renaissance downtown in which black-led businesses got virtually a zero share.

Most critically, the old manufacturing plants to which

poorer educated blacks traditionally looked for high-wage jobs and social mobility had all been relocated or restructured so that the norm now was minimum-wage sweatshops. Meanwhile, young blacks, especially males, were being locked out of the more attractive service sector jobs, for example on the sales force in regional shopping malls.

The net result was 45 per cent youth unemployment in a country which had, until that time, seen unbroken growth. Finally, this all slotted into a broader environment in which public spending cuts had left 50,000 homeless, with black infant mortality rates approaching Third World levels.

If these factors were the incubus, crack was the spur. Denied other options, ghetto youth regrouped around one of the few social organisations that gave them clout: the street gang. And crack was the commodity that gave the gang its terrible momentum.

Similar stories were to be told in Seattle, Dallas, Detroit, Miami, Chicago. If not the gang, then freelance corporate units were processing and dispensing the drug, and securing their territorial claims over particular patches of 'turf' in the manner historically resorted to by their own and other governments: through violence and terror.

The US war against cocaine, domestically and overseas, was intensified throughout the latter part of the eighties.[30] It took the form of crop eradication/substitution programmes in the producer countries, ever-more spectacular seizures of the finished product (tons at a time), the arrest of thousands of distributors by the Tactical Narcotics Team, and stiffer enforcement measures against users.

Coke Use Declines

By 1990 the official indicators were pointing to good news.[31] Fewer people were reporting using, 'cocaine-related' emergency room visits were down, and the numbers calling the National Helpline had more than halved (from 40,000 in 1988 to 18,162 in 1990).

Had the Reagan/Bush Just-Say-No War on Drugs worked?

Ansley Hamid, assistant professor in the anthropology department at New York's John Jay College of Criminal Justice, thought there were other, more credible explanations.[32] He believed 'natural limits' had probably been reached. 'Inasmuch as crack operated as an instrument of capital depletion of low-income neighbourhoods [the successful dealers don't stick around; they take themselves and their money out] . . . a limit may have been reached which would not tolerate the movement upwards and out of any more dollars or resources.'

The target consumer group was also depleting. A new generation, alerted by the example of what the drug can do, had steered away from it. Crack users were now being treated with revulsion and gangs of youths, as young as sixteen, were making a new pastime of ridiculing or beating up crackheads who, they believed, disgraced neighbourhoods and were nuisances and thieves.

Existing customers – those aged twenty-five and over – were also on the decrease, Hamid noted. Many had bolted to escape problems. Tens of thousands were in prison or had dropped from sight to the city's shelter and relief systems for the homeless. Others were in hospital or were dead.

The Freak House

Those who remained were more marginalised and more reckless in every facet of their daily lives. Whereas once the scene operated through crack houses and kerbside transactions, now the mode was the 'freak house' – first observed in June 1990 in several 'low-income minority neighbourhoods' in New York City. Hamid describes how they functioned.

An older man – established with his own apartment – receives sexual services and gifts of crack from a core group of five or six young crack-using females. In return, the women get sanctuary and a place to earn a living. They promptly attract several other females and the combined 'harem' draws in young male users, drug distributors, and working men of all ages – the latter to 'freak'; that is to say, use any and all of the females sexually. 'A favourite pastime,' says Hamid, 'is "flipping" – the male going from one to as many females as are present in continuous succession.'

For these sexual favours and other services, such as the provision of beer, cigarettes, and a private space, a fee is charged: cash or crack.

Whether the freak house is to be regarded as the ultimate in urban degeneracy, or an ascent to new heights in resource-fulness for a social category whose status is that of human refuse, is a matter of taste. But, as Hamid observes, fewer crack users does not portend the end of the story for the wider population. 'As crack use declines, it functions as a high risk factor for AIDS. And violence related to its distribution may increase, as distributors compete for fewer sales, or as consumers commit more desperate acts to pay increased prices.'

Crack in the UK

The American picture of urban desolation has been mirrored here in the UK – for instance, in the 'de-industrialised' regions of Tyneside, Merseyside, and the West Midlands. And so are the crushing disparities between rich and poor, this last feature perhaps even more pronounced on home soil.

One survey[33] revealed that the top 1 per cent of income earners had received no less than 93 times as much per head in tax cuts between 1979 and 1992 as the bottom 50 per cent. 'The gap between the highest and lowest paid,' it was said, 'has increased to a level last seen in 1886.'

And the government's own figures showed that the poorest tenth of the population suffered a 17 per cent fall in real income between 1979 and 1991/92, with their relative position continuing to worsen. The richest tenth, meanwhile, had seen a 62 per cent income jump in the same period.[34]

Target Europe

Alarm in official circles about cocaine began to surface in the early 1980s, triggered by the US 'epidemic'. A 1984 House of Commons Home Affairs Committee paid a visit to the US where they found '. . . cocaine is turning respectable people into criminals to satisfy a craving which dominates all other appetites.' Within five years, they feared, we'd get the same here, and recommended 'intensified law enforcement against drug trafficking by HM Customs, the police, the security services and possibly the armed forces.'[35] Soon after came the Drug Trafficking Offences Act 1986, which allowed for the freezing of the assets of convicted drug traffickers and the confiscation of what are identified in court – not always on the best evidence – as the proceeds of drug dealing.

While there was still no data to suggest that the full cocaine terror had reached the UK, more warnings were sounded to the effect that the North American market was becoming saturated and cocaine traffickers were beginning to target Europe. Supporting evidence turned up in Customs seizure figures. Then came the seminal visit in April 1989 of former US Drugs Enforcement Administration official Robert Stutman, who gave a guarantee to a meeting of chief constables that 'two years from now you will have a serious crack problem.'

A special Crack Intelligence Unit was set up by the Metropolitan Police and, soon after, the media began reporting stories about Yardies – gun-toting Jamaican gangsters and crack dealers who, it was said, were so fearlessly ruthless they scared even the hard cases of the American ghettos. The Home Affairs Committee paid a second visit to the States, where they collected more crack-related horror tales. On their return, they heard evidence from the police that 'crack misuse is an escalating problem and one which . . . is spreading into the shire counties of England.'

It was against this background that the Home Office commissioned an extended survey into cocaine use, one that included three annual investigations in ten cities and towns involving the clients of drug agencies, as well as cocaine or crack users who were not currently in touch with any agency.

211

The most politically sensitive findings emerged from the Home Secretary's own Nottingham constituency, which was found to have a 'highly visible crack street dealing scene . . . dominated by Afro Caribbeans.' With the growth in crack dealing, the researchers reported, came guns and violence. A black crack user said, 'It's messing up the black community, they're shooting each other . . . stealing from each other.'[36]

But still the Home Office remained sanguine. In response to the Nottingham and other findings it remarked: 'It seems very likely that the number of people who are using cocaine or crack in this country has increased since 1989 but there is certainly no evidence from the research reported here that use has reached anything like epidemic proportions.'[37]

Perhaps the tone was inspired by the drug professionals who actually conducted the research. There was, throughout the drug treatment industry (composed mostly of liberal, practical-minded individuals), a resistance to the idea that a crack epidemic was taking hold. There is always resistance within these circles to any kind of drug-generated moral panic, since history shows that such panics lead to punitive, knee-jerk responses which make matters worse.

There was also a concern that fears about crack would soon translate into a bout of racist scapegoating (another lesson of history), whereby the drug habits of the white, indigenous population and whatever harm befell it would be laid at the door of the darker-skinned *aliens within*. Added to these concerns was a third: for nearly thirty years there had been a proliferation of drug treatment services, research programmes, and a host of peripheral activities. But in all this time there had been little sustained effort – certainly little success – in attracting black and other ethnic minority drug users into making use of what was on offer.

Overwhelmingly, treatment was geared to the white male opioid user, especially if he was an injector. For injectors are potential contaminants of 'decent' society.

And so, for a combination of noble and self-serving reasons, the notion of a crack epidemic was resisted. There were 'pockets of serious use', one leading analyst told me in the winter of 1993, but nothing remotely comparable to the American picture.

But this analysis failed to impress a young black researcher,

Janaka Perera, who had recently completed a series of investigations on some of the more deprived estates of South and West London. I met him at the Centre for Research on Drugs and Health Behaviour in South London. 'This person is right,' said Perera, 'when he talks about pockets of use and it not being an epidemic in the proportions you see in the States. But those pockets of serious use are within the black communities and that's fucking serious. It's destroying the communities, devastating them. I did a lot of work on the Mozart estate [in north Westminster] just before the police busts in the summer of 1992. I hung out with dealers and users. I saw the despair and hopelessness. A lot of those people were burnt out already at 18, 19. A lot of them were beginning to hide away because they'd begun chasing heroin and were scared of being seen as "junkies".'

Cocaine use, said Perera, signalled success when he was a youth in the late seventies. 'I was very impressed to see a man put a bit of charlie in his spliff. It said the man must be doing well. In that sense it's always been around. Crack came on the scene, in the late eighties, purely as a currency. It was a means of getting self-esteem when you'd been rejected from any economic opportunity. The hustling's not attractive but the outcomes are for a few people – a nice car, lot of gold, nice clothes.

'After all the hype with [US special agent] Stutman's visit in 1989, the authorities said there was no epidemic, but then that's because they were looking in the wrong place. They were looking at the treatment demand indicators, which are 95 per cent related to opiate use. We haven't got a crack cocaine problem, they said. If we did, these people would be presenting. But there *was* a crack problem and it was exploding.'

From Peckham in South London, the problem spread east, west, and north of the city. 'We had Stonebridge estate over-run, Harlesden, Chalkhill.'

The major dealers, says Perera, are white. This is because they can more easily import and make connections with the South American producer cartels. But, as far as crack went, the majority of consumers were black – that's until 1991/92 when the black customer base began getting saturated and the scene spilt out into traditionally white drug-using areas.

'You can see that happening,' says Perera, 'all over South and East London.'

While he supported the kind of 'tough' and focused policing that would take the most destructive dealers off the streets, he believed the only way real progress could be made was to 'stop tackling crack use as exclusively a crime problem and wake up to the health and social perspective.' That meant more responsive treatment programmes, ones that answer not just to *drug-takers*, but to a whole person and all his/her needs.

Inevitably, Perera's depressing view of crack's inroads into black inner-city areas is not shared by all black drug workers, even of his own twenties/early thirties generation. Some question the thoroughness of the research. Anita Hayles, based at the South London Stockwell Project, told me (summer 1994) that she thought crack was 'rife but it hadn't taken over the black community. It was causing tremendous harm but to what extent wasn't clear.' In other words better research was needed. She praised the good work of church people, black ex-users and black workers within the field. The task, she said, was educational – 'going into youth clubs, prisons, initiating groups, empowering young people with information.'

Yardie

Where there was a co-ordinated, official response to crack in the UK, it was directed at the ogre of the moment: the Yardie. Yardies, in the orthodox formulation, as we've seen, were gun-toting, drug-dealing criminals from the slums of Kingston, Jamaica. They moved freely between London, Bristol, New York, Washington – vanishing within the bosom of the settled Caribbean community whenever the authorities got close. They dealt summarily with their rivals: shooting, mutilating, throwing them from high-rise buildings. They were fearless and incomparably lustful in their appetite for wealth and status.

True?

The term Yardie itself has been misunderstood. People

214

who know the scene tell you it means, simply, a Jamaican – someone who comes from 'the Yard'. But it also denotes a transference of culture from the West Indies to foreign shores, often an uneasy transfer.

How crack and guns entered the picture is disputed. The roots seem to lie in the Jamaican sound-system culture of the mid-seventies in places like the run-down ghetto areas of Kingston. It was a hierarchical set-up involving operators (who dealt with the mix, the turntable and amp), the selector (who chose the tunes), and the crew of sound boys (who looked after the system). It seems the sound boys started taking over security and hustling weed at dances. The thing became territorial.

Politicians of the rival Jamaica Labour Party and the People's National Party moved in. It's said they sensed political advantage in the territorial carve-up. They manipulated the key figures, supplied guns, stoked the divide during the bloody 1980 general election, a campaign that left 800 dead. Alternatively, the venal mischief-makers are said to be the CIA: *they* introduced the guns and/or cocaine. They did so because America was troubled by Jamaican Premier Michael Manley's 'recognition' of socialist Cuba. They believed that the best way to thwart his re-election was to destabilise the country.

Whoever were the prime manipulators, after 1980 cocaine, guns and violence were linked indissolubly for a section of Jamaican ghetto males. Some, pressed on home shores or seeking better opportunities overseas, set up in American cities where they cornered a healthy share of the new crack market. Later, they established themselves in the UK.

'They saw the UK as easy,' according to Janaka Perera. 'Having been brought up in the ghettos of Kingston, your coping strategies for survival are very attuned to that environment and it more than equips you for survival in this country. You can be over-rough. For instance, someone else will be more patient when there's been transgressing on a drug deal. But with crack, it's going to be seriously dealt with that one time. It's predominantly the way it's been dealt with in Jamaica.'

Inevitably, a grand mythology about the Yardie enforcer/avenger grew up among a proportion of black British youth. This was especially so before the kind of hurt that crack could cause their own communities became apparent. That the Yardie figure was able to perplex and traumatise the commanding figures of white society – the police and politicians – became a source of pride. Every bloody escapade, every tabloid denunciation, caused a pleasurable frisson. If being a Yardie brought status and gold then they too would become Yardies. Or they would act the part.

Gun Play

A detailed survey[38] of the drug economy of Brixton, South London showed that few truly made the grade. While the author identified a drug *culture* (people using and dealing) he could find no discernible drug *economy*, whereby illegal proceeds are laundered and encouraged to grow by being invested in legal enterprises. The work of street dealing, he found, was small-scale, boringly repetitive and without real reward. Because of Brixton's reputation, police were everywhere and most drug-dealing youth were sooner or later jailed. The major dealers lived in less troubled parts, and they took their money with them.

As to the violence, the general view of those he canvassed was that it was more associated with alcohol than drugs and it reflected the increasing level of violence in society as a whole. Said a local drug worker: 'Among my clients, I don't see any Dillinger or Al Capone, but they all think they are gangsters. Somebody made them think they are – perhaps the media or the police. In fact they delude themselves: they think they are making a career, but they . . . are vulnerable and obvious, they'll never make it to the top.'[39]

A local social worker commented: 'What we see here is a few big cars and some portable phones. But this is not big money, as some are inclined to think. What annoys me is, all right, drugs are producing a lot of money, but none of that money is then invested in this community. All we've got left here is some gold and gaudy clothes for a few dealers.'[40]

This was in a borough where one in four of the workforce was unemployed (and the number rising rapidly), where homelessness nearly trebled between 1980 and 1992, but where financial aid from central government had declined during that same period.[41]

Though the daily grind of the user/dealer is apparently remorseless, the alternatives on offer might seem no less so. 'If they [the dealers] are able to pay rent,' says Lewis, the aforementioned twenty-eight-year-old West London man, 'and they can get a down-payment on a BMW, and they've got nice shoes on their feet, then it beats selling hotdogs. It also beats getting constantly pulled over by the police when you're in your own cab that you've maybe saved years to get. But in the end I don't know anybody who made some money, stayed straight and did well out of it.'

The first 'true Yardie' London-born Lewis ever met was in the late eighties in Earl's Court – a friend of a remote family member. 'He'd come over from Jamaica and married an English girl but he had only one thing in mind: to get to America with some money. He carried a gun but never used it. He was a sweet-natured guy who didn't use himself. He brought the coke with him, washed it [converted it into crack] and worked it through his own network in Earl's Court. We were his soldiers. We sold it. In fact, we ran Earl's Court for a while in those days. But we started to bleed him because we were all major users and, in the end, he had to move to another patch.'

The function of guns on the scene, says Lewis, is straightforwardly functional. 'Perhaps you've spent £300 on rocks with someone and you're still out of your mind for more, but now the money's gone. So you go back to him. You ask for one more rock and he refuses so you take it from him. You go through his pockets and take his rocks. I've done it countless times. But a gun is the great equaliser. You don't do it if you know he's packing. People used to have bird-scarers [shotguns] or just knives. Now it's sophisticated, sleek-looking designer pistols.'[42]

Lewis has come back from the brink. He's taken some degree courses and now helps vulnerable youngsters understand what it means to let crack run away with them. 'Everything I learnt was by discouragement from an early age,' he recalls. 'And everything that ever happened to me reinforced the suspicion that I was a piece of shit. But I'm learning to love myself bit by bit.'

Anita's Story

Lack of self-esteem was 'Anita's' problem. She was one of eight children, the first three born in Jamaica. Dad worked at Ford's in Dagenham and for London Transport. But he frittered away his earnings on the cards and horses. Supper might mean a shared bag of chips.

'They bought their own house,' says Anita, 'but it was taken away through his gambling and we were put into a slum in Stratford [East London].'

She developed asthma and eczema. Her skin, she says, looked like that of a crocodile. School was her great comfort. But, aged fifteen, she met a young man and with a child on the way her schooling came to an end.

'They warned me about him but I didn't listen. He was a man and he was interested in me – this is at a time when my eczema had only just cleared up.'

He turned out to be obsessively jealous, timing her when she went to the shops, dishing out regular beatings for giving men the wrong kind of look. He was also a gambler, like her father. Her mother helped her make the break. At this stage – the early eighties – she was using only cannabis.

Cocaine and crack started with the father of her second son, a nightclub bouncer who also dealt in weed, hash, cocaine, and stolen chequebooks and cards. Her house was safer than his so it would be from there that the dealing was done. Regularly, it would be full of people and money – thousands in cash, just lying around. Anita says that he betrayed her by having affairs, some of them with 'the opposite colour'. So she'd slip bundles of cash from under his nose. 'He'd say, "Count that", and five hundreds would go down the settee and he wouldn't know cos he'd be out of his box anyway.

'The very first time I touched crack was when he was getting ready to go to work and he'd just washed up some powder. There were some of his friends round. I saw the effects on them. They looked all right. I was curious so I

218

tried it. The euphoria made me feel powerful and talkative and happy. I'm naturally a quiet kind of person, so *that* I liked. That night we smoked a whole four ounces. He came back from the club and found us still sitting there at six in the morning, and couldn't believe the amount we'd got through.

'So now he used to come home instead of going out with his friends and we'd do it together. Things felt better for a while.'

But then he lost interest in her and she too started having affairs. When he found out he nearly killed her. By this time – 1986 – she was a 'full-blown crack addict'. Another man came into her life, a 'good man', who only smoked cannabis and drank. He had his own garage business. She carried on with her habit, supporting it with dead-end jobs in shops and factories. For a year she 'falsified the truth' of her situation. Then she acknowledged her drug habit. The truth didn't save them. 'All I was interested in was the coke. I couldn't care less whether a man came or went, not while the coke was in front of me.'

She finished with her partner in 1990 and met a thirty-nine year-old Venezuelan big-time fraudster who, as well as dealing, had had women on the street.

'He said he'd been smoking for fifteen years and it was obvious the drug had affected him mentally. He was crazed, especially when the stuff was finished. He'd turn on me. He would barricade me in the house and accuse me and the kids of plotting to nick his stuff, and my kids would have to jump through the windows. It was the crack.

'But I didn't care whether he was or wasn't in love with me. I just wanted the drugs. I just wanted someone big enough and well placed enough to guarantee it.'

In 1991 she broke down and sought help from her mother. Through her GP, she was referred to Newham Drugs Advice Project and then on to City Roads residential service for what should have been a twenty-one-day treatment.

'It was my first time away from my family. I also felt uneasy because most of the residents were white smackheads.'

Her Venezuelan friend reeled her back in with a series of phone calls. He picked her up with gear already in his pocket and took her home. One of her brothers eventually got rid of him. 'My brother beat the shit out of him. He didn't like the fact that he was putting me deep, deep down and that I was staying away from my home and kids. That's what got to him – even though my brother's a crack dealer himself.'

Her own use soon escalated to the old levels. 'I was getting through ounces and ounces, thousands and thousands of pounds. I could be smoking for twenty-four hours, feeling physically weak but still carrying on.'

A new boyfriend chased away her one remaining drug-taking crony and now she was smoking on her own. The pleasure was gone but the drug bills, without a wealthy benefactor around, were more difficult to meet. She worked two straight jobs, borrowed where she could, and performed the odd sexual favour for male friends.

By this time her oldest son was sixteen and telling her what a lousy job she'd made of mothering him. 'He started to support himself financially, doing God knows what. He's been in trouble a couple of times with the law – all because I wasn't around to give him what he needed. At that age they're interested in girls and going out, so he'd steal and whatever, and all those things got to me. Academically, he's fine, and so is my twelve-year-old; he plays football for the borough. But it's the behavioural problems.'

In the summer of 1994, she recognised that if she didn't want her boys to walk out for all time, and if she wanted to keep her new, sober, decent boyfriend, changes had to be made. She went back to Newham Drugs Advice Project who this time referred her to the Maya Project in Peckham, a residential unit with a strong bias towards black female clients. New entries are supposed to be straight for twenty-four hours before admission, but she'd smoked that same morning.

I met her five weeks into a four-month course. She'd been through the sweats, diarrhoea, depression, self-enforced isolation, and was already beginning to reconstruct a new life for her family and new boyfriend. They would live together, far away from her old haunts and cronies. 'I know if I go back there I'm going to have people non-stop knocking on my door.'

How and why did drugs run away with her?

'It was me the person, the person I am, that caused me to start taking drugs. I lack esteem. I think I really always wanted to be somebody, achieve something. I loved school, I topped the classes, but I didn't take the exams due to being a mother so early and having that creep in my life so early.

He wouldn't even allow me to go to evening classes. If ever I wanted to he swore blind I wanted to see a man. He knocked the confidence out of me. I became really shy. Coke was a drug that made me verbal.'

Moss Side

Whereas the major race-turmoil dramas of the 1980s were acted out (as far as the media were concerned) in Brixton, during the first years of the 1990s the locale was Manchester's Moss Side. Suddenly, we were reading about gunfights between hooded youths less than two miles from the city centre. A pub is sprayed with submachine-gun fire; a fourteen-year-old boy (Benji Stanley) is gunned down, maybe in error, in a fast-food takeaway. Some months later, a twenty-year-old is murdered on his mountain bike. He was wearing a bullet-proof vest but the shot was directed at his head. A witness protection scheme is set up – the first outside London – after nine trials collapse in the region because witnesses refuse to testify, change their stories, or fail to appear in court. It is all drugs-related, we are told: dealer rivalry between gangs known (after streets on the estate where they live or hang out) as the Dodingtons and Gooches.

Journalists, politicians and social pundits flood the place. A hard-nosed black American cop is brought over by Granada TV's *World in Action* to make some dread predictions about how Moss Side is about to get American-style inner-city wipe-out unless it mends its ways. Liberal Democrat leader Paddy Ashdown promenades through the danger estate and subsequently complains that he was threatened with a gun.

What is happening? Is this not England?

As one more pundit, I paid a visit to Moss Side and adjacent Hulme in March 1994, having spent some time in the area roughly ten years earlier while researching the first edition of this book. During that earlier visit the seeds of the present troubles were already evident. I wrote about Hulme's shooting galleries where social rejects gathered together in cheap tower-block apartments and filled their veins with heroin.

The impression that imprinted itself this time was one of

demolition. In Hulme, two of the four giant high-rise crescent blocks had been knocked down and the other two were empty and about to be flattened. Also demolished were thousands of surrounding maisonettes. The whole district was to be eradicated as part of a giant project in social engineering.

A new Hulme would rise from the rubble but the new inhabitants – according to local opinion – would be more prosperous and socially 'conventional' than the previous occupants, most of whom had been dispersed throughout the city. It was all a repeat of events of the mid-1960s when the area's pre-war back-to-back terraced houses were trashed to make way for the ultra-modern crescent blocks that were now coming down. Their undreamt of failure is now attributed to the cut-price materials and construction techniques employed; also to the policing difficulties presented by a confusion of interconnected blocks and landings.

As the fabric of post-1960s Hulme disintegrated, it turned into last-resort housing for city-wide residents who often brought with them more problems than solutions. There followed the familiar spiral of decline, with crime, drugs and vandalism becoming a daily feature.

The much smaller Moss Side is just across the road. In fact the boundaries between the two have never been clear. With its large, attractive park at the centre, Moss Side had always been a fairly up-market area, composed of a combination of back-to-backs and larger Victorian houses. The latter were knocked down in the 1960s and 1970s and in their place came the Alexandra Park Estate, scene of the 1990s 'gang wars'. Whereas Hulme was always predominantly white, Moss Side is regarded as a black area; even though whites and blacks continue to live together without tensions on the estate.

The killings and maimings we've read about have been black on black. Usually youth hurting youth. The 'sociological' explanation I heard locally from various well-placed individuals (who, like everyone I spoke to, preferred to remain anonymous) was related to a lack of any opportunity for the young to advance themselves in the legitimate economy. People felt ghettoised, driven low, cornered by the hostility of the outside world. So they charted their own course towards wealth and status. The young, in particular, were not going to play by the standard rules if those who ran the game were never going to let them win.

Beyond that, there were the usual conceits of young males: guns, gold, flash cars, expensive clothes, aggressive posturing. As to the weapons, young men around the world – with or without good reason – love to fire them off (in Serbia, Palestine, Rwanda, Belfast . . .) while older men will always be ready to keep them supplied and to bury the dead. The police propound all kinds of theories about sources of weapons. They range from the opening of the European Union borders to illegal shipments from the US to 'under the counter' deals in UK gun shops.[43] The Police Foundation, a non-government research institute, claimed that just a few dollars could buy sophisticated weapons in Eastern Europe, and pointed out how 'very easy it is to smuggle bits of guns into this country.'[44]

But in Moss Side, I was assured more than once, the killings were not over drugs, as was habitually declared. Said one young woman who knew the area from birth and continued to do community work there: 'People have got personal arguments. It starts off between two people and a few friends and then it's blown out of all proportion. But whereas at one time you might have gone round and given them a good kicking, the gun is how things are dealt with now, the tariff's got up that high.

'The first time someone's shot it's like, hit me and you've got to hit all my twenty friends.' And soon, she says, kids are growing up getting drawn into sides and territories and alliances. It's the Sicilian vendetta syndrome. The badlands reputation of Moss Side grows, which attracts more media, more police, and more hustlers from other parts of town. Added to all this is the juice of disappointed expectations. 'If you completely cut off a community of young people,' says a local youth worker, 'if you say to them you haven't got any legitimate place in society, then the only strong self-image on offer is that of the gangster. On the estates you wear your bandanna and you skank about a bit, and what goes along with that is that you tote a gun. If you don't tote that image you're going to lose what you have got.'

Yes, there are a lot of drugs on offer in Moss Side: cannabis, heroin, cocaine and crack. Buyers come from all over town, white and black. Junkies from other parts might shoplift downtown and come up to Moss Side to score. Some big money has been made but there's little sign of it in the vicinity. The big players seem to live outside, or they're in jail. The police, with their rapid-response armed units, their special investigation team and helicopter sorties, have been busy.

Until the mid 1980s, dealing in Moss Side was discreet and centred mostly on cannabis. Then, simultaneously, a lot of brown heroin arrived and trading moved out on to the street. It was during that period that a lot of money began to be made and there was a noticeable increase in GTis, gold chains, and other pricey paraphernalia.

The new shopping precinct became the centre of action, with lots of brazen dealing going on. People would draw up in taxis, purchase their gear, and drive off. Night and day the scene was busy. There were some police raids, surveillance cameras were established in empty shops, but it was easy enough to elude them. Dealing moved inside the shops themselves or on to the nearby Alexandra estate, which was even more 'unpoliceable' than the precinct owing to its intimidating dead ends which the police would have to traverse on foot.

It was decided to apply the Hulme solution: remove the buildings in which the trouble occurred. The entire shopping precinct – so new the council hadn't yet paid for its construction – was gutted, leaving just a shell. The bridge linking it to the Alexandra estate was ripped away. During my visit I saw the ragged end of it hanging in mid-air. And the same was done within the estate itself. Though the blocks of single-deck brick houses looked to be in good shape, where they presented a policing problem they were flattened. The school where most of the kids had gone was also flattened.

'They've taken the heart out of the community,' complained one resident of ten years, a white woman. 'Maybe it will be better when it's rebuilt but for months people have had nowhere to shop – no electric board, no chemist, no post office. They've taken it all away. If it wasn't Moss Side they'd never be able to get away with it.

'The rest of the world thinks we spend our time here ducking bullets, but this is a well-integrated community with a lot of very straight, upstanding, church-going families who are fed up not having their thoughts taken into account and fed up with having the place more and more ghettoised by all the media attention. A few are spoiling it for the majority and the press is making everything worse.'

Meanwhile, the feuding was continuing, as was the street dealing – now conducted in old Moss Side among the back-to-backs. The favoured spots were where 'sleeping policemen' and other traffic-calming devices had been installed. These brought the customers to the dealers on foot, which meant less chance of being covertly filmed, and no chance of a rapid vehicle approach by the police.

By the summer of 1994 the national media had gone quiet on Moss Side and some believed that the worst of the area's guns-and-drugs traumas were over. But not all local people I spoke to were convinced. While the surface activity may have been suppressed or displaced, the old poison hasn't yet been drawn.

Getting it here

Despite billions of dollars spent on interdiction, crop destruction/substitution, the seizure of 'precursor' chemicals, the trashing of laboratories, and even full-scale military sorties against the trafficking enemy, the cultivation of coca crops continues to rise. It comes, ready processed, by ship, truck and plane via a bewildering zig-zag of routes taking in Argentina and Brazil, the West Indies, Florida, North Africa, Spain, and Holland; or via North Africa and central Europe.[45] Wherever the heat is on, necessary route adjustments are made. Much of the proceeds are passed through legitimate business fronts and end up residing in accounts in countries such as the US, Switzerland, the Cayman Islands, and Panama. But the Colombian Central Bank has estimated that between $1 and $2 billion comes home to Colombia every year.[46]

Peru tops the world league in crop production (up from 6,000 tons in 1980 to 275,000 in 1991), followed by Bolivia (totalling 100,000), and Colombia (80,000).[47] The latter country retains its dominant position in the processing sphere and as the main exporter to world markets, although Peru and

Bolivia have for some time been diversifying into manufacturing, just as Colombian interests are reported to have moved in on the heroin trade.

Having reached saturation point in the huge American market by the early 1990s (up to 1,100 tons of finished cocaine are smuggled there from Latin America each year[48]), the Colombian drug traffickers seemed to have turned their attention to Europe, striking distribution deals with the Italian mafia[49] and with criminal groups in Russia, Ukraine, and Belarus.[50] Warsaw and Prague are also reported to be important new 'hubs' in the Colombians' distribution machine. This is due to the relative security they afford.[51] The Colombian cartels, according to Jan van Doorn, head of the central Narcotics Bureau of the Dutch National Criminal Intelligence Service,[52] look on Western Europe as one single market which they supply with increasingly large shipments. These are concealed within legal cargo bound for the likes of Southampton and Rotterdam. Hence, seizures of shipments exceeding 1,000 kilos in several European countries.

Van Doorn believes that the Colombians 'make use of Europeans' because of the import and storage facilities they have at their disposal. But once landed, the South Americans take charge of the distribution at wholesale level across the continent.

Leaf Production

An article in the *Scotsman* newspaper[53] described leaf production and transshipment in and from Peru, where 60 per cent of the world's cocaine originates. The centre of activities was the Huallaga valley, which the author considered 'one of the most dangerous places in the world.' Operating within it were Colombian and Peruvian drug traffickers, guerrillas from the Maoist Sendero Luminoso, corrupt police and army officers, and US drug enforcement agents mounting helicopter sorties from a jungle fortress.

The leaf is grown in the valley, collected and converted into coca paste, often using swimming pools as giant refining tanks. Peasants take the paste in small quantities to a central point – and it is these small-timers rather than the better-connected big operators who suffer the majority of arrests. When about 1,000 kilos have been gathered, a deal is struck with a Colombian processor and a small plane is sent to collect the material.

The Peruvian government's anti-trafficking measures failed to impress the author of the *Scotsman* article. The police station in Tarapoto, which supposedly co-ordinates the battle against the powerful and wealthy drug barons, does not even have a roof at present. And the badly paid Peruvian policemen not only have to buy their own uniforms, they have to purchase their own bullets.

'It is hardly surprising that so many of them are corrupt, believing they have a right to supplement their low wages. The same is true of the army.'

Nor is it surprising that, despite major US operations targeting the Huallaga, coca production has substantially increased since the 1980s. The peasant growers are now experimenting with the production of heroin.

Should the US win full co-operation from the Peruvian authorities, elimination of the coca menace still seems unlikely. The growers, it is predicted,[54] will move deeper into the jungle or to an entirely different, equally inaccessible region of the country

The Colombian Cartels

Colombia, according to some estimates,[55] is the most violent country on earth, with 10 per cent of the world's murders occurring there. Yet, despite the headlines, drug trafficking is believed to be only 'minimally' involved. 'Killing is often an accepted way of achieving justice,' according to a 1994 *Guardian* article,[56] 'where there is no legal means of redress. Fewer than 3 per cent of reported crimes lead to a conviction.'

Violence was the daily lot of Pablo Escobar, fabulously wealthy head of the so-called Medellin cocaine production and distribution cartel, who finally reached his end-point when fifty men from a special government task force stormed his suburban hideaway and shot him dead. His personal fortune was judged by *Forbes* magazine in 1990 to be $2.6 billion, and while, during the course of his war with the authorities, he was held to be responsible for the slaughter of three presidential candidates, hundreds of policemen, officials, judges and civilians, many of the people of his home town of Medellin regarded him as an incomparably generous champion of the poor. In Medellin Escobar had built homes and soccer fields. The government 'vendetta' against him, he believed, was precisely because of such philanthropy.

In its mid-1980s heyday, the 'Medellin cartel' – a loose alliance of drug-dealing groups of which Escobar was the most prominent leader – was said by US drug enforcers to control up to four-fifths of the world's supply of refined cocaine, including the majority entering the States.[57]

But whereas the Medellin's key Cali cartel rivals were content quietly to buy influence among Colombia's politicians and élite, Escobar (who was said to have cut his criminal teeth stealing gravestones from cemeteries and reselling them with fresh inscriptions) sought to enter politics directly as a representative from Medellin. Inevitably, he was drawn into a confrontation with the state, one that reached a crescendo of high farce when, in 1991, he permitted himself to be incarcerated in a prison of his own luxurious design. Known as Hotel Escobar, it was equipped with two jacuzzis, a sauna, an exercise machine, and the latest in office equipment, permitting free contact with the outside world. Unnerved by what was going on behind his back, Escobar is said to have ordered the murder of 50 of his own associates while 'inside'. Before long he 'escaped' with several lieutenants and at this point began the manhunt that ended on 2 December 1993 on a rooftop in a Medellin suburb known as Las Américas.

Escobar's assets included a fleet of 250 aircraft, 200 apartments in Miami, hotels in Colombia and Venezuela, and a private zoo.

In the end, Escobar made too many enemies and died abandoned by those he had enriched. But while his destruction was a useful symbolic victory for the authorities, it produced no change in Colombia's pivotal role in the world's cocaine trade. Escobar's rivals had for some time been moving in on the territory he was forced to cede during his long struggle for survival. Such individuals were now 'expanding their hold on the banking, justice and political systems and with far greater sophistication than the violent pioneers from Medellin.'[58]

The Right Stuff

What has been submerged under world headlines about the illegal killer-cocaine trade is the licit industry in leaf products and the essential part this has played in Andean culture and economies for thousands of years. Aside from leaf-chewing, there are coca-based chewing gums, toothpastes, and a highly regarded tea known as *maté de coca*.

In Bolivia, some 30,000 acres of shrub are legally harvested each year for these products. The remaining 74,000 acres are diverted into the drugs trade. In Peru, most of the 200,000 coca hectares are grown by cocaine producers.

'Our real enemy is prejudice,' said Evo Morales, president of the Andean Council, which represented the 200,000 families who cultivated coca in the Andean-Amazonian region. 'Once people understand that coca is delicious and good for you, the whole world will be sipping Andean maté.'[59]

Double standards as well as prejudice troubled Morales. Western pharmaceutical companies can husband and profit handsomely from the coca crop, as can Coca-Cola, which is permitted to export eight tons of coca leaf every year for use in its beverage. But the indigenous people of the Andes are barred.

Morales was speaking at the launch of a campaign to lift the international ban on coca-based products, imposed by the 1961 Vienna Convention on Narcotic Drugs. It applies even to maté tea because an average serving is said to contain a microscopic 4.42 mg of cocaine.

Some US researchers are not only untroubled by an amount that can have no possible psychoactive impact, they recommend it for digestive problems, arthritis, obesity, fatigue, and anxiety.[60]

Help

Tip-off signs

The habits and disposition of dependent coke/crack users are not unlike those of the amphetamine lover. Fresh calculation should be made to account for the shorter duration of cocaine's effects and, therefore, its reduced tendency to cut into sleep.

Coming off

Again, comparisons with amphetamine can be made, including the rebound depression, fatigue, and mood swings. More intense disturbances are likely to result from injecting or freebasing than from the intranasal use of powder. The question of the prescribing of a substitute drug during the critical early weeks of cocaine withdrawal and/or for a period after that (the equivalent of methadone for ex-heroin users) is a contentious one. The British treatment establishment – preoccupied with opioids to the virtual exclusion of stimulants – has never seriously considered it, let alone undertaken a sufficient number of pilot studies which might establish the sense or otherwise of such a programme. There have been scattered projects where cocaine powder was offered (in Halton, Cheshire, for instance) but they often attract strong criticism from people who feel that substituting one strong drug for another is a trap; that total abstention is the answer.

Acupuncture, relaxation, and confidence-building are now the favoured strategies of a number of drug agencies – especially when fed into a 'holistic' view of the individual and his/her needs and residual strengths.

Life-saving

Should the Casey Jones Reaction take hold of a companion (see page 192), immediately try artificial respiration, and call an ambulance fast.

Notes

1 Mark Gold, 'Cocaine (and Crack): Clinical Aspects', in *Substance Abuse, a Comprehensive Textbook*, Williams and Wilkins, Baltimore, 1992, p. 205.

2 Many thanks to Ciaran O'Hagan, a University of North London social research degree student, on whose first-hand experience of the Garage, Progressive House, Jungle House, and related scenes I have drawn.

3 Peter White, 'Coca: An ancient Indian herb turns deadly', in *National Geographic*, January 1989, p. 11.

4 L. Osoria Bryson, 'Environment and drug trafficking', in *Bulletin on Narcotics*, Vol. XLIV, No. 2, 1992.

5 Helen Pickering *et al.*, 'Crack Injection', in *Druglink*, January/February 1993, p. 12.

6 Ibid.

7 Gold, op. cit., p. 206.

8 *Drug Notes: Cocaine & Crack*, ISDD, p. 12.

9 Ibid.

10 Michael Gossop *et al.*, 'Cocaine: Patterns of use, route of administration, and severity of dependence', in the *British Journal of Psychiatry*, 164, 1994, pp. 660–4.

11 C. Van Dyke and R. Byck, 'Cocaine', in *Scientific American*, April 1982, pp. 109–19.

12 Ibid.

13 Gold, op. cit., p. 210.

14 J. Philips and R. Wynne, *Cocaine: the Mystique and the Reality*, Avon Books, New York, 1980.

15 'Dangerous lies in the delivery room', in *New Scientist*, 18 December 1993, p. 15.

16 *Drugs, Pregnancy and Childcare*, ISDD, 1992, p. 17.

17 Mary Hepburn, 'Drug use in pregnancy', in the *British Journal of Hospital Medicine*, Vol. 49, No. 1, 1993, p. 51.

18 C. Medawar, *Power and Dependence: Social Audit on the safety of medicines*, Social Audit Ltd, 1992, p. 33.

19 Ibid.

20 Gold, op. cit., p. 206.

21 *Drug Notes: Cocaine & Crack*, ISDD, p. 3.

22 White, op. cit., p. 32.

23 A Home Office committee, appointed in 1916 and reporting a year later, said that it was unable to find evidence of 'even noticeable prevalence of the cocaine habit amongst the civilian or military population of Great Britain'.

24 T. Parssinen, *Secret Passion, Secret Remedies: Narcotic Drugs in British Society 1820–1930*, Manchester University Press, 1981, p. 121.

25 Marek Kohn, *Dope Girls*, Lawrence & Wishart, London, 1992, p. 97.

26 Gold, op. cit., p. 207.

27 White, op. cit., p. 34.

28 See Mike Davis (with Sue Ruddick), 'War in the Street', in *New Left Review*, No. 170, 1988. By 1994, senior Bloods and Crips gang members were touring the UK together, celebrating their truce and exhorting British youth to act positive and eschew violence.

29 As charted by Davis and Ruddick, op. cit.

30 Ansley Hamid, 'The decline of crack use in New York City', in *The International Journal on Drug Policy*, Vol. 2, No. 5, p. 26.

31 Gold, op. cit., p. 205.

32 Hamid, op. cit., p. 27.

33 Andrew Glyn and David Miliband (eds), 'Paying for Inequality: The Economic Cost of Social Injustice', Rivers Oram Press/ Institute for Public Policy Research.

34 From *Households below average income*, HMSO, 1994, as quoted in the *Guardian*, 15 July 1994, p. 5.

35 Jay Mott (ed.); 'Crack and cocaine in England and Wales', Research and Planning Unit Paper 70, Home Office, 1992, p. iv.

36 *Druglink*, January 1993, p. 5.

37 Mott, op. cit.

38 Vincenzo Ruggiero, 'Brixton, London: A drug culture without a drug economy', in the *International Journal of Drug Policy*, Vol. 2, 1993, p. 83.

39 Ibid, p. 87.

40 Ibid, p. 86.

41 Ibid, p. 83.

42 There were at least ten London murders and twenty attempted killings linked to the crack trade during 1993, according to the Metropolitan Police. Assistant Commissioner David Veness announced in July 1994 that 'several hundred' crack dealers had access to guns, including automatic weapons; a scene he described as 'ultra violent . . . treacherous and unstable'. Reported in the *Guardian*, 2 July 1994.

43 Peter Hetherington, 'Doubts over armed officers despite gun crime rise', in the *Guardian*, 17 May 1994.

44 Ibid.

45 'UK Drugs Situation', presentation to the House of Commons All Party Drugs Misuse Group by Stuart Wesley, National Criminal Intelligence Service, 1993.

46 Ken Dermota and Noll Scott, 'Going, going, gone', in the *Guardian*, 4 December 1993.

47 Jan van Doorn, 'Drug trafficking networks in Europe', in the *European Journal on Criminal Policy and Research*, Vol. 1–2, p. 100.
48 Dermota and Scott, op. cit.
49 Committee of enquiry into the spread of organised crime linked to drugs trafficking in the member states of the European Community, draft report, rapporteur Patrick Cooney, 28 October 1991.
50 That's according to the UN's International Narcotics Control Board, in its annual report published March 1994.
51 Leonard Doyle, 'Cocaine trade surges in Europe', in the *Independent*, 2 March 1994.
52 Van Doorn, op. cit., p. 101.
53 Ewen MacAskill, 'Into the valley of death', in the *Scotsman*, 8 October 1993.
54 Ibid.
55 Timothy Ross, 'Little to choose in neck and neck presidential race', in the *Guardian*, 7 May 1994.
56 Ibid.
57 Dermota and Scott, op. cit.
58 Ross, op. cit.
59 Carl Honoré, 'Coca addicts fight to end ban on a forbidden fruit', in the *Observer*, 10 October 1993.
60 Ibid.

HALLUCINOGENS

Intro

The hallucinogens are a group of substances of great chemical and structural variance – some concocted in labs, others plucked from the ground – which have the common ability to shake up the user's internal world. While experiences vary, the typical hallucinogenic trip involves visual and auditory distortions, leaps of the imagination, introspection, mood changes and moments of intense excitement and, perhaps, panic.

Some hallucinogens have strong stimulant effects. Ecstasy, the most famous member of the 179-strong MDA family, falls into this category and is usually classed as an hallucinogenic amphetamine. LSD and the peyote cactus are at the other end of the spectrum, producing a purer experience of the head rather than of the body.

Citizens of the United States probably have the world's broadest choice of hallucinogens, for not only are the Americas rich in naturally occurring mushrooms, roots, seeds, and other psychoactive vegetation, but the US schooling system produces high-grade chemists from whose ranks – since the mid-1960s – have sprung many an unlicensed back-street druggist. Altogether some two dozen natural, synthetic, and semi-synthetic products are in common use there. But with *How To* manuals now available[1] the variety as well as total consumption looks set to expand.

Here in the UK, the Acid House/rave/dance scene greatly amplified what was a flagging hallucinogenic movement. Acid House started in 1988 with LSD and Ecstasy, but the search for novelty and purer substances led to an extraordinary mixture of items being sucked into the clubs. By the mid-1990s, these ranged from the supposedly safe, all-natural E alternative known as Cloud 9 to LSD's powerful chemical cousin,

235

DMT. Also on the menu were some highly disorientating human and veterinary anaesthetics and sedatives (ketamine, 'GBH', Tiletamine/'Breakfast Mix'), and this was in addition to the countless variations on the Ecstasy theme, achieved by shifting a molecule from here to there, or by 'cutting' the product with anything from the following list: speed, LSD, Temazepam, heroin, antihistamines, decongestants, caffeine, worming tablets, crushed lightbulbs, and rat poison.

On a purer note, other indigenous options include the ever-popular psilocybe ('Liberty Cap') mushroom and the red-capped, white-flecked toadstool of fairy tales – *Amanita muscaria*. Another 'organic' group of domestic hallucinogens are those belonging to the 3,000-strong *Solanaceae* family, which includes the common potato. It also numbers some of the most potent and deadly plants in existence. Species of mandrake, henbane, and belladonna were all important agents of European sorcerers and witches, who used them, depending on dose, for healing or mystical excursions. An ointment rubbed into a receptive mucous membrane, such as the vagina, is said to have produced wild, often sexually ecstatic hallucinations. In more moderate doses these drugs would have been used as medicines, and in slightly higher ones (only slightly higher because the difference between the therapeutic and lethal measure is not great) to despatch enemies. Just as the mystics were ultimately dealt their mortal blow – killed or forced underground by a rampant Christian orthodoxy – so their favourite preparations fell into disregard. Given their great potential for harm in uneducated hands, it is probably just as well that mandrake and the rest haven't enjoyed the kind of revival among Western recreational users that other traditional magical plants have.

LSD

Properly called d-lysergic acid diethylamide, LSD is part of a chemical family called the indolealkylamines which bear a structural resemblance to a neurotransmitter substance (5-hydroxytryptamine) found in the brain. Its close relatives include LSA (d-lysergic acid amide, which is found in varieties of morning glory seed), psilocybin (found in certain 'magic' mushrooms), and DMT (dimethyltriptamine).

LSD itself is derived from the fungus ergot, which grows on rye and other grasses. In its unmolested state ergot has been used for centuries as an aid to childbirth. It constricts the blood vessels in the uterus, so preventing or stopping haemorrhaging after delivery. Ergot from infected rye bread was also the likely cause of the medieval affliction St Anthony's Fire, which periodically struck the inhabitants of European villages where rye bread was a staple. Sufferers developed convulsions and hallucinations as well as black 'charred' limbs that were actually gangrenous. The cure was to desist from eating the ergot and so allow the constricted blood vessels to widen out again. Many sufferers did desist in the course of their pilgrimage to the shrine of St Anthony. Naturally, it was St Anthony, not their ergot-free diet, who took the credit.

The first ergot alkaloid in pure chemical form was isolated in 1918 by the Swiss-based chemist Dr Arthur Stoll. His work was carried forward by his young associate, Dr Albert Hoffman, who, in the 1920s, began to synthesise a number of compounds closely related to ergot at Sandoz Pharmaceuticals in Basle.

Several of Hoffman's ergot analogues were explored in relation to migraine, obstetrics, and geriatrics. The twenty-fifth in his series was d-lysergic acid diethylamide. It was made by mixing lysergic acid with diethylamide and, after freezing, extracting the resulting LSD by distillation or evaporation. Animal tests followed, revealing nothing of the true character of the drug, and it was not until April 1943 that Hoffman himself discovered LSD's almighty mind-altering properties when accidentally ingesting a tiny amount, either by breathing in the dust or by absorbing it through the pores of his skin. He describes pedalling home on his bike and becoming 'transported into other worlds'. There were several more trips, and of one he wrote:

I lost all account of time. I noticed with dismay that my environment was undergoing progressive changes. My visual field wavered and everything appeared deformed as if in a faulty mirror. I was overcome with fear that I was going out of my mind. Occasionally I felt as if I were out of my body. I thought I had died. My ego seemed suspended somewhere in space from where I saw my dead body lying on the sofa. It was particularly striking how acoustic perceptions such as the noise of water gushing from a tap or the spoken word were transformed into optical illusions. I then fell asleep and awakened the next morning somewhat tired, but otherwise feeling perfectly well.

Hoffman's experience must indeed have been terrifying, not only for the dry, sure world of pharmacology that was his environment but because in 1943 he was alone with these sensations. Sandoz performed further tests on volunteers, after which it was concluded that what had been discovered was a most powerful psychomimetic – in other words, a drug that could produce a 'model psychosis' whose study might unlock the secrets of schizophrenia and other mental illnesses.

The therapy years

The war interrupted distribution of the drug, but by its close it had been sent to numerous psychiatric researchers. Often they worked in large teaching hospitals, which meant LSD could be tried out on both healthy volunteers as well as the sick.

A similar dispersal job was performed in what were then Warsaw Pact countries by Spofa of Prague, Czechoslovakia. An Italian company and then Eli Lilly in the US also manufactured LSD using their own processes. A key attraction of the drug in those early days was the concussive effect it could have on memory. For a repressed neurotic eluding his/her Freudian analyst's attempts to probe at the roots of the disorder, LSD seemed capable of delivering the big bang. The problem, as it later emerged, was what to do with the stream of discordant information that poured forth.

It was LSD's big-bang effect that also appealed to the military and intelligence communities. It appears that the US Army tried it as a possible incapacitator of enemy troops and as a means of reversing the brainwashing of liberated prisoners of the Korean War. The CIA also spent some twenty years looking at the drug – as a disabling, brainwashing device that could be mobilised on behalf of the Free World or (in their nightmares) by its enemies. Many of its tests were on prisoners and servicemen. Among the most bizarre, according to an article in the *Observer*,[2] involved members of the public who were picked up by prostitutes, taken back to CIA-run brothels, and given LSD-spiked drinks. As the subjects flailed in panic or fumbled their way through sex, agency men watched and took notes through two-way mirrors.

Outside the intelligence sphere there were also some dubious applications. Too often, medical practitioners failed to understand the extraordinary 'violence' of the LSD experience and so would have no qualms about, for instance, attaching electrodes to their subjects and putting them through some very icy scrutiny in a setting that was itself sufficiently bleak to induce a panic. To compound such gaucherie, the drug, according to Terence Duquesne and Julian Reeves in their book *A Handbook of Psychoactive Medicines*,[3] was often administered by injection – a method wholly unsuitable since it slams the recipient straight into the intense hallucinogenic phase without even the shortish run-up that is provided when swallowing the drug in pill form. Peter Stafford states in his *Psychedelic Encyclopedia*[4] that all manner of doses were tried, from small, cumulative amounts to one-off combustive attacks at around 1,500 micrograms. It was tried in one-to-one therapy and among whole mental wards. It was also used on prisoners, such as the black American narcotic addicts who were given escalating doses over a period of some two weeks, cut off dead, and then reintroduced with a massive dose that sent them through the prison roof. (From this it was learnt that LSD ceases to have any psychoactive powers when used daily over as little as three or four days; a break is needed for its potency to return.) Many doctors reported patients being cured of debilities such as arthritis, partial paralysis, headaches, hysterical deafness, and skin rashes. It was also used enthusiastically on alcoholics, often hard-core 'incurables'. A review of 800 treated in a Canadian LSD programme indicated that 'about one-third remained sober after therapy and another third benefited.'[5] Where schizophrenics were excluded the results were substantially better than that.

'There are no published papers', claimed psychiatrist Abram Hoffer in relation to the Canadian programme, 'using psychedelic therapy which shows it does not help about 50 per cent of the treated group . . . Even more important is that this can be done very quickly, and therefore economically.'[6] Sceptics weren't so sure: couldn't the success rate also be attributed to the keenness of psychiatrists working with such a chic new tool?

Another important area of LSD research, one tackled by the respected Czech physician Stanislov Grof, was with the terminally ill. Grof found that LSD was not only a more effective pain reliever for cancers than traditional opiates but that sufferers passed on their way with less anguish. In the US too Dr Eric Kast of Chicago reported better pain relief than from traditional analgesics and, again, an ease of passage. 'It was a common experience', wrote Kast 'for the patient to remark casually on his deadly disease and then comment on the beauty of a certain sensory impression.'[7]

Methodical analyses of LSD's disparate, often unruly early use are few. A classic survey was Cohen's 1960 review of the work of forty-four American clinicians.[8] It embraced 5,000 experimental subjects as well as patients who between them ingested 25,000 LSD or mescaline doses. The survey revealed two trip-related suicides and eight psychotic reactions lasting more than forty-eight hours. As would be expected, the psychiatric patients rather than the healthy volunteers were more prone to upsets.

A similar though clearer report (in that it didn't involve mescaline) was produced for the UK by Nicholas Malleson.[9] It aimed to sum up the experiences of all seventy-four clinicians who by 1968 had dispensed LSD. This time there were 4,500 recipients who between them had received about 50,000 'therapy sessions'. Three people killed themselves close to their therapy. 'There were 37 cases of psychotic disturbances lasting over 48 hours, ten of which became chronic. Two deaths, a small number of superficial injuries incurred during therapy and the birth of one abnormal child were also noted.'

In response to this study and others like it the government's Advisory Committee on Drug Abuse concluded that 'there is no proof that LSD is an effective agent in psychiatry. Equally there is no proof that it is an exceptionally hazardous or prohibitively dangerous treatment in clinical use in the hands of responsible experts and subject to appropriate safeguards.'[10]

Nonetheless, by the early 1960s, the bulk of the clinical work was finished and in psychiatry its uses were becoming confined to two basic groups of cases: chronic alcoholics and those suffering psycho-sexual problems. This work too was to dry up as recreational use of the drug flourished and the authorities took fright.

The former Harvard professor Timothy Leary is inevitably cited as the high priest of the psychedelic era for having broadcast more vehemently than anyone else the alleged spiritual and sensory benefits of LSD. But some reports identify 'Captain' Al Hubbard, an ex-spy turned 'nuclear businessman', as the first acid evangelist.[11] After discovering the drug in 1951, Hubbard is said to have bought a vast cache from Sandoz and, urged on by Aldous (*Doors of Perception*) Huxley, began dispensing it to his élite friends in the worlds of art, industry, science, and the priesthood

Among the drug's early, not to say surprising, converts were Time-Life president Henry Luce, who said it gave him a glimpse of God; and Hollywood's Cary Grant, who felt 'born again' after a protracted period of misery.

Leary arrived on the scene in 1961, having discovered 'the divinity within' during a psilocybin mushroom trip in Mexico a year earlier. Conventional academia bored Leary. To the chagrin of his Harvard employers, he set up various experimental communities devoted to mind exploration (the most famous being at Millbrook in New York State), and in the teeth of growing disquiet on the part of the political authorities continued proselytising on the drug's behalf. In 1963 he was relieved of his teaching post and, together with men like *One Flew over the Cuckoo's Nest* author Ken Kesey, embarked upon his mission with unrelieved zeal.

Initially Leary was for the democratisation of the psyche-delic experience – *turn on, tune in and drop out* – but later recanted, calling this exhortation naive.

We failed', he wrote, 'to understand the enormous genetic variation in human neurology. We failed to understand the aristocratic, élite, virtuous self-confidence that pervaded our group. We made our sessions wonderful and expected nothing but wonder and merry discovery.' Not only did Leary recant,

he is also alleged to have 'finked' – according to the San
Francisco underground paper *Berkeley Barb* – on his former
psychedelic cohorts. He appeared as a prosecution witness
in a drug case against his own lawyer[12] and is said to have
been used by the authorities in their attempt to mount a case
against those who actually helped him escape from the prison
where he was serving a term in the mid-1970s for marijuana
possession.

After the authorities were finished with him, Leary toured US
clubs and halls as a 'stand-up philosopher and comic', and later
surfaced in England partnering on stage the man who was in
charge of Richard Nixon's dirty tricks department, the man who
in the 1960s led the raid on Leary's psychedelic idyll: G. Gordon
Liddy. Such was the dismal pass the psychedelic movement
had come to.[13] But then Leary and his Harvard colleague
Richard Alpert, Ken Kesey, and others of their prestigious
ilk were untypical of the average 1960s 'tripper' and in the end
unessential. Mostly they were handy protuberances by which
media people could haul themselves up (or down) to inspect
what for them was a mysterious new generation of long-haired
deviants.[14] The idea that there ever was a homogeneous
acid-swallowing 'youth culture' is largely, but not entirely, a
delusion. It was fed by the adepts themselves because they
felt more powerful as a great uniform wave, and by such forces
as the music, clothing, and film industries which could enhance
their bottom lines if their customers all wanted to look, sound,
and be like each other. In reality there were the ever-familiar
diverse tastes among 1960s youth, both within and without
the long-haired ranks. The drugs, together with the faddy
routines, simply helped to mask the divergencies. Later, those
homogeneous hippies were to splinter off into drug-dealing,
computer programming, and 'straight' jobs wherever they could
be found, the notion of communal youth put paid to.

Even after the flower-power bubble burst at the turn
of the 1970s, there was still plenty of high-grade LSD
around, particularly in the UK where an illicit multi-limbed
manufacturing operation, said to be the world's largest, was
established around a former chemistry student called Richard
Kemp. In concert with members of the American pseudo-
religious and drug-dealing group (established by Leary) called
The Brotherhood of Eternal Love, Kemp and his cohorts
managed to turn out enough LSD for 6 million tablets. And

this was done in just three bumper runs between 1970 and 1973. The following year, after a laborious undercover investigation called Operation Julie, Kemp and his team were pinched and jailed.

As is the way of the marketplace, the dearth of LSD following the Julie raid didn't so much persuade users to quit their mind-juggling as to find an alternative to do the job. This alternative, it turned out, was not only free of charge, it was free of the unpredictable adulterants that could be present in any and all drugs trafficked on the streets. They were those members of the *Psilocybin* and *Amanita* mushroom families containing psychoactive acids and alkaloids. They were easily picked, dried, or boiled for an experience that, depending on species, could be as profound as LSD. The fungi habit persisted and grew, even after acid stocks were again plentiful from 1982.

In the 1990s, the acid experience has been more democratised than Leary could ever have imagined, with smaller, more manageable doses on offer (down from 250 micrograms in the 1960s to around 50 mcg). The drug is cheap, sharply marketed under famous-brand icons of the moment – from Bart Simpson to Saddam Hussein – and has been taken up by all shades of young people whether in schools, dance clubs, village greens, or housing estates. Today the drug is as often eaten for a straight 'laugh' as for any Learyesque excursion of the mind.

Magic Mushrooms: What Are They?

As part of the Old World, the UK is endowed with considerably fewer hallucinogenic plants than the Americas, where some hundred-plus species have so far been identified. And yet these isles do offer a dozen types of mushrooms capable of giving a jolt.

Magic mushrooms can be divided into two distinct groups – one for species containing the drug psilocybin and the 50 per cent more powerful psilocin, and the other much smaller Amanita group which have ibotenic acid and its derivative muscimol as their main psychoactive ingredients.

243

Psilocybe semilanceata (Liberty Cap)

There are ten native species containing psilocybin and psilocin, but the drug content in most of them varies markedly depending on soil, weather, and the age of the fruit. Some lose their potency from the moment they are picked, notes Richard Cooper in his *Guide to British Psilocybin Mushrooms* (Hassle Free Press, London, 1977). By far the most reliable in that it contains roughly predictable amounts of the two drugs is *Psilocybe semilanceata*. Known as the Liberty Cap, it is also the most readily available and the most appreciated by mushroom heads for the distinct yet measured effects it conjures up.

The lethal dose of Liberty Cap is estimated to be around 8 lbs of fresh specimens, but an amount considerably less than that will do damage. Though the drug content of Liberty Cap is comparatively reliable, there is still some variation between different fruits – not least because they vary in size. Working out a suitable dose not only has to account for this, but for additional factors like the user's body weight and contents of the stomach: in a hungry mushroom eater the effects will be greater. They will also be heightened if taken with alcohol. These factors considered, an effective dose usually ranges from between ten to thirty mushrooms.

Usually seen growing in groups of long lines, they are a tiny, elegant species with a yellow-brown conical cap that often comes to a sharp point. This cap sits on a wavy, lighter-coloured stem which is 4–8 cm tall. But since this is a generalised description and one that can fit others of the UK's 230-odd common fungi, it is vital for anyone who decides to eat this or any other species to establish its identity beyond question. This can be done by taking along a mushroom guide and then studying the fungus – once it has been brought home – against a checklist of clues. Important signs are found in the type of gills, spores, and the presence of a volva, a veil or a ring. Recommended are Richard Cooper's book and the standard pocket companion to all types of British fungi, *Collins' Guide to Mushrooms and Toadstools*. At the very least, any mushroom hunter should be able to recognise the dangerous specimens.

Amanita muscaria (Fly Agaric)

The Amanita genus is the most feared of any fungi native to Britain because it includes the Death Cap (*A. phalloides*) and Destroying Angel (*A. virosa*). Both these lethal fungi should be noted well. Like most of their relatives they grow through a 'cracked egg' volva and bear a skirt-like ring on the stem just beneath the cap. *A. phalloides* is 8–12 cm tall with a 6–12 cm cap that ranges from white to olive green and is to be found in a range of habitats, but mostly in oak or beech woods. *A. virosa* has roughly the same height and cap width, and has a similar bag-like volva and skirted ring at the top of a shaggy stem. But it is disturbingly, enticingly white. Both have white spores, and between them are responsible for 90 per cent of all UK mushroom deaths. Fifty per cent of those who eat them will die.

Cooper identifies two other members of the domestic Amanita genus that deliver a psychoactive punch. One (*A. pantherina*) is so rare that the Collins guide doesn't include it. Cooper warns of its high toxicity.

The other major Amanita species mushroom eaters go for is *A. muscaria*, known commonly as Fly Agaric. This is the toadstool of gnomic fairytales and the most visually extraordinary of all the British fungi. It is 10–22 cm tall and sports a bright red cap speckled with white warty spots. As it ages the cap widens to about 22 cm, fades to an amber colour, and the warts begin to vanish. It has a ring at the top of the stem, but not a volva. It is found principally with birch, and can be seen growing directly beneath the trees either alone or in scattered groups. Because of its proximity to trees any user has to consider the possibility that a dog might have lifted a leg on the specimen s/he is about to pick. Its fruiting season starts in late July and ends in early December.

Amanita muscaria should not be consumed raw, but either cooked in a low oven or hung up to dry. A maximum of three mushrooms is usually the 'recommended' upper limit, although one is a safer dose.

The first Western reports of Fly Agaric's intoxicant effects came from eighteenth-century visitors to Siberia who noted its use among the tribesfolk. These 'primitives' were nothing if not thrifty; knowing that the mushroom's active alkaloid was quickly shed from the body – unmetabolised – via the urine, they made a habit of drinking their own or another's urine in order to extend the period of the high. (Vodka has since taken over as the favourite intoxicant in that part of the world.) But these hardy souls stopped short of drinking their reindeer's waste, even though these creatures are believed to be partial to the fungi.

Mushrooms and the law

In regard to Fly Agaric mushrooms the law does not intrude. Neither the fungi themselves nor their main active ingredients are controlled under the MDA and so, until established otherwise in court, it would seem that they may be lawfully consumed.

Liberty Cap's active ingredients, psilocybin and psilocin, are, however, controlled. Despite this, the authorities have not yet found it legitimate to penalise possession of the mushrooms themselves. To do so would call into question the legality of a host of otherwise innocuous items containing the controlled substances. Among them would be certain species of toad and even the human animal itself. For we too are alive with naturally occurring analgesics, stimulants, and hallucinogens. So for an offence to be committed the controlled drug must first be 'separated' from its host. The Misuse of Drugs Act also penalises 'preparations' of these fungi. 'Preparations' has been interpreted to mean any tea, soup, omelette, cake, etc. But there is still no clarity on the question of dried mushrooms. Convictions for possession of a class A drug have taken place where defendants have been found with dried and crushed psilocybe mushrooms. Similarly, if the police find a panful of cooked fungi or a line of them strung across a bedroom wall, then that would not look too good in court. However, dried mushrooms per se don't rate as a preparation since they could have been collected after drying in the sun.

After separation and preparation the third possible illicit activity is the actual growing of the mushroom. This was tested at Snaresbrook Crown Court in March 1983 when a North London man was charged under the Misuse of Drugs Act with 'producing a product' containing a Class A drug – namely psilocybin. He was arrested in May 1982 when two ounces of fungi were found growing in his flat. The species was *Psilocybe cubensis* whose spores the defendant was said

246

to have bought through the US magazine *High Times*. (Magic mushroom kits are popular in the States.) In answer to an investigating constable who had asked him, 'What's going on here, then?' he is said to have replied, 'I am trying to grow a health food. I am trying to make the world a better place.' When asked if his mushrooms were a narcotic he replied, 'No, they are sacred.' And got himself arrested.

The critical ruling by Judge Clive Callman was that despite the paraphernalia 'the production of *Psilocybe cubensis* up to the time they are fresh and free from preparation is outside the scope of the Misuse of Drugs Act 1971.' And with that he ordered the jury to acquit the accused.

Ecstasy

Its chemical name is 3,4, methylenedioxymethamphetamine or MDMA, and it is one of the 179-strong MDA family thus far 'discovered' and promoted by California renegade chemist Alexander Shulgin. The structure and effects of each family member vary according to how the component molecules are shifted around. But even Shulgin in his lab must depend on nature – the starting point for his drugs being the oils of nutmeg, sassafras, crocus, saffron, and the like.

While Shulgin was the first to describe Ecstasy's effects in humans and has published the simplest and most elegant method of synthesis,[15] the Ecstasy story long pre-dates Shulgin's mid-1960s discovery. It starts in 1910 with the synthesis of the parent drug, MDA (methylenedioxyamphetamine), by two German chemists. Nothing much happened on the MDA front until the late 1930s when it went through a series of, ultimately, aborted trials as a remedy for Parkinson's disease and as an appetite suppressant. In 1957 an American researcher, Gordon Alles, described to a scientific meeting the drug's potential for heightening perception and producing strange visual distortions. Enter the military – which added MDA (codename EA1299) to the host of other substances it was exploring as potential brainwashing and chemical warfare tools.[16] By 1968, MDA had made the journey from the war labs to the streets of California (where it was dubbed the

Love Drug) only to be outlawed as a dangerous substance two years later.

Its more famous offspring, MDMA, followed a similar course, having first been formulated in 1914 by Merck and Co. as an appetite suppressant. It was thereafter the subject of experiments by the Army and chic psychotherapists, especially those dealing with battling marriage partners, before reaching the American 'abuser' around 1981. As its popularity grew, so did the storm warnings from toxicologists and neurologists who produced a series of reports outlining the drug's alleged devastating physical and psychological impact.

The furore was at once reminiscent of the 1960s LSD panic. Back then there were legends of acid heads staring unblinking at the sun until their retinas fried. In respect of Ecstasy the accounts were of adepts locked in foetal positions for three full days (and of a psychiatrist user who ended up in the wrong town directing traffic).

At a more scientific level the 1960s LSD fear centred on split chromosomes and malformed babies (the grisly after-effects of thalidomide were just being witnessed). Subsequently, the chromosome panic was acknowledged to have been misplaced, not least because the significance of chromosome breakdown was not properly understood (still the case today). With MDA the initial scare was that the drug caused Parkinson's disease. Then the focus shifted to a 'messenger' chemical in the brain known as serotonin – believed to be responsible for affecting mood. Ecstasy was said to deplete serotonin stocks as well as damage serotergenic nerve terminals in certain locations: i.e. cause brain damage. By 1985 it joined MDA on the banned list, after which more health worries surfaced relating to the drug's impact on the liver, its capacity to induce lingering depression and anxiety, and – most dramatically – cause death in the parched, sweaty environment of a rave through heatstroke and hyperthermia (extreme fever).

E culture

The story of Ecstasy's coming of age in the UK is the story of the modern dance scene. The starting point is 1985 Chicago when House music (a DJ-concocted sound combining synthesised percussion tracks, high-energy Europbeat sounds, and selections from early 1980s soul and disco hits) came of age. The name House derived from a club called the Warehouse where much of the experimentation was done. Soon the Warehouse Djs were in the studios producing tracks from scratch and making the national charts. The sound and the success crossed to the UK.

Back in Chicago, House was given a new twist – the addition of a 'deep', highly synthesised trance-inducing sound that broke through pop's traditional literalism. This was the start of Acid House, a theme taken up in late 1987/early 1988 in Ibiza, the sunny holiday retreat for London's smart set. Under the high-energy influence of Ecstasy, the Ibiza crowd partied for days at a time in what came to be known as the Summer of Love. The Ibiza mood was brought back to England where for some years the clubs, especially in London, had been tyrannised by strict notions of what was musically and aesthetically hip.

The 'right' clubs began filling up with young people of every disposition – hard nuts and soft nuts – who brought with them a new style of dressing down that made use of jokey T-shirts, head bands, smiley symbols, even hippy flares and kaftans. The mood was overwhelmingly peaceful and co-operative. Even DJs got hugged instead of ignored after their sessions – the start of the jock cult that, within five years, would elevate the most successful of them to the status of wealthy pop icons.

Having begun as the secret obsession of hip insiders, Acid House was now rushing down-market causing a magnificent upheaval of London and suburban nightlife. Where E wasn't yet available, old-fashioned LSD was swallowed, perhaps in combination with amphetamine. The clubs, with their restrictive opening hours, proved too small to contain the phenomenon and demand grew for underground warehouse parties, often in shabby Docklands venues. The parties got bigger, began attracting 10,000 or more people, as well as the interest of a disapproving tabloid media. A series of police raids was launched, but these simply precipitated some highly inventive evasive tactics by the major organisers, calling for secret ticketing arrangements that hooked up hundreds of phone lines to a computer system. As many as a thousand cars full of young people would gather at a meeting point – typically somewhere on the M25 orbital motorway. Once a critical mass had been reached they would receive word of the party venue and rush to get there in large enough numbers ahead of the police. The vast gatherings became unstoppable.

Tired of being outwitted, the police resorted to road blocks, phone bugging, and mass detentions. At one party, 836 people were detained overnight at thirty police stations; only twelve of them were charged.[17] Anti-youth hysteria grew, as did the hunt for the evil, drug-peddling figures at the centre of the party craze. A special anti-rave police unit was established, phone companies were pressurised into preventing party organisers from using their systems, while pirate radio stations that had been guilty of broadcasting rave location details were raided and shut down.

'Civil liberties were crushed,' according to one right-wing, pro-rave campaigner, 'in order to stop young people committing the heinous crime of dancing all night without a licence. If that was not enough a draconian new law was introduced in July 1990 which meant that party organisers could face up to six months in prison and confiscation of all profits.'[18]

The centrality of Ecstasy to the rave phenomenon arose from its specific pharmacological effects (it delivered dance energy, feelings of blissful empathy, and a sideways, absurdist angle on the world) which, in turn, united adepts in a shared esoteric rite. In a similar vein, LSD had brought together a nation of 'heads' some twenty years before. And just as the 'democratisation' of the acid experience led to a coarsening and disentangling of that scene, so rave was ultimately beset by bad drugs, bad undercurrents, and even a series of dance-floor deaths caused by heatstroke. The common musical theme also unravelled as the original Chicago House went through a thousand mutations[19] – Garage House, techno, Belgian New Beat, hardcore techno, breakbeat, Ragga, Jungle and – by way of a respite – trance and ambient. In London, seasoned ravers retreated to their niche clubs where they could fix on their select sounds. By now there was more bad E around than good (see above for details of the imposters and the adulterants used) and the general clubland pharmacopoeia had expanded to include temazepam (often to cope with the jarring effect of bad, speedy Ecstasy), cocaine/crack, amphetamine, and anabolic steroids (to produce a rippling torso and/or counteract the

wasting effects of the relentless expenditure of energy).
Booze was also back.

One twenty-two-year-old East London rave veteran told
me (in 1994) how he fell out of love with a scene that had
long since emerged from abandoned warehouses and secret
outdoor locations into leisure centres, sports stadia, and the
more traditional clubs: 'Before rave, it was cooler and posier.
You dressed to impress. In raves you've got 8,000 people
going off their heads, screaming and shouting, everyone in
a world of their own and violence the last thing on anyone's
mind. Then, starting in 1990, it went a bit sour. After you've
been going out twice a week dropping four or five a night,
people started realising what it really was and what it wasn't.
You start getting paranoid in a group of people. You clam up,
don't like to speak. You start to lose weight. More people I
know are going to cleaner clubs now, often out of town. In
London, it's all jungle – fast *bleep-beep-winnick*-type music.
You've got the roughnecks coming out, people with attitude.
I go to Tots in Southend. It's a more conservative sort of
place where people dress up to pull a bird. That's the bottom
line. And you drink. Pure Buds. That's what most people are
drinking.

'We used to go out fifty-handed, you'd see little mobs all
over the place. The current sixteen- to eighteen-year-olds,
they're all puffing draw in each other's bedrooms, playing the
Sega. I don't think they're going anywhere.'

Rave new business

But someone was going. By 1993, the rave business was
said to be worth at least £2 billion a year, with a million
youngsters spending £35 million every week.[20] The calculation was done on the basis of a £15 average admission
charge and the same amount going on drugs. Not included
in these rave-expenditure calculations were such essentials
as laser, slide, and video shows, smoke machines and the
rest. The drinks trade was said to be hurting badly, with pub
visits having fallen by 11 per cent in the five years to 1991.

But it was more than just money. It was a sensibil-
ity, a different kind of take on the world. The attitude
started feeding into TV advertising (Tango, Skol, Golden
Wonder), into chart music, high-street fashion, lifestyle

magazines, television programme graphics and backing music. The Ecstasy death cult which just a few years before was being publicly excoriated through most popular channels of communication was now responsible for rejuvenating those same media; the old story of youth condemned then appropriated.

Rave, according to one notable commentator,[21] allowed 'young women to occupy their social space with confidence.' Many of the participants whom she surveyed spoke of a sense of joy and belonging and of feeling free of sexual threats. This obliged drug workers to abandon the old boiler-suit feminist notion of young women caught up 'in a male-dominated drug-taking world 'which cast them either as victims or in a deviant (often sexually deviant) light.'

The dance drug culture 'offers a view of women as active participants in drug use, instead of the more usual image of passivity and powerlessness.'

The appropriation of a large slice of rave by the country's traditional economic powers was joined by a further political assault on what remained of the original renegade spirit. This came in the shape of the 1994 Criminal Justice and Public Order Act, containing measures specifically targeting unlicensed outdoor raves, festivals, and parties.

A spokesperson for the Advance Party, whose free festivals were threatened by the anti-rave measures, declared: 'Some of us might have bizarre haircuts and want to dance all night but why should we be criminalised for it? Personal freedom is a right that should never be compromised.'[22]

For others there was no going back: 'Five years of rave in Britain has culminated in a scene which has unleashed a cultural wave of spiritual positivity, social responsibility, intergenerational co-operation and wild fun. Sound, light, music and global communications are all part of this accelerating evolutionary process – creating space for discussion, breaking down of barriers and shifting of consciousness. It can only focus the youth into an appreciation of their environment. How else can we precipitate eco wisdom other than creating mass events that are "fashionable"?'[23]

Choice of a Thousand

Ecstasy, LSD, Liberty Cap and Fly Agaric are the clear UK market leaders but there are a host of other synthetic and organic substances capable of producing bizarre effects which sometimes show up domestically. Notably, there are the other members of the MDA (phenethylamine) family that have been frequently passed off as E. These include MDA itself (a more hallucinogenic trip), MMDA, MBDB, and MDEA (known as Eve). These last three are all at the comparatively mild end of the spectrum. More potent compounds are PMA (another MDA offspring), DMT (a currently trendy LSD-family hallucinogen that is injected, sniffed, or smoked, and whose effects rarely last more than two hours), DOM (which has been reported to trip people out for more than twenty-four hours), and PCP. This last is better known as *Angel dust* or *peace pill* and was massively popular in the States through the 1970s and early 1980s though – as I write – has little currency in the UK. American peak use was associated with a high level of reported cases of schizophrenia-like psychotic states, severe anxiety, panic, rage, aggression, and delirium – such outcomes being mostly confined to higher doses.

There are, in fact, already more than a thousand compounds in the hallucinogenic amphetamine category with more on the way. The move to 'totally organic' pill highs had begun by the turn of 1994, a front-runner being the so-called 'herb-derived' Cloud 9 – made to an 'oriental formula' and sold in ten-dose bottles.

Still rare in this country is the peyote cactus (*Lophophora williamssi*) together with its alkaloid derivative, mescaline. Native to Mexico, peyote's hallucinogenic properties were discovered in the late nineteenth century by raiding parties of northern Mescalero Apaches who transported it back to their American homelands, employing it there in religious and healing rites. A cult grew up around the drug. This cult developed into a formalised church, and after several court battles the US federal government finally upheld its members' rights to use peyote. Mescaline – recognisable as a white crystalline powder – is obtained from the spineless 'buttons' that range across the head of the peyote cactus. It can additionally be synthesised in a laboratory.

An important enthusiast for the mescaline experience was the English writer Aldous Huxley, who described its mystical and 'cleansing' qualities in his influential 1954 work *The Doors of Perception*. US demand for the drug (and its organic parent) was further stimulated by the writings of Carlos Castaneda who, in a series of enigmatic books, set adrift a young white novice among some crafty Indian shamans. Here in the UK, many people know of the drug, but few have experienced it first-hand. Bogus mescaline, however, has been in fairly plentiful supply at various times.

LSD: Sensations

Whether or not enlightenment is sought from the LSD experience, it is a drug to be treated with care or else it can produce a miserable, stormy passage known as a 'bad trip'. While the experience depends on the amount consumed, the problem users face is knowing how much each little paper square contains. The dose can run from a mildly affecting 35 micrograms to over 400 mcgs. Just 100 mcgs is sufficient to provoke the most dramatic effects lasting up to twelve hours; it is one of the most potent hallucinogens ever made – some four thousand times the strength of mescaline.

Most experienced users will establish a comfortable setting free from harassment or unwelcome dramas. Another key to the experience is the user's mental condition. Is s/he able to withstand the inevitable sensory buffeting a 100 mcg-plus dose will bring? Can s/he deal with and steer through the maelstrom of visions and emotions, some of them corresponding to concrete reality, others a figment of the drug's chemistry? Even when mood and setting are right there is still an unfathomable factor X that is going to shape what takes place. The drug, in short, cannot always be contained.

Despite all this, users report that getting a balanced frame of mind in a secure place and in the company of a friend who knows the drug will help to avoid a bad trip.

Effects will usually come on in about forty minutes, but could take as long as two hours. The first sensation will be excitement, perhaps agitation, an awareness of the body and its motor functions. The external world might now start looking unfamiliar, crooked, misshapen. The room has sludgy-coloured walls, though in reality they are white. The absurdity of manufactured style might be noticed – that pompous chair, the guzzling, moaning television set straining to exhibit life, perhaps *is* life. The visions need a backdrop to grow from, something as simple as a square inch of carpet or the grain in a wooden table. They can evolve from almost anything the eyes alight upon and can be stopped by simply swivelling the eyes. Although the user's own flesh can look curious to him/herself, like putty or meat, it will appear perfectly normal to everybody else. There will be a distortion and heightening of sound, warped reverberations and moments of piercing clarity. Much of today's post-rave dance music is wise to the drug's effects and plays on them.

'In almost the same breath', reports one user, 'you will feel elated, scared, wonderful, ridiculous – part of the universal hoax, and then all these swirling certainties and uncertainties will break into fragments and begin and end again.'

In the early stages of a 100 mcg-plus trip – the first two or three hours – events can either move rapidly or hang so motionless the user is put on the edge of panic. Activity can help. LSD is not an immobilising drug, which is why it has proved popular in the dance clubs. The more tasks undertaken, the less opportunity the drug's sensory effects have to entrance. But driving and other mechanical functions are not going to be handled effectively: driving and operating machinery of any kind can be dangerous.

Ego death

Of this initial period, when sensory bombardment is at its strongest, some people talk of the death of the ego (the drug's discoverer, Albert Hoffman, for one). By this it is meant that the experience can be so overpowering that the self is forced to retreat in the face of it. This retreat is not so much a defeat as a learning of proper humility. The 'self' – the drug seems to instruct – is an invention. Not only is it meagre in the context of the whole of creation, it cannot even withstand the battering afforded by some near-invisible grains of rye fungus. And yet this meagre self, together with the bodily organism that houses it, *is* part of the universal whole, and fittingly so. This constructive lesson passes many trippers by. They attempt to assert the primacy of their own position by staying rigid and attempting to fight off the drug's effects. They will more than likely come off worse in this war and in so doing suffer the vaunted 'ego death'. This could mean a shattering of inner confidence from which it might take some time to recover.

The later stages

After the early sensory bombardment it is usual to become deeply reflective. Now is the time to sift and sort the experiences of the first few hours. Alcoholics treated with LSD frequently achieved the vital 'realisation' at this stage. They saw what their shrivelling lives amounted to and resolved to free themselves. But it is at this stage that other kinds of ideas can get reinforced. Charles Manson and his devotees were LSD adepts and came to believe than the divine hand was on their bloody work.

In the final stages of the trip it is typical to feel a sense of melancholia. This is emphasised if friends who have been tripping together part abruptly. Some people turn to a favourite CD, others call upon cannabis to ease them down.

A long sleep is now in order, following which there will be no hangover, although flashbacks in which an acid vision is thrown up without warning are fairly common. These might return over the next few days or even weeks. Cannabis or some other kind of sensory input might trigger them. The medical profession makes a great fuss about the flashback syndrome, but for the vast majority it seems to be of no consequence and, rather than interfering with normal functioning, acts as an ironic counterpoint to the formalities of daily life.

What's described above is a substantial LSD experience. The current demand is for a far less concussive 'hit' of around 50 mcg, from which most users will be seeking a laugh as opposed to an excursion into deep inner orbit.

Magic Mushrooms: Sensations

The Liberty Cap experience is related to LSD but milder and less frenetic. 'Bad trips' are possible, but rarer since there tends to be less of a pressing psychological dimension to the experience – more one of wonder and a soothing euphoria. The effects start within half an hour and pass their peak within three or four hours, after which there is a tailing-off, followed by sleep. The head is clear on awakening.

A teenage schoolgirl described the experience like this: 'You start off feeling sick and giggly. Then your senses take over from your mind. It's like not conforming to society. Like being a child again.'

An older hand, a high master of the vanishing art of hippy-speak, described his recent Liberty Cap experiences in these terms: 'It has a Mayan magic to it. My wife characterised it as going home. I would sit and do nothing but *be* and it was very, very reassuring that *being* is all there really is and I was very conscious of *is* as the ultimate *ism* which is just to *be*. And it was such a wonderful feeling and I was *being* but *being* on a level of pure consciousness, very connected to the universal being . . .'

Not many users care to mess with Fly Agaric more than once owing to its tendency to provoke nausea, puking, and other untoward effects. Fewer still want anything to do with the more toxic *A. pantherina*. While Liberty Cap is like – as a third mushroom head put it – 'sipping wine in a punt with fairy lights, Fly Agaric promotes a drunken feeling, stiffness in the joints, unco-ordination.' After the initial immobilising phase a light sleep is common, accompanied by vivid imagery. Upon waking comes the more psilocybin-like euphoria, a sense of increased mental and physical energy, and self-absorption. Strong doses will produce great animation – perhaps derangement and convulsions. The entire episode lasts anything from two to eight hours (longer if urine is consumed).

Ecstasy: Sensations

The effects start after anything from twenty to sixty minutes. The body tingles, the mouth goes dry, and there can be an amphetamine-like stiffening of the limbs and jaw-clenching. The ensuing trip is a cross between amphetamine and one of the less explosive hallucinogens such as mescaline. The drug's popular nomenclature relates to its ability, during a four- or five-hour trip, to encourage users to shed their inhibitions and hostility, to become joyful, mystic, appreciate the tactile and aesthetic pleasures of everyday surfaces such as skin, hair, cotton, or a pine table. In the dance clubs, the drug has allowed users to dance with freakish, locked-in energy and to believe in a oneness of spirit and flesh. It even succeeded in taking violence off many of the football terraces. While it tends to make people feel more empathetic and sensual, it doesn't seem to have any aphrodisiac qualities. In fact the dance clubs – at least to start with – were a virtual sex-free zone.

Some experienced users, however, feel that it compares unfavourably with some of the purer psychedelics. One described it as 'the white bread' of the field. 'It hasn't got the depth of most of the other psychedelics. It gives you the ecstatic feeling and does take you into different dimensions but not as richly veined dimensions as LSD or mescaline. But it is a lot safer. You're not going to find anything on E that's going to freak you out. You're not going to go deep into your past and realise something awful about yourself that's always been hidden.'

It can, though, produce paranoia, anxiety, and confusion, depending on the user's mood and the setting in which the E has been taken.

Health Effects

This is an especially difficult area to make clear-cut statements about because the hallucinogens on offer are almost never as advertised. Something called Ecstasy will be manufactured to all kinds of formulas and will then usually be heavily

258

adulterated with anything from antihistamine to ground glass. The quality of what's sold also constantly changes, and so people who do intend to swallow something should check for up-to-date 'intelligence' from their local drugs agency, or from the national advice organisation Release.

LSD: Physical effects

LSD is not an inherently toxic drug. Just four LSD-linked deaths between 1982 and 1992 are reported in Home Office statistics,[24] and all these are classed under the sub-category of 'accident', suggesting the tripper was involved in a fall, a traffic accident, or something similar.

Of all the early scares associated with LSD, the one that caused the most worry was the drug's apparent ability to inflict genetic damage and thereby give rise to malformed babies. Its impact on brain tissue was also a worry. Today, most of those concerns have dissipated and one research team was able to report in 1992, 'There is no generally accepted evidence of brain cell damage, chromosomal abnormalities, or teratogenic [literally: *monster-causing*] effects after the use of the [LSD-type] hallucinogens and mescaline.'[25] Which is not to say that this view won't subsequently be revised after further research.

Mental effects

The phenomenon of the 'bad trip' is described above in the 'Sensations' passage. Stressful external circumstances (e.g. being arrested and slung in a police cell), too much self-control, negative expectations (based, perhaps, on some dread description seen in a newspaper) can all be factors leading to a miserable outcome.

Ignorance of the drug and how to steer through the trip is another important predictor. As one young Edinburgh clubgoer put it to me: 'With kids of fourteen and fifteen chucking acid and Es down their throats without a thought, it's not surprising some are coming to grief.'

The anxiety, paranoia, and panic reactions of a bad trip are best dealt with by moving out of any stressful situation and, ideally, by a friend or some other trusted individual who is experienced in the ways of the drug offering calm

259

reassurance. Such support can produce results in a few minutes, or the 'guide' might be needed for several hours.

In vulnerable people adverse psychological effects can persist after comedown. They might suffer mental and emotional instability, depression, loss of confidence (see Ego death above), paranoia, and unpleasant flashbacks. The idea that the drug can cause a lasting schizophrenia-type psychosis is one that has been much discussed though it still presents 'serious shortcomings'.[26] But in someone predisposed to schizophrenia (itself a not-too-clearly understood term) LSD may do one of the following: a) cause the psychosis to manifest at an earlier age; b) produce a psychosis in someone who might never have fallen sick if not for use of the drug; c) cause relapse in a person who had previously suffered a psychotic disorder.[27]

Such LSD-linked psychoses accord with what is found in people who were once known, among the drug laity, as 'acid casualties', but who are these days said to have 'lost it'. These are individuals who have dosed up on so much LSD (or Ecstasy) that they have never quite returned from orbit. It's as though a fragment or more of their brain has ceased to function. The processing of sensory data is more difficult and unreliable, and there are gaps in logic: a mental lopping off.

Tolerance

Tolerance of LSD's psychoactive effects builds rapidly so that a normal dose taken three or four days running will, by the fourth day, produce no trip. Only by abstaining for several days will the sensitivity return. Also, a cross-tolerance operates with other members of the LSD family – morning glory seeds, LSA, psilocybin, and DMT (this last is a product of the laboratory but can be found in plants that have for centuries been used by South American Indians as hallucinogenic snuffs).

The nature of this cross-tolerance is such that however the LSD family members are interchanged it is not possible to trip using any one of them for more than a handful of days consecutively.

Addiction/dependence

No true physical addiction to the drug develops whereby the body suffers trauma when deprived. But psychological dependence, as with any mood-altering drug, can occur. It is comparatively rare with the LSD family because its members are too mentally combustible to be regular companions.

Magic Mushrooms

Because of psilocybin and psilocin's close chemical relationship to LSD, much of what has been written above about LSD's low toxicity, its effects on mental stability, tolerance, addiction, and so forth, can be extended to magic mushrooms. However, there are the additional factors of accidental poisoning, and the other material components of fungi which have so far been little studied.

Avoiding the killers

As a general rule, mushrooms that emerge from the ground through a volva (like a broken eggshell) should be avoided by the novice. Avoid also those a dog might have pissed on. It is also important to stay away from old, wet, dirty and bug-infested specimens, and not to store any away fresh – particularly not in a plastic bag. The sealed environment encourages them to convert into an extremely unpleasant dark slime.

Dried mushrooms should *never* be bought on the street. The purchaser will have no idea what they are.

Sudden deaths

Deaths have occasionally resulted from an overdose of Fly Agaric, and more rarely still from *A. pantherina*. A lethal dose triggers delirium, convulsions, coma and heart failure. In terms of Fly Agaric's longer-term impact on the body, this has not so far been analysed in any detail.

Addiction/dependence

Liberty Cap and Fly Agaric are not physically addictive, although like LSD they can give rise to psychological dependence.

Poisoning

If trouble is taken to select healthy specimens of the 'recommended' species in sensible doses there will be no trouble with poisoning. However, mishaps do occur and, while relatively few, they are increasing each year with the rising popularity of magic mushroom eating. In 1978 the National Poisons Information Service could trace just 33 cases. In 1981 the figure was 142. By 1992, the Poisons unit at Guy's Hospital was dealing with 130,000 emergency enquiries. Most of these involved quickly resolving symptoms, and there were no fatalities. Mushroom poisoning can mean a quick vomit or it can mean death where the wrong species has been chosen. The longer the symptoms take to appear the more serious the likely outcome, since the toxins will have had time to percolate through the system. Release put the case straight in its 1979 guide, *Hallucinogenic Mushrooms*: 'If you become ill a day or so after eating the mushroom you should get medical advice at once, even if you begin to feel better after a while. It is characteristic of serious mushroom poisoning that the person affected has periods of recovery but may nevertheless die some days later. Remember, since mushrooms are legal there's no problem about calling a doctor. You won't get busted.'

Many symptoms of mushroom poisoning can be difficult to distinguish from the early effects of a trip on Fly Agaric. They will include vomiting and diarrhoea, cramp, watery eyes and mouth, twitching or fits, respiratory problems, a yellow pallor, and unconsciousness. Obviously a person in the extreme condition needs emergency treatment. Call an ambulance or get them to the hospital yourself. Take samples of the offending fungi with you and, if available, specimens of your friend's liquid or solid waste. Release offer the following additional tips: if the fungus has been eaten recently and the symptoms are just beginning, help your companion vomit up the poison by feeding him/her hot salty water and then burnt toast to soak up the remaining toxins. But don't try this if they are semi-conscious or spark out. They will choke. If they do pass out lay them on the floor in the coma position – on the side with the knee nearest you bent up and the near elbow and forearm on the floor. Ensure the throat is not obstructed by the tongue or by vomit and check for breathing. If there is none apply artificial respiration.

If a fit or a convulsion starts stick a soft wad of cloth like a hankie in the mouth to prevent chewing or swallowing of the tongue. Lie the victim down in a place free from hard, sharp objects so s/he can thrash without risk of injury.

Ecstasy: physical effects

The less serious unwanted effects of taking Ecstasy can include teeth-grinding, jaw-clenching, increased muscle tension, blurred vision and – the day after – a type of hangover that might produce an inability to sleep, tiredness, sore jaw muscles, loss of balance, and aching head.[28]

More disturbing is a phenomenon known as a 'head rush' – usually occurring at a rave where, for up to three minutes, dancers experience a blanking-out of sights and sounds.[29]

Because of Ecstasy's appetite-suppressing effects, long-term users run the risk of experiencing a range of problems associated with malnutrition. See amphetamine chapter.

Some long-term users have also reported an increased susceptibility to colds, 'flu, sore throats, and the like, suggesting that the drug (or the life that goes with it) suppresses the body's natural immunity to disease.[30]

Women and E

Some women E users report that their periods have been irregular and heavier than normal; others say they have no periods at all.[31] While there is no evidence that MDMA damages the foetus or causes problems in the newborn, the general view among physicians is that all drugs (legal and illegal) should be avoided during pregnancy, unless there is no alternative.

Heatstroke

Ecstasy causes body temperature to rise. When the drug is taken in a hot, crowded place (a rave), and the consumer then dances frenetically for several hours, body temperature rises more dramatically. Pints of fluid are sweated out and – in susceptible individuals – a fatal heatstroke can follow. Convulsions and widespread blood-clotting accompany the sudden rise in body temperature and victims can go into a terminal coma. Between 1988 and October 1993 there had been at least fourteen such cases reported. Why some people come to grief in this way, even on comparatively small doses, while others can withstand far more severe 'abuse', remains a puzzle. The technical cause of most of the deaths has been respiratory collapse caused by blood clotting in places where it shouldn't, notably in the lungs – a syndrome known as disseminated intravascular coagulation (DIC). With the lungs congested in this way, air cannot get through and death results. It is believed that MDMA can precipitate DIC by somehow reacting with the chemicals responsible for the proper coagulation of blood.[32]

In October 1993, a further possible explanation for the sudden death syndrome was put forward.[33] This suggested that the fatalities were linked to the absence in the vulnerable individuals of an enzyme called cytochrome P450 246, which is responsible for breaking down Ecstasy in the body. With the enzyme missing, so the theory went, the drug remained in the system long enough to produce its fatal toxic effects. About one in twelve people were said to be missing the key enzyme – which still left open the question: why so few deaths when a million young people go raving every week, a good proportion of whom will be consuming Ecstasy? The team responsible for the theory admitted that more exploration was needed.

Liver

There is some evidence that Ecstasy might harm the liver, there being reports of jaundice and liver inflammation in E users. More seriously, a team at Guy's Hospital's National Poisons Unit reported in a 1992 article in *The Lancet* seven cases of severe liver damage associated with Ecstasy use.[34] Most made a partial recovery, but one died and another received a liver transplant. The authors said that none of those affected had any history of heavy alcohol or injecting drug use and none had signs of infectious hepatitis – factors that might otherwise explain their condition. The team believed that such cases were increasing and 'may be related to repeated exposure to MDMA . . .' But they also suggested that the damage could have been done by a contaminant or additive rather than by the Ecstasy itself.

The same Guy's team had published in *The Lancet* details of other Ecstasy-linked deaths and injuries, but in a subsequent issue of the same journal an Oxford neurologist complained that the group had failed to report these dire outcomes in the context of how often the drug was being used. Without doing so, he wrote, 'one cannot determine if MDMA is any more dangerous than aspirin. For the public to make rational decisions about recreational drug use the incidence of death and serious morbidity [disease] needs to be known. When medical scientists allow their data to be uncritically used they reduce the chances of more serious messages being listened to.[35]

Brain

Fears of Ecstasy-linked brain haemorrhages were raised following a 1992 report of four such cases from Scotland[36] – although amphetamine as well as MDMA was consumed by the victims. Three made a 'good recovery', one died. The authors thought that impurities in the drugs may have played a major role given that the four cases came in a cluster.

A far greater controversy relates to MDMA's supposed capacity to damage brain cells, related to the production and transmission of a chemical messenger in the brain known as serotonin (or 5-HT). Although what is known about the function of serotonin and the system that processes it is still largely guesswork, the best guess to date is that they are involved in the control of sleep, food intake, sexual behaviour, anxiety, and mood generally.[37]

The arguments centre on the 'suitability of extrapolating results using laboratory animals to human MDMA users, the way in which neurotoxicity [brain poisoning] is defined, and the degree to which the neurochemical changes caused by exposure to MDMA diminish over time.[38] An additional problem is that the animals concerned were usually injected with the drug rather than receiving it orally, as do ravers.

According to one medical sceptic, Ecstasy damages the fibres of serotonin brain cells but has little effect on their cell bodies.[39] And that, he believes, could mean that the cells have the ability to repair themselves. 'It's too simplistic to say that Ecstasy kills neurons.'

Human experiments subsequently showed that one group of Ecstasy users appeared to have reduced levels of serotonin in the fluid bathing their brains. But again, this reduction might be temporary and does not demonstrate brain damage – only the possibility of such damage.

In personality tests, the group concerned were 'less impulsive and hostile and showed greater constraint and control. These were all aspects of behaviour thought to be mediated by serotonin.'[40]

Psychological

Another researcher found similar mood changes as long ago as 1986.[41] In a letter to the *British Medical Journal* (complaining that a senior British physician had looked only for the bad news in his ecstasy research), a Santa Fe, New Mexico doctor noted that 'eighteen of my 29 subjects reported positive changes in mood after their sessions; 23 reported improved attitudes, such as toward self and life in general; 28 reported improvement in interpersonal relationships, and three of the five couples reported improvements in their working life; 14 reported diminished use of abusable substances (alcohol, marijuana, caffeine, tobacco, cocaine, and LSD); 15 reported beneficial changes in their life goals; and all nine subjects with diagnosable psychiatric disorders reported considerable relief from their problems . . .'

But such benefits, pharmaceutical history shows us, will probably be temporary, only to be followed by a 'rebound' condition wherein precisely the opposite effects to those desired are experienced. Speed starts off producing increased energy and confidence but ultimately leaves users exhausted and shaken. Tranquillisers sedate at first but then produce great agitation. Heroin induces a pain-free, carefree condition, but in the end delivers the opposite.

There are already plenty of signs that some heavy E users

are suffering some very un-ecstasy-like feelings: depression, loss of confidence, shakiness, anxiety – all of which persist for varying lengths of time.

Says Manchester's Lifeline drug agency: 'We knew people who, once the life and soul of the party, were stuck in the house anxious, confused, tired and depressed . . . What had started out as the drug to end all drugs – the perfect drug – was leaving behind it a sorry catalogue of people in jail, people in mental hospitals and shady people selling snidey drugs to eager young recruits looking to start on the honeymoon period. More and more reports come to Lifeline about long weekends being brought to a close with a handful of diazepam, Temazepam and (God forbid) even heroin. People who started taking drugs to make them feel good were having to take other drugs just to stop them feeling bad – sad!'[42]

It is the impact of E on the emotional stability of young users which will undoubtedly prove its most important health legacy (and probably the most neglected). The drug's capacity to strip some users of their psychological defences, to encourage them openly to trust and empathise, can prove costly in the long term. Whether the 'mechanism' at work is psychological, neurological (to do with serotonin and the like), or a factor of the communal rave culture is a question that's unlikely ever to be settled definitively. But that some young people are coming to emotional harm is beyond question.

Tolerance addiction

Tolerance develops to the effects of MDMA, so that increasing amounts are needed to get high. While there are no major physical withdrawal symptoms associated with the drug (of the sort experienced with barbiturates and heroin), depression, fatigue, anxiety, and the like can follow cessation. This can lead to more use in an attempt to alleviate such symptoms.

With other conditions

Research to date suggests that Ecstasy can cause additional problems in people already suffering heart disease, high blood pressure, glaucoma, epilepsy, or who are generally in poor physical or mental health. Women with a history of genito-urinary tract infection are also warned against using the drug.[43]

With other drugs

Mixing any drugs can have unpredictable and potentially dangerous results. Because hallucinogens are often something other than as advertised (they are made to unknown formulas and include unknowable adulterants), there is greater potential for grief than usual. Anaesthetics (ketamine and GHB included) are worth a special mention.

This class of drug can react especially badly with Ecstasy.[44] Therefore, if someone who's taken Ecstasy needs to go to hospital to be resuscitated, or for accident damage to be repaired, the doctors should be told that E has been used.

Help

Many constructive initiatives have sprung up around the rave scene, designed to minimise the negative effects of E and other drugs. Clubbers themselves have established groups that produce easily digested educational material, and they also meet with their peers. Front-runners in this field are Edinburgh's Crew 2000 (well supported by local professional drug worker Willie McBride). Manchester's Lifeline, the Swansea Drugs Project and Bradford's Drugs Prevention Team have also produced packs for ravers which include everything from educational comic books to videos and free condoms.

For some of these agencies it has reached the status of (fairly) big business. Lifeline, during 1992/93, sold over a million items of literature directed at young people, bringing in profits of nearly £35,000. Witty, raw-edged characters like Peanut Pete and Granpa 'Smackhead' Jones might have aggravated some of the town's elders, but they hit the spot with the drug consumers themselves. Similar material emerged from Merseyside and elsewhere.

A number of agencies have set young workers trained in emergency resuscitation techniques loose in the clubs, and some of the club owners (who were once guilty of turning off water taps in the toilets to boost bar sales) now let the water flow and even have paramedics of their own standing by.

Coping with a bad trip

Ecstasy users sometimes need to be talked down from a bad, panicky trip in the same way as someone 'freaking' on LSD. If in a turbulent environment (a rave, a party), they should leave (or be encouraged to do so by a friend) for somewhere quieter. Anyone offering help should avoid actions that could be interpreted as being shifty, for this could raise the paranoia level (e.g. whispering to a third party, making 'strange' arm gestures). Talk to the bad-tripper in a calm manner, using uncomplicated language.

Avoiding heatstroke

Manchester's Lifeline lists the following warning signs that something drastic might be about to happen:[45]

Failure to sweat; heat cramps in the legs, arms, and back; giddiness; headache; fatigue; vomiting; fainting; suddenly feeling exceptionally tired and irritable; being unable to pee very much though the desire is there, and what comes out is highly coloured.

The advice for all ravers is to drink a pint of water every hour or so – but not alcohol because this causes further dehydration. Also, take regular rests from dancing and allow the body to cool down – preferably somewhere away from the hubbub. In short, *chill out*.

Ketamine

Ketamine is a powerful anaesthetic, used mainly on child hospital patients, which has found its way into the clubs in recent years. Medical textbooks warn of its potential for causing hallucinations and other 'psychotic' outcomes, and that's precisely what the experience has been for recreational users. Few who have tried it have any favourable words on the subject. A London man told me: 'When you're coming down from E it's supposed to take you right up. Everything's swaying and moving. Your heart skips a beat and you can feel your head filling up and your blood pressure rising. I've see people go over on it and stay out for five minutes. It feels like your blood is boiling and something is trying to get out of your head.'

A Birmingham man said he had taken it by accident 'and felt like he had been raped by the drug, like someone had abused my body against my will.'

GHB/'GBH'

This is another anaesthetic – used in the US for its sedating rather than painkilling effects; British pharmaceutical text-books don't list it. From around spring 1994, it began showing up on the UK club scene, starting with London gay venues. While some call it GBH (signifying the potential 'violence' of the experience) others know it as *Liquid E* or *Liquid X*. Its chemical name is gammahydroxybutyrate. It's a salty tasting, colourless, odourless liquid that comes in small bottles. The potency of the contents varies, since it will be home-made to various consistencies. Ingredients include solvents and caustic soda. Some people down the whole bottle (£10–15 at the time of writing). Others regard the 40 ml or so it contains as three separate hits. Rarely, it is injected.

GHB's effects, at lower doses, are a cross between alcohol and the now-defunct euphoriant downer methaqualone. Inhibitions are lowered, leading to a quirky calm feeling or, perhaps, to a darker mood. At higher doses, it causes sedation, nausea, vomiting, muscle stiffness, confusion, convulsions and – at the top end – coma and respiratory collapse.[46] One man described how he 'felt like I was drifting away in my own little bubble of consciousness but my friends said I was puking and out of it.'[47]

By May 1994, the National Drug Intelligence Service was reporting that around two hundred people had been hospital-ised after taking the drug, and there were accounts of two Scottish men dying 'at a club where GBH . . . was being sold.'

Apart from clubbers, the other category of GHB user is

body-builders. They are attracted to its apparent ability to promote 'slow wave' sleep, during which muscle-building growth hormone is secreted.[48]

While there have been no confirmed GHB-linked deaths, either in the UK or the US (from where recreational use originated), media lore has it the late American actor River Phoenix was killed by the drug.

Questions of tolerance and physical and psychological dependence are not properly understood, although given what's already known of the drug's character, there is the probability of all three developing in some individuals. Long-term impact on physical and emotional well-being are also not yet understood.

In 1990, the US Food and Drug Administration declared GHB 'an unauthorised new drug' and several states subsequently outlawed it. In the UK, possession is not illegal (at the time of writing) but unlicensed manufacture or distribution is an offence under the Medicines Act. Importation is also prohibited, unless for 'personal use'.

Notes

1 Alexander Shulgin, the Californian chemist who discovered Ecstasy, has published – with his wife Ann – *Pihkal: A chemical love story* (Transform Press), which details the contents of 179 members of the phenylethylamine family (Ecstasy included), as well as methods of synthesising them.

2 J. McClellan, 'Tripping down memory lane', in the *Observer* magazine, 21 March 1994, p. 44.

3 T. Duquesne and J. Reeves, *A Handbook of Psychoactive Medicines*, Quartet, London, 1982, p. 328.

4 P. Stafford, *Psychedelic Encyclopedia*, J. P. Tarcher Publishing, Los Angeles, 1983, p. 78.

5 Ibid, p. 80.

6 Ibid.

7 Ibid.

8 'The amphetamines and LSD', report by the Advisory Committee on Drug Dependence, HMSO, London, 1970, p. 36.

9 'LSD – recurrence of a communal nightmare', ISDD, London, p. 2.

10 ACDD, op. cit.

11 McClellan, op. cit.

12 D. May and S. Tendler, *The Brotherhood of Eternal Love*, Panther Books, London, 1984, p. 276.

13 In 1990, by now in his late seventies, Leary was refused entry into Britain by the Home Office. He was due to give a talk on virtual reality computer software.

14 Bus-loads of tourists would cruise hippy HQ, San Francisco's Haight–Ashbury, during the 1967 'Summer of Love'. In response to having cameras pointed at them, some Haight residents would hold up a mirror.

15 P. McDermott, in the *International Journal on Drug Policy*, Vol. 3, No. 2, p. 109.

16 'Ecstasy: Drug Notes', ISDD, 1993.

17 This is according to Paul Staines, a right-wing libertarian writer and campaigner, whose voluble critique of the government's crackdown on the rave scene was given vent in his 'Acid House parties against the lifestyle police and the Safety Nazis', Libertarian Alliance, London, 1991.

18 Ibid.

19 Thanks to Crew 2000 in Edinburgh for helping an old dog like me understand something of the evolving club scene; and to Ciaran O'Hagan, a University of North London social research degree student, on whose first-hand experience I also drew. Other important sources for this section include *Eternity* – self-billed as 'the most important controversial underground dance magazine', No. 14, Wakefield.

20 According to a survey by the research and forecasting organisation the Henley Centre.

21 S. Henderson, 'Fun, fashion, and frisson', in the *International Journal of Drug Policy*, Vol. 4, No. 3, 1993, p. 122.

22 'New Lords threat to Howard', in the *Guardian*, 26 April 1994, p. 6.

23 The word of 3T & Desmondo, of rave organisers Evolution.

24 'Statistics of drug addicts notified to the Home Office, UK, 1993', in *Home Office Statistical Bulletin*, Table 17, 22 June 1994.

25 J. Thomas Ungerleider and R. Pechnick, 'Hallucinogens', in *Substance Abuse, A Comprehensive Textbook*, Williams and Wilkins, Baltimore, 1992, p. 280.

26 Ibid.

27 Ibid, p. 287.

28 Ibid, p. 286.

29 ISDD, op. cit.

30 Ibid.

31 Ibid.

32 ISDD, op. cit. John Henry, consultant physician at the National Poisons Unit, was the first to suggest that rave deaths were due to heatstroke. He also made the early ground in trying to explain the mechanism.

33 'One in twelve Ecstasy users risk death', in the *Independent*, 15 October 1993; 'Death risk to one in 12 Ecstasy users', in the *Yorkshire Post*, 16 October 1993. The research was by a team from Sheffield University's department of medicine and pharmacology.

34 J. Henry *et al.*, 'Toxicity and deaths from 3, 4-methylenedioxymethamphetamine', in *The Lancet*, Vol. 340, 15 August 1992, p. 384.

35 Simon Ellis, of the Department of Clinical Neurology, Radcliffe Infirmary, Oxford, in a letter to *The Lancet*, Vol. 340, 19 September 1992, p. 726.

36 D. P. Harries and R. De Silva, 'Ecstasy and intracerebral haemorrhage', in the *Scottish Medical Journal*, 37 (5), 1992, p. 150.

37 Ungerleider and Pechnick, op. cit., p. 287.

38 Ibid.

39 Marcus Rattray, biochemist with Guy's Hospital, as reported in *New Scientist*, 29 August 1992, p. 34.

40 'How Ecstasy blows your mind', in *New Scientist*, 20 November 1993.

41 G. Greer, 'Ecstasy and the dance of death', letter to the *British Medical Journal*, Vol. 305, 26 September 1992.

42 *Ecstasy and Eve*, booklet published by Lifeline, Manchester.

43 ISDD, op. cit.

44 D. Rittoo, letter to *The Lancet*, Vol. 340, 19 September 1992, p. 725.
45 'Too Damn Hot', Lifeline, Manchester, 1992.
46 *Druglink Factsheet No. 8: GHB ('GBH')*, ISDD.
47 'GHB', in *The Big Issue*, 10 May 1994, p. 6.
48 ISDD, *Druglink Factsheet No. 8*, op. cit.

HEROIN

Intro

Historically, heroin has taken turns with cocaine in inspiring the most zealous drug-related rhetoric (pro and anti), and in drawing the big socio-medical research money. Drug libraries are stacked full of unread tomes on this narcotic *par excellence*. Poets and musicians can't be kept quiet on the subject.

Britain's whole drug treatment strategy is tailored with heroin in mind, to the neglect of other 'hard' substances which are consumed in far greater quantities (amphetamine) and which are capable of causing just as much harm to individuals and their communities.

So what is this strange *romance* with heroin? Why, when people discuss it, do they leave their shoes and talk in symbols and metaphor? The heroin experience, for those who don't let the drug run away with them, is warm, woozy, and carefree. Nothing matters any more in their beautiful bubble. For everyday users who have lost control, the experience is ultimately a mediocre one. The drug does not open doors to other worlds (as with LSD) but closes them. It stupefies and kills feeling.

Perhaps the key to understanding heroin is to recognise that, for most of these compulsive users, it serves as an antidote to a wretched existence – lives that might be full of pain, might be too complicated to manage, or – conversely – empty of any meaning whatsoever. Heroin promises neutrality. It promises *nothing*.

Why, then, won't governments allow such people their *nothing*, preferring all the crime, ill-health and social dislocation that follow from a policy of prohibition? The substitute drug methadone is handed out instead of heroin, even though it appears to be more addictive, less effective, and kills more people through overdose. Perhaps the logic is that if you start

275

handing out free tickets to oblivion on the carrier of people's choice, everyone will want to go.

But heroin doesn't always deliver people where they want to go. It holds out the promise of escape but, for those who return to it too often, it makes matters worse. Or it kills.

Hello there again my old friend
Always there to count on 'til the end.
Bathing me in warmth like a wave,
Who says heaven is after the grave,
With your magic trance, I shut this world out
Forget my troubles and cast away doubt,
No more searching for society's golden crown,
Now that I have my powder brown.
Like everything else it has its price
It's demanding and cruel but sure is nice.
There are various ways it can be done
To chase your dragon on a tainted sun.
If your body first seems to reject
You'll find your high when you inject.
If you want to keep that monkey on your back,
Just keep taking the good old smack.
So hello again old friend
My companion and compatriot 'til the end.

T. Clinton (first published in the Scottish edition of *The Big Issue*, 4 March 1994).

What Is It

Heroin is one of a class of drugs known as narcotic analgesics, narcotic from the Greek *narcotikos* meaning benumbing, and analgesic from the Greek meaning without pain. Heroin itself belongs some way down the line of the family of narcotic analgesics known as the opiates. They are called such because they all derive from the opium poppy (*Papaver somniferum*). The most straightforward extract from the poppy is opium itself, which starts as a milky juice oozing from the poppy's seed pods. A few days after the petals drop, a series of

276

shallow incisions are made in the pod. The juice exudes and a day later, when it has turned a gummy brown, it is scraped off and left to dry in a shaded area, all the while darkening and hardening. Once firm it is shaped into bricks ready for the consumer. Getting smoking opium out of these crude bricks requires repeated boiling and sieving until all impurities are removed and a black, sticky paste results at the bottom of the cooking pot. This paste is then dried and smoked. Pharmaceutical opium comes in tablet or injectable form.

Morphine

Within opium are more than a dozen alkaloids, yet only a few of them have any medical utility and fewer still are of interest to the recreational user. Principal in both recreational and medical categories is morphine – a product up to ten times more potent weight for weight than its parent opium. In fact morphine is the opiate pain killer against which all others are compared, though among its drawbacks is a propensity to cause nausea and vomiting. In its pharmaceutical format morphine comes as a pill, a suppository, a hydrochloride solution, and in an injectable ampoule. The stuff found on the streets in one of these forms is probably the product of a chemist or hospital break-in; or else it will be pills or powder smuggled in from India, which supplies most of the licit opiates required by the world's pharmaceutical companies. Tasmania is also an important producer of poppies for licit products.

Codeine

Another major alkaloid of opium is codeine, used in the main to deal with coughs and mild to moderate pain. Having about one-sixth the kick of morphine, its street value is limited to a hit of last resort or thereabouts. It can be found in countless across-the-counter preparations, often in tiny quantities mixed in with aspirin, ephedrine, and the like. In its pure formulations it appears as a tablet, syrup and ampoule. Used long-term it is powerfully constipating.

Heroin

Heroin is something of a bastard child of mother opium and the laboratory chemist. It is made by boiling equal amounts of morphine with acetic anhydride, a colourless heavy liquid used in the manufacture of synthetic fibres and celluloid film. The combination produces a raw base. To get heroin itself, this product then goes through several more stages calling for hydrochloric acid, strychnine, caffeine, and much drying, sieving and other processing – depending on the quality of the heroin required. In its purest form the drug is up to three to four times more powerful than morphine. Medical heroin (whose proper chemical name is diamorphine) comes as a tablet, a linctus, and as ampoules of powdered solution.

Dominating the street scene is a heavily adulterated product known as 'brown'. Originating in Pakistan, purity levels generally range from 25–45 per cent. Brown's basic ingredient is diamorphine base, an insoluble material devoid of the hydrochloride salt found in the medical version. This makes street heroin smokeable but not injectable. It must first be dissolved in an acid (usually citric) before being administered via a syringe. Added to the diamorphine base are various cheap 'cuts' designed to maximise the dealer's profits. Typical adulterants include lactose (a milk sugar), glucose, and the laxative mannitol. Less friendly additions include chalk dust, talcum powder, and even battery acid – anything that looks the part.

Rarely seen in the UK these days is 'Chinese' heroin, a product grown and processed in South-East Asia. The best example of Chinese is the so-called Number 4 type – a white crystalline powder resembling pharmaceutical heroin in appearance and purity. Lesser grades take on a shading reflecting the dilutants used.

Street names for heroin include *skag, brown, junk, horse, H, boy* and *smack* – the last being a corruption of the Yiddish 'schmeck', which means to sniff.

Others

Other opium alkaloids with clinical value are papaverine, noscapine, and thebaine. These too are used, in various combinations, to deal with pain and coughs, as well as diarrhoea, impotence, colic, and wayward behaviour of the muscles. The question of their 'abuse' has rarely arisen.

Synthetics

Heroin and the other drugs listed above fall into the opiate category, in that they are wholly or largely derivatives of the poppy. Other drugs have similar effects but are made from different materials. The collective name for the pure opiates as well as their close relatives is *opioid*. There are scores of substances falling into this category, but just half a dozen have been adopted in non-medical circles. These are:

Pethidine – a painkiller of shortish action made without recourse to the poppy and which comes as a tablet or injectable ampoule. Some users report getting a hallucinogenic buzz. Prescribed for pain relief during childbirth and after surgery. Branded as Pamergan.

Dextromoramide – a far stronger analgesic that comes brand-named Palfium, in tablet or suppository format. The effects, according to expert street opinion, are short-lived, 'artificial', and often include feelings of grogginess.

Dipipanone – comes as a pink tablet brand-named Diconal and with the addition of an anti-nausea drug called cyclizine hydrochloride. This pukeless element, together with the high-quality 'rush' the drug imparts when injected, once made it a revered hit among hard-core users. Doctors, during the 1970s and early 1980s, prescribed Diconal with fairly witless abandon, believing, or affecting to believe, that it would not go into feeding a needle habit. But it did. The dangers of injecting Diconal – rich in silicon – were finally recognised by the Home Office and the drug can no longer be prescribed by medics unless they are specially licensed. Current street stocks derive from chemist break-ins or – according to one Manchester consumer – from certain cash-starved cancer patients to whom the drug is issued for pain relief. The perils of silicon-rich Diconal were neatly summarised by seasoned drugs pundit Peter McDermott: 'After a couple of hits your veins become filled with sand and get as hard as glass. Keep on injecting and you end up with abscesses and ulcers at best, and amputated limbs if you are unlucky.'[1]

Dihydrocodeine – one of the most widely prescribed painkillers in the UK, it is judged to fill the slot between the opioids and milder solutions such as paracetamol. It comes as a tablet (some branded DHC Continus), an ampoule, and elixir. The brand name DF-118 was formerly used for some of these products. Produces particularly severe constipation problems and, one user told me, 'is horrific to inject. You go red all over and scratch and get pins and needles from head to foot.'

Pentazocine – once oversold as a painkiller of morphine's stature (though with supposedly minimal side effects) its prescription is now semi-officially discouraged[2] owing to the extra stress it places on the heart and its tendency to create 'hallucinations and thought disturbances'. It is still, however, issued for moderate to severe pain, and comes in tablets, capsules, amps, and suppositories under the brand name Fortral.

Buprenorphine – like pentazocine, this is both an opioid *agonist* and an *antagonist* – which means, respectively, that it can substitute for other drugs detailed in this chapter, and yet might precipitate withdrawal symptoms when someone dependent on opioids takes it. Scottish doctors during the late 1980s/early 1990s saw buprenorphine as *the* wholesome 'cure' for heroin addiction, issuing it with such unstinting generosity than the drug came to dominate the Scottish street scene, often outselling mother heroin and figuring in many of the 100 or more annual overdose deaths. Brand name is Temgesic.

Methadone – the official state fix for heroin addicts and endlessly controversial. Clinics and other agencies prescribe it as a substitute for smack, then usually try to reduce the dose down to zero, the goal being abstinence. Where abstinence can't be achieved the addict might be 'maintained' on a stable minimum dose. In different parts of the country and at different times over the last twenty-five or thirty years the severity of the prescribing regime has varied – anything from dizzyingly rapid reduction scripts to long-term maintenance on 'generous' doses where a habit is thought to be deeply ingrained.

Ultimately, prescribing policy has reflected the tensions between what is considered a) good medical treatment for the actual user, and b) a desire to protect the wider community from what are seen as predatory, infectious, and potentially subversive junkies. For more on this subject, see below.

The anti- and pro-methadone camps make their arguments with unreserved passion. The pro camp insists that the drug draws people into treatment and reduces the level of crime, disease, and general harm to users as well as to the broader community.[3] Opponents fall into two broad camps: the *say-no-to-all-drugs* abstentionists, and those who are convinced that methadone is even more addictive than heroin, produces more protracted withdrawal symptoms, leads to many more overdose deaths (nineteen times more according to consultant psychiatrist Dr John Marks who ran clinics in Widnes and Warrington until his funding was cut), and is so boring that recipients often top up with more interesting street substances. And anyway, this faction argues, if people want heroin, why not give it to them? Why is it inherently more 'moral' to dispense methadone than diamorphine?

The drug comes in four basic formats: 5 mg tablets (brand name Physeptone), 10 mg ampoules, a 2 mg/5 ml linctus (usually prescribed for severe coughing), and a 1 mg/1 ml 'mixture' that is two and a half times the strength of the linctus. The mixture is the format most universally favoured by treatment agencies. It comes as bottles of brown, yellow, or bright green liquid, the colour depending on how much of which sort of food dye the pharmacist uses. Tartrazine (also known as E102) is a yellow substance commonly used in chewing gum, mint sauce, and fizzy drinks. It is associated with hyperactivity in young children and in adults might cause symptoms such as skin rashes, hayfever, tight chest, and blurred vision.[4] The mixture also contains a large dose of glucose syrup (to make it palatable) and chloroform water, intended to dissuade users from taking their hit via the needle. If it is injected, the chloroform burns and damages the lining of the vein, leading to blood clots and the vein's eventual collapse.[5]

If requested, the mixture can be formulated without the tooth-rotting syrup and the colourings. But it is not just the syrup which teeth take a battering from. Methadone hydrochloride is a strong acid which attacks tooth enamel. The drug also restricts production of saliva – a natural defence against plaque.[6]

Routes of Admission

There is a well-observed pathway to heroin addiction that starts with sniffing or smoking, graduates to skin-popping, then on to mainlining via intramuscular injection, and often back again to skin-popping when all good veins are used up. This is not to say that everyone who begins sniffing or smoking will become an addict, or that you can't be an addict unless you inject. Any route of admission can lead to addiction.

Sniffing

Heroin is sniffed in the same manner as cocaine – chopped with a blade on a hard surface, drawn into lines, and snorted up one nostril at a time. Because of heroin's bitter flavour and the presence of adulterants, many find this method unappealing.

Smoking

A dose is placed inside a strip of tin foil and a flame run underneath it. As the heroin heats up it turns black and wriggles like a snake – hence the term Chasing the Dragon. The rising fumes are sucked up through the nostrils via a tube.

Skin-popping

This is where the fatty tissue just under the skin is targeted. The medical term is subcutaneous injection. Forearms, thighs, buttocks, and stomach are probably the safest zones.

Intramuscular

The big muscles are usually targeted – top of the arms, mid-thigh, and buttocks. Breasts should be avoided.

Mainlining

Mainlining means targeting the large vein running the length of the inner arm. It is the most thrifty method of disposing of junk and also affords a rush, at least before a big habit builds up. Repeated injections can cause veins to become scarred or thromboid (they get lumpy and collapse), and so others must be sought out in the neck, wrists, feet, behind the knees, etc. The last resort is to return to skin-popping. When seeking out deep veins there is always the danger of hitting an artery, especially in the groin or stomach area. This can lead to damage requiring limb amputation, or even to death.

To prepare powdered heroin for injection it is placed in a teaspoon with a small amount of water (preferably boiled and allowed to cool). If heroin in base form is used (the ubiquitous 'brown') it will need the addition of citric acid or vitamin C powder (ascorbic acid) to ensure that the powder dissolves. Lemon juice and vinegar are sometimes used but these can cause fungal infection. The solution is next warmed by running a flame underneath the spoon (to help dissolve remaining particles) and the solution is then sucked into the syringe and injected. Cleanliness of the injection site and all the paraphernalia is a prerequisite if infection is to be avoided. To filter out any impurities a clean cigarette filter can be placed on the end of the needle and the solution drawn through it. A dab of cotton wool is sometimes used but this can result in fragments of fibres being plunged into the bloodstream where they cause vein damage. Two useful, unpretentious quick guides to safe injecting are: *What Works*, from the Exeter Drugs Project, and *Back to Junkie School with Grandpa Jones*, from Lifeline in Manchester.

Syringe Safety

Needles and syringes should be used only once. Used works should not be carelessly dumped. Someone – e.g.

a child, a refuse collector – could hurt and infect themselves. Needle exchange schemes provide special 'sharp-safe' plastic containers which can then be returned for safe disposal at the agency, or at certain chemists.

If you find it impossible to get to your needle exchange, make sure your used works are securely disposed of in a coffee jar, a tin can or some such.

Sharing injecting gear is best avoided, but if you see no alternative, the following tips can help you avoid infection.

Method one: put a generous squirt of washing-up liquid in a cup and add cold water. Draw the liquid up the needle and into the syringe. Flush it all away (not back into the cup). Draw some more soapy liquid right up and flush that away. Then thoroughly flush the works through with cold water three or four times.

Method two: draw concentrated bleach (e.g. Domestos) from a cup up the needle into the syringe, and flush it away (not back into the bleach bottle). Repeat. Then flush the works through with cold water three or four times.

Where bleach and washing-up liquid are not available, flush the works through with cold water four or five times – although this is a poor third best.

The safest method of all is to take the works apart and boil them in a pan of water for five minutes. But some syringes collapse under this treatment. Check with your syringe exchange agency which type is boil-proof.

By Mouth

This route is seldom used because the drug – which in the stomach is rapidly transformed into morphine – must first pass through the liver before reaching other parts of the body. A great deal of it never reaches other areas, so effective is the liver in breaking the morphine down.

Combinations

Not many opioid users are purists, but will often use other drugs either to heighten the effects or to cope in periods of abstinence. Falling into the latter category are alcohol, barbiturates, and tranquillisers. But while these three depressants might ease the craving, they are of limited use during the actual crunch period of withdrawal. Stimulants such as speed and coke work as anti-soporifics and users often pair up their opioid with a stimulant and inject them together. The archetypical combination is heroin plus cocaine – a *speedball*.

Crack cocaine has also become a favourite with the opioid set in recent years. This is because too much heroin over too long a period kills the buzz and so users need to look elsewhere; and/or they might feel less sordid smoking crack than injecting heroin. Among British blacks of Caribbean origin there has been something of a reverse syndrome at work. Needles and heroin have traditionally been regarded as a degenerate white junkie phenomenon, and where a strong kick was sought coke, then crack, were resorted to. But the jabbering paranoia of too much crack often delivered them to smack – a much *quieter* experience.

Sensations

The effects of heroin are ultimately the same whether snorted, smoked, skin-popped, or mainlined. The special element obtained from the last two methods – especially mainlining – is the *rush*; a climactic sensation at the moments during and shortly after the stuff is pumped into the bloodstream. As with all drugs, the variety of responses to heroin is considerable. Some people get nothing from it, others find it nauseous and repugnant. In fact retching is not unusual for novice users. Practically all who try it must learn how to steer on to a pleasurable track. The experience usually starts seconds after administration (perhaps a minute or so with sniffing) with a warm feeling in the belly which flows throughout the body producing an overall calm, warm, dreamy, self-sufficient feeling. Inevitably, the talk is of 'returning to the womb' or of being 'wrapped in a cocoon'. It is not a euphoric drug in the sense that it sticks a grin on the face, but it does place the troubles of the world at some distance, producing contentment. Some users get drowsy, others become garrulous. One user tells me that he used to enjoy a stiff bicycle ride with his club. At higher doses, it is typical to slip into a dreamy dozing state where the eyes fall shut mid-sentence and the head rolls in a routine known as *gouching*. While gouched-out, users are quite capable of accidentally scarring their bodies with lighted cigarettes, the narcotic powers of the drug dimming any experience of pain. Other more physical effects include sweating, itchy skin, a runny nose, extra peeing, constipation, slowed-down breathing and heart rate, and a lower body temperature. Despite this literally run-down state, the heroin user's brain – at moderate doses – generally remains clear and active. Some claim that because the mind is uncluttered with everyday worries it can go to work – between gouching – more effectively.

As with all things methadone-related, there is no agreement about whether or not there is a useful 'buzz factor' associated with this drug. This is partly because everyone reacts differently but also due to the innate resistance to a substance that is the state's authorised solution to bad habits. One man told me of the 'blinding buzz' he got the first time he used but that subsequently there was only drowsiness. A keen observer of the scene[7] has referred to blind trials in which users given oral doses of heroin and methadone, but not told which was which, were unable to distinguish between the effects of the two drugs. The consensus view, if we search hard enough for one, seems to be that methadone does usually produce a high but not an injecting rush and that the high, while less intense than heroin's, lasts considerably longer.

Pain and the Pleasure Principle

Knowledge of the extremely complex interactions involved in the body's natural defences against pain is still in a primitive state. In recent years much attention has centred on how what turns out to be a painful experience (e.g. a pinch or punch) translates from the initial 'stimuli' into the unpleasant experience. The present state of knowledge suggests that the pinch travels along nerve cells as waves of electrical signals and, upon reaching the brain, these signals are converted into molecular groupings known as neurotransmitters. The best-known neurotransmitter is dopamine. Neurotransmitters next convey the sensation to specialised nerve endings known as receptors.

Found chiefly in areas of the mid-brain, receptors are said to govern the individual's responses to pain by reacting with or binding to a host of natural opiate substances located in and released from other parts of the brain. Claimed to be the most important of the natural painkillers (probably because it has been the most studied) is the so-called 'endorphin'. It gets its name through the combination of the words *endogenous* (meaning originating from within) and *morphine*.[8]

In simple language, the current thesis is that the body has its own chemicals for dealing with pain and distress. They lie in wait, chiefly in diverse parts of the brain, ready to lock on to the site where the experience of pain is registered. As far as opioids are concerned, these too are believed to seek out and lock on to the pain receptor sites. It has been surmised that addicts are people with a low volume of natural opiates, and thus an inadequate natural remedy for pain. They seek out narcotics as a solution. But whether the natural pain-relieving stock runs down as a result of opioid use or whether the individual starts out with a low base can only be guessed at.

But, of course, the whole business is even more complicated than I've just outlined. Addiction is not just about physical pain relief; it involves questions of pleasure, escapism, and all manner of inner torments and urges. Thus, while early scientific attention focused on the brain's own natural opiates (the latest thinking is that authentic morphine and codeine are present in the brain, not just substances similar to them[9]), the big money is now on chasing down the brain's internal chemical messengers, the neurotransmitters – especially the one known as dopamine. Some believe dopamine is 'the substance that helps convert the neurochemical spells of drugs into the brain's own language of habit and pleasure'.[10]

According to a recent *New Scientist* article[11], 'addictive drugs share the ability to hijack a neural pathway in the brain . . . that makes eating, having sex and mothering infants seem pleasurable and worth repeating. In cold biological terms, the threat of addiction is the price we must pay for having evolved the capacity to respond to pleasure; or, if you like, for not being bored to death by sex and food.'

Antagonists

As already indicated, drugs of the opioid family are known as agonists because they are compatible with each other – one being able to relieve the misery of withdrawal from another. A drug that blocks the action of opioids – in other words, stops users getting stoned – and which also precipitates withdrawal symptoms is called an antagonist. One such is naltrexone (brand name Nalorex), an orange-coloured tablet that is sometimes given to recovering addicts to discourage them from old habits. Since it offers no comfort on its own account, it is not especially popular.

Some drugs work, somewhat unpredictably, as both agonists and antagonists. Buprenorphine (Temgesic) and pentazocine (Fortral) are the main examples.

A third category worth noting are the drugs used to bring a person round following opioid overdose. Naloxone is the chosen remedy – a short-acting substance administered by repeated injections in amounts governed by the respiratory rate and depth of coma.

Casual Use

It must be said that heroin use does not automatically equal addiction. The one-hit-and-you're-a-junkie myth is just that. Some people manage to engage in controlled recreational use for years, consuming precisely when they choose to. But it is also true that virtually every addict started out believing s/he could boss the drug.

Problem Use

It is an unpalatable irony that the most cost-effective means of taking heroin is by mainlining it into a vein. This is because the needle route takes the drug straight into the bloodstream and on into the brain with no loss in stray smoke or from material sticking to the nasal passages. It is the stomach which is usually the centre of the injecting experience; the words used to describe the feeling often being of a sexual flavour. For others, the analogy is with death. As the drug is pumped in, the feeling is so overwhelming it is as though they are sinking into oblivion. The joy comes from the relief, moments later, when they discover they are still alive. It is these sorts of melodramatic notions – the sense of running with life-and-death forces, the commingling of deprivation and succor, not to mention the daily panic of ensuring a hit – which keep some addicts engrossed in what in reality is a mundane obsession. And it is from these sources that addicts derive their sense of potency. Normal drug-free living appears too scary, or too scarily empty of meaning, and so a private sensory world is created in which 'normal' human experiences are received in reverse. For the straight citizen, joy is effervescence. For the addict joy is the suppression of such feelings: it is the suppression of sex, hunger, physical vitality, even the need to defecate and cough (though not, interestingly, to piss). The addict's life clearly does more closely resemble death than orgasm, and not surprisingly, some addicts say of themselves that their habit is a long and deliberate suicide.

High-Tech 'Solutions'

Who, then, is most likely to launch themselves into problem heroin use? The vogue these days is to search for genetic explanations. There is, for instance, the so-called 'Al allele' gene – said to 'code' for a particular kind of receptor in the brain which has an affinity for the above-mentioned chemical dopamine. Anyone with Al allele, according to its discoverer, is not only more vulnerable to alcoholism but also to a whole gamut of 'compulsive diseases' including crack and heroin addiction, Tourette's syndrome, unrestrained gambling, and carbohydrate bingeing. The gene's discoverer, Ken Blum, a pharmacologist at Texas University in San Antonio, believes that carriers have a 75 per cent chance of developing some kind of addiction in their lives.[12]

Blum's fellow bio-sleuths are divided on such matters. Some believe the theory to be noodle-headed crap, some cheer him on, others look to the chemistry of the brain itself rather than to the genetic material that 'codes' for it.

What will inevitably follow (and is probably already happening as you read these pages) is a move towards screening of the newborn for the suspect gene – either at the embryo stage, or at some time during childhood. Such screening will at first be for those who can afford it. But if Blum and Co. make their case ardently enough the public might be encouraged to demand screening at the state's expense – an enormously profitable enterprise for those who hold the patents for the equipment and methodology.

Prior to birth, the bad gene – it will be claimed – can be 'fixed'. (Never mind the potentially catastrophic foul-ups.) After birth, different kinds of genetic 'therapies' would be involved. Other options for children with the 'wrong' genetic equipment include aversion counselling and/or special drugs designed to kill off any incipient appetite for mood-altering substances.

A recent *New Scientist* article[13] envisaged multi-disciplinary Dependency Diagnosis Centres where those who harboured fears of innate weaknesses could submit themselves or their offspring to neural (relating to the nervous system) scans, DNA profiling, psychological questionnaires, and life history analysis. The significance of the outcome of such tests would be considerable in terms of the reception the subjects can expect from a school, a medical insurer, or an employer. And, as such tests become commonplace, those who decline to take them might not only be regarded with squint-eyed suspicion, they will probably find all kinds of penalties, subtle and otherwise, falling upon them.

Who *Is* Vulnerable?

So why does one person turn out a 'junkie' and his brother, growing up in the same house, become an abstemious success in the City? Clearly, geneticists prefer genetical explanations, psychologists psychological ones, sociologists believe it's a matter of social discontinuity, while the law-and-order lobby thinks the whole thing can be licked with a lick of discipline. Taking all things together, and in no particular order, we can credit luck, the company that is kept, availability of the substance, inborn vulnerability to these influences, and ignorance about the likely outcome of certain types of use. There is even a suggestion that the way a child is delivered affects his/her chances of developing obsessional tastes in later life.

The records of 200 opiate addicts born in Stockholm between 1945 and 1966 were studied and it was found that the nitrous oxide used to ease their delivery may have played a part in them developing a taste for heroin later in life.[14] The same was true where barbiturates and opiates were given to their mothers during childbirth. These conclusions held fast even after allowing for the social status of the parents and various other factors. (For more details see amphetamines chapter.)

Addiction and Tolerance

Once a person does start succumbing to whichever influences are at work, the drugs have their very own momentum leading towards addiction. The novice will most probably have come to the drug without any specific pain. The odd thing about heroin is that it will soon provide it. (And though some drug professionals reject the idea that pain is experienced during withdrawal, preferring terms like discomfort, pain is how addicts usually perceive and describe what they are going through.) Pain, as the writer Richard Lingeman points out,[15] is heroin's antidote. And vice versa. This pain can develop in mild form after just three or four weeks' use. In other words, the body's molecules can be altered to such an extent, in such a short time, that if the supply is cut off it signals its dismay by ordering pain. If the use has been for a longer period and in larger quantities, then the magnitude of discomfort after withdrawal will increase accordingly. Also speeding up will be the onset of these distress signals relative to the time of last taking the drug. The novice will get high for about four or five hours and experience no distress in the aftermath. The veteran won't get high at all, but merely use the drug, perhaps through a syringe, half a dozen times a day to put the pain at a safe distance. In a real sense the addict gets into the same condition as some terminally ill cancer patients who are also never without pain or distress unless cushioned with an analgesic. One addict put the formula like this: 'Once hooked you're never straight. You're either stoned, or you're ill. I'd say 60 per cent of the time you're sick, 20 per cent of the time you're racing around trying to get the stuff, and the last 20 per cent you sleep.'

How long it takes to get into such a state varies; someone shooting up 30 mg of pure heroin a day will have acquired a reasonably handsome habit within two or three weeks. A daily snorter or chaser of perhaps a quarter-gram of adulterated *brown* will have to work at it longer. More typically, people drift into addiction, taking weeks, months, or even years, and thereafter dropping in and out of dependent use. But once caught in the addiction spiral there are formidable obstacles to quitting. The actual physical withdrawal is not especially awesome – although it can appear so from the addict's perspective – and not in the least physically threatening. It is often compared with a stiff bout of gastric 'flu (an analogy that rankles most of those who have gone through it), and as with that ailment can be faced out if a good, comfortable environment is found with nourishment and rest. Many addicts face it. Many times. The reasons for slipping back are various.

On a *social* level there are the obvious reasons of same old environment, same old drug-using crowd. And if there's no job, what else is there except drugs, and the time-filling scramble to score them? Boredom defeats many recovering addicts. Family and straight friends have maybe exhausted their patience, so there isn't even a warm hearth to come home to. Extending from these social factors are a number of political circumstances such as the government's faltering commitment to pick-up-and-mend facilities, the failed strategy of most treatment options, and the continuing persecution through the courts of ordinary users.

On the *psychological* level there is the user's own innate 'defects' of character or those that have been inculcated during the course of addiction. The individual probably feels weak, scared, guilty, useless, lacking in substance, or perhaps filled with powerful inadmissible drives. The heroin has provided relief from these feelings by laying a cloak over them. To remove the cloak without dealing with what's underneath is to invite relapse.

On a *biological* level there is the relationship between pain, pleasure, sex, and the actual fabric of the body and the various chemicals swimming around it. Is addiction predetermined? Or is the attachment freely entered into? Whichever the case, former addicts will often experience vague miseries for many years. They will feel the cravings return when simply passing through an old drug haunt or seeing a familiar face. Equally, addicts making a fresh start in new territory invariably do better than if they had remained subject to the old drug-taking cues and prompts.

Health

Impact on the body

There is little evidence that heroin causes serious physical problems in itself, even when taken for a lifetime. The problems come from unstable patterns of use, from adulterants, from the hypodermic syringe, the company an addict keeps, and the general run-down in health caused by poor eating and rest which results from a drug-fixated existence. Regular users often find themselves breathless, deeply constipated, and for ever coughing up phlegm. They also lose their appetite for food and sex and, because there's an increased risk of respiratory problems, this, in turn, can lead to various lung ailments. Pneumonia is especially common among users, whether or not they inject. Friends might recognise growing use by a marked weight loss, a pale or jaundiced complexion, and a constantly dripping nose.

Risks of injecting

There are health risks common to injectors of any substance. These include vein damage and inflammation and infections at the injection site. Hitting an artery instead of a vein can lead to the loss of a limb or worse. Arteries take blood under high pressure away from the heart to the far corners of the body. Veins bring the blood back to the heart. You know you've hit an artery if the plunger is forced back by the pressure of blood or if, when you pull back, the blood comes out frothy. If this happens, pull out the needle, raise the limb, and apply firm pressure for at least ten minutes. If bleeding continues, get help.[16]

HIV/AIDS

The sharing of the paraphernalia associated with injecting[17] can lead to the transmission from person to person (via traces of blood) of a whole range of bacterial and viral infections, the most discussed and feared being the Human Immunodeficiency Virus (HIV). Other ways of transmitting HIV are through semen and pre-ejaculate fluid, menstrual blood, vaginal secretions, and breast milk.[18]

The role of HIV in causing a range of infections leading up to the devastating Acquired Immune Deficiency Syndrome (AIDS) is still disputed. Some believe it to be just one of several 'co-factors' that produce a breakdown of the body's immune system and the cluster of opportunistic infections and malignancies that follow. Others[19] go further and suggest that HIV is merely a harmless 'passenger' virus, antibodies to which happen to turn up in most *but not all* cases of AIDS. (Whether this theory is right or wrong, whether HIV is a plague or a phantom, it still makes sense to go safety-first during sex and when injecting drugs.)

The very existence of AIDS is doubted in some quarters. It is argued that AIDS is merely a new name for a collection of old conditions, as witnessed by the tendency of the medical authorities to revise and extend, from time to time, the list of defining ailments whose presence calls for an AIDS diagnosis.

But the clear consensus view is that AIDS does exist and that it is caused by HIV. Many people who test HIV antibody positive will remain essentially well for ten years, some for twenty years, and others will never get sick. But most who test 'positive' will eventually succumb to various of the defining diseases and tumours drawn up by the US Center for Disease Control and Prevention. They include protozoal infections (e.g. cryptosporidiosis), tuberculosis, cytomegalovirus, herpes simplex, Kaposi's sarcoma, lymphoma, neurological conditions such as dementia, and HIV wasting disease.[20]

In women, three gynaecological conditions are linked to AIDS: vaginal candida (thrush), cervical cancer, and pelvic inflammatory disease. Children are prone to a form of pneumonia known as lymphatic interstitial pneumonitis.

Hepatitis

Hepatitis, a viral infection affecting the liver, long predates AIDS in the drug-injecting community. It is also far more easily transmitted than HIV. There are three main hepatitis viral strains. Hepatitis A is associated with poor hygiene – especially infected food and water. The two versions most relevant to drug injectors are B and C. Although both are most easily transmitted through blood, B is also found in semen, urine, and saliva. This opens the possibility for transmission through such household items as razors, unwashed cutlery, toothbrushes, flannels, etc. The question of transmission within families through items like Hep C has become more a cause for worry since 1989 when an antibody test was first developed.[21] By 1993 it was being suggested that as many as 60 per cent of the injecting drug users in Britain might be infected with it.[22]

As to the disease progression, Hepatitis B incubates for about three months, during which time the carrier is highly infectious to others. There then follows a range of symptoms – typically fever, flu, and jaundice. A small number of people will suffer liver failure but, more typically, a full recovery is experienced within about six months. In about 10 per cent of cases, however (more in women), the virus persists. These individuals not only remain infectious to others, they run the risk of developing cirrhosis of the liver and/or liver cancer.

The evolution of Hepatitis C disease is less well understood but there appear to be two phases:[23] the first, covering the six months after initial infection, results in the kind of mild symptoms associated with the B version. Then comes the chronic phase, experienced by about two-thirds of cases. This is when the virus grows in the liver, killing off some cells, leading ultimately – perhaps after twenty years – to cirrhosis. By year twenty-five or thirty, liver cancer can result. Immoderate booze consumption will make both these outcomes much more likely. It seems Hepatitis C carriers are always infectious.

All three versions of hepatitis can be passed on by pregnant women, via the placenta, to their offspring, with a suggestion that transmission of Hep C from mother to child occurs in about 16 per cent of cases.[24]

The only available treatment for Hepatitis C is interferon alfa – given by injection three times a week for up to a year. The cure rate is said to be about one in four. While there have been calls for widespread screening and administration of the drug for those affected, some have criticised the proposal for the 'astronomical' costs that would be involved and the detrimental impact this would have on medical care as a whole.[25] Known side effects[26] of interferon alfa include flu-like symptoms (a common occurrence), lethargy, depression, heart problems, liver toxicity, thyroid abnormalities, and skin rashes.

A further complication in dealing with Hepatitis C is that there are actually six types of this one main virus, three of them found in the UK. And each of these six can be further broken down into at least three more sub-types.[27] In fact, as with HIV, it is quite likely that a constant process of mutation is taking place.

Overdoses

The term overdose (OD) simply means the ingestion of a quantity of drug that the body hasn't built a tolerance to. Once overloaded, the body reacts in a number of ways, some of them fatal. The 'classic' overdose that ends lethally takes from one to twelve hours to run its course. It starts with slow, shallow, or simply irregular breathing. The pupils reduce to a pinpoint, the skin turns blue (hence the street name – 'bluey'), blood pressure is severely diminished; then comes coma. Pure antagonists (see above) can immediately reverse these effects, but since they set off potentially dangerous withdrawal symptoms they should never be taken without medical supervision. Death, when it does occur, usually results from respiratory failure and complications in the region of the heart.

Why ODs happen

Over-indulgence by an addict who is insecure about supplies is a common cause of ODs. Another pitfall is where tolerance to the drug's respiratory depressant effects is allowed to fall as a result of a period of not using. When the old high dose is suddenly administered the body can't cope. Addicts who have gone into hospital or prison are particularly vulnerable to this fate when they return to old levels of consumption. Another OD cause is the use of street heroin purer than the user anticipated.

For safety's sake it's best not to fix alone (or in the company of people who are out of it) and certainly not in a place where you're unlikely to be found should you get into trouble.

ODs and Methadone

As previously indicated, methadone is now associated with many more overdose deaths than heroin, even though some claim there to be perhaps 200,000 heroin users as against only 20,000 on methadone.[28] The state's fix, according to Dr John Marks, Merseyside consultant psychiatrist, 'is more addictive, more dangerous and more deadly than heroin itself. It's toxic muck and should be banned.[29]

Sudden Deaths

A more dramatic outcome that is often called an OD is where the user dies with the works still hanging in his/her arm. Why such deaths happen isn't known. The bodies of victims don't always show a high drug count, nor is it necessarily the fault of an adulterant. Some doctors put it down to shock, others to 'acute allergic reaction'.

Pulmonary oedema

This is a particularly horrifying way of perishing. The victim more or less drowns from bodily fluids that surge into the lungs. The problems start with heart failure, causing the pulmonary arteries (those leading to the lungs) to become congested with blood. As pressure builds and the heart can no longer pump away the blood, fluid is forced out of the capillaries (tiny blood vessels) straight into the lungs.

Suffocation

This happens because of blockages to the air passages by (most commonly) vomit that under normal circumstances would be sicked up. OD victims who have also been drinking are especially prone to this sometimes fatal complication.

With Other Drugs

The simultaneous use of opioids and certain other drugs can be problematic. Heroin and alcohol together may cause vomiting – especially dangerous if the combination has caused unconsciousness. Opioids used with any of the central nervous system depressants (barbiturates, major and minor tranquillisers, as well as drink) accentuate respiratory depressant effects.

Serious, sometimes fatal, reactions have occurred following the administration of pethidine to patients receiving a type of anti-depressant drug known as monoamine oxidase inhibitors (MAOIs). Pethidine and related opioids should not be taken within two weeks of stopping MAOI therapy. Indeed, the use of any opioid with an MAOI seems to present a 'special hazard'.[30]

Complications can also result when opioids are taken

with certain anticoagulants, anti-epileptics, and antivirals (eg AZT).

In Association with Medical Conditions

Opioids can also cause problems for individuals with severe respiratory ailments such as those found in asthmatics and cyanosis sufferers; also for those with illnesses related to alcohol problems, hypothyroidism, low blood pressure, liver disorders, certain prostate conditions, and anyone suffering with obstructed or inflamed bowels.

Opioids and Women

The repeated use of any drug places a strain on the liver, but because women's livers are usually half the size of men's they are more susceptible to harm.

Habitual use commonly stops ovulation and a woman may not see a period for several months or even years if her habit continues. The cycle usually returns to normal when the drug is stopped. Other women will not have a period, but ovulation will continue sporadically. This masking of the cycle makes it easier to get pregnant unwittingly. Diarrhoea during withdrawal might render the contraceptive pill ineffective.[31]

Pregnancy[32]

For pregnant drug users of whatever substance there is an increased risk of giving birth to underweight babies, either as a result of retarded growth in the womb or through premature delivery. There is also a higher incidence of perinatal mortality (death within the first week of birth) – being born early increasing the risk of such deaths. More congenital abnormalities also turn up in the offspring of dependent drug users.

Many of these depressing outcomes cannot necessarily be

tied directly to the effects of one drug or another, but to their combined use; also to the kind of poor diet and chaotic living conditions generally associated with heavy drug use.

But the constant statistical association between opioid use and low birthweight, premature deliveries and stillbirths is to be taken seriously – even though some experts suggest that the 'mechanism' at work is not the drug itself but the woman's erratic on-off drug consumption leading to the developing foetus going into repeated episodes of withdrawal and, quite often, being born prematurely.[33]

Though many women wish to quit drug use when they find themselves pregnant (in an effort to protect their child and 'make a fresh start), abrupt withdrawal should be avoided. Some women can be helped to withdraw slowly. For others it's better to be maintained on a steady dose of methadone whose supply will at least be guaranteed.

Junkie babies

The spectre of junkie babies is a lip-smacking one for the tabloid media. That some babies of drug-using mothers do go through a withdrawal syndrome when born is undeniable – although it can often be minimised where doctors are properly trained and prepared. Symptoms vary from mild to serious. Typically, the infant is irritable and hyperactive. S/he does not sleep or feed well and has a characteristic high-pitched cry. In extreme cases, twitching and spasms might lead to convulsions. The general constitution of mother and baby are important in determining how severe any withdrawal might be. In the past, mothers were encouraged to blow opium smoke into the child's mouth to alleviate withdrawal symptoms. Today, chlorpromazine (the 'liquid cosh' major tranquilliser) is commonly used, although some physicians favour benzodiazepines, with opiates employed as a last resort.

Pregnant users can be reluctant to disclose their habit for fear of social services stepping in and removing the child. But even where hospitals have no forewarning, distress to the baby can usually be greatly minimised if the medical team has had the proper training (a rarity) and refrains from taking a panicky, moralistic line.

Breastfeeding

Most drugs do not pass into the breast milk in quantities that will have a major effect on the newborn. But breastfeeding is not advised for mothers on a methadone regime exceeding 80 mg.

Morality and medicine

Where drug-using pregnant women get the right antenatal care and social support the outlook for them and their child is greatly improved. It is far better, notes Dr Mary Hepburn, consultant obstetrician at Glasgow's Royal Maternity Hospital, to 'objectively identify the real problems and distinguish early between medicine and morality . . . Using this approach we found that of the first 200 babies born to women drug users attending the service, only seven per cent required treatment for withdrawal symptoms while even fewer required admission to the special care nursery.'[34]

Earliest Use

Opium, the mother plant of both heroin and morphine, has proved a seductive and often scary proposition from the time humankind first incised the poppy pod and saw its milky juice ooze out. It is not known exactly when that was, although there are written references to the poppy as the 'joy plant' in Sumerian texts judged to be 6,000 years old. The Sumerians occupied land in what is now southern Iraq, and it seems that most of the peoples of the Middle East were familiar with poppy juice as a balm for both body and spirit. The first clear-cut reference to the plant's pharmacology is in the third-century-BC writings of the Greek philosopher and botanist Theophrastus. Contemporaries were already warning about the drug's addictive potential.

Though opium smoking is firmly affixed by folklorists to 'Chinamen', it was many centuries before the Chinese developed their taste for the drug and they probably hadn't even glimpsed opium until Arab traders brought it to them in the seventh or eighth century AD. It was used by the Chinese chiefly as a medicine until the seventeenth century, when a fad developed for warming globs in a candle flame and inhaling the fumes. The practice alarmed the Emperor who, in 1729, ordered all imports to be stopped (China was manufacturing virtually none of her own) unless under licence. But the decree had little impact and the drug continued to flow into the country, largely though the Portuguese who had a settlement in Macao. The Portuguese did well enough from opium, but it was the British who really stepped up trade and in the process became the world's largest peddlers of the drug. Her stocks came from the newly conquered land of the Bengals in the Indian subcontinent. Her agent was the East India Company, which owned the monopoly on the Bengal poppy harvest. Though already selling a portion to the Chinese, under licence, the company saw the chance to do far better out of China's 300-million population. As Brian Inglis notes in his book *The Forbidden Game*,[35] there was a snag: foreigners were permitted to trade with China only though Canton.

The East India Company enjoyed a monopoly of British trade there. If the company shipped in more opium than allowed under licence, it might lose that monopoly.

The solution was to sell the drug in India to Indian merchants who could then smuggle it into China. That way the British stayed legal. By these means, and ignoring Imperial edicts to cease the trade, the drug had reached deep into the interior by the early 1800s. It reached Peking and into the palace itself, enslaving members of the Emperor's bodyguards and his court eunuchs. Back home in England a rumbling started over the correctness of pushing so much of what was now considered a destructive drug. A House of Commons Committee of Enquiry was set up in 1830 to scrutinise the East India Company's affairs, but this was easily disarmed by lies and bogus moral posturing. The company line of argument was that it had to retain its opium monopoly in order to ensure prices remained high enough to restrict 'non medical' demand. An even more decisive argument was the economic one. The opium trade with China was worth over £2 million which, as Inglis notes, was almost half the amount it cost annually to service the Crown and the civil service in Britain. If not from opium sales, where would the revenues come? From British taxpayers?

The Company was deprived of some privileges and allowed to retain others so that, in effect, it was the British government itself which emerged with the direct responsibility for future opium trade between India and China. The true impact of that trade on the eighteenth- and nineteenth-century Chinese is open to argument, but it is believed to have bitten particularly sharply into the army and into the children of the wealthy and powerful. The Chinese Emperor himself (Tao-Kwang) is said to have lost his three eldest sons from opium addiction.

So what were the Chinese to do? They tried flogging and the *cangue* (a sort of mobile stocks). They tried exile and capital punishment. They seriously considered, in the late 1830s, legalising the drug so as to abolish any need for the black market, but the legalisation lobby lost the argument and in its place the Emperor went to the root of the problem or at least as much of that root as was visible. Most traffickers lived in Canton. It would therefore be sensible to arrest them there, send all their ships home, and forbid more trade of any kind until opium smuggling ceased completely. The man placed in charge of executing the new policy was one Lin-Tse-hsu, and he had barely taken office in 1839 when he ordered British merchants to surrender 20,000 chests containing approximately 140 lbs of opium each. The chests were polluted with salt and lime and flushed into the sea. Lin-Tse-hsu had then intended to purge the Customs service, but ran into the kind of blanket resistance anti-dopists have encountered throughout history. The drug was simply too much in demand and the trafficking structure too sensitive for prohibitory moves to make headway. If the authorities lunged at imports, bigger bribes were paid to bent officials to account for their extra risk. The additional margin was acquired from the customer who, if addicted, would pay almost any price and simply turn to crime to get money for new supplies. And if the authorities clamped down with more stringent penalties, the participants would get even more desperate, more likely to kill to hide their traces.

Even as Commissioner Lin Tse-hsu was learning this baneful lesson the British were sounding off about 'the most shameful violence' that was the destruction of their opium stocks. In June 1840 an expeditionary force was despatched, and two years later a miserable capitulation had been extracted from the Chinese, under the Treaty of Nanking. The island of Hong Kong was ceded, trading and residential rights were gained at several more ports, and there was an indemnity of £60 million China was obliged to offer Britain as compensation for the loss of her opium and the cost of conducting the war. Within a few years other Western powers moved in to claim their portion and the long-dreaded 'Invasion of the Barbarians' became a reality.

In the decade following the Nanking Treaty, opium trade with China (not all accounted for by the British) doubled. A new emperor made more stout moves to prevent the drug's consumption (beheading for persistent users, their families sent into slavery), but he hadn't the muscle to make it stick, even in friendly parts of the empire. Finally another commissioner was sent to Canton to take up the cudgel once wielded by Lin Tse-hsu. The new man, Yeh Ming-Chen, was more circumspect, but the British were once more on the look-out for grave insults and thus an excuse to undertake a new military excursion. There were issues beyond opium now. Along with France and America, Britain was unhappy with the general level of trade that had resulted from concessions under the Nanking Treaty. If more ports could be opened up, she believed, the situation would be righted, and the only way to effect such a rupture was militarily. The pretext came in 1856 when a Chinese-crewed smuggling ship was apprehended off Canton. When Commissioner Yeh Ming-Chen refused to apologise for seizing this 'British' vessel (it ran a British flag in the hopes of deterring searches) the British navy shelled his official residence. Back in England a public row broke out. But when Lord Palmerston called a general election on the issue of the grave Chinese insult to the Crown, he found an electorate boiling up with patriotism and could thus claim a mandate for a second war.

The second opium war opened up eleven more ports to Westerners. In addition, the drug was made legal in return for a modest duty payable to the Chinese authorities. Opium trade rose briskly from about 60,000 chests in 1859 to more than 105,000 in 1880 – most of it derived from British India. The Chinese addict population is said to have been in excess of 15 million.

At this point the Chinese authorities finally absorbed the lesson that it is better to take a yen than a beating. They now permitted, even encouraged, the growing of Chinese opium, to try to reduce the strain on their currency. The British resisted by forcing import duties down in order to make their own Indian supplies more competitive, but within a few decades Chinese home-grown production had outstripped British imports from India. The wheel had turned full circle: the drug Britain and other Western powers had pushed on the Chinese under force of arms was beginning to travel in the reverse direction amid sounds of terrible panic and indignation. The West had long been consuming tinctures of medical opium and, later on, therapeutic shots of morphine, but this smoking of the drug . . . this was considered a filthy, entirely foreign habit.

The European Experience

Though Europeans are on record as having used opium as far back as the ancient Greeks (who also used to smoke it) it wasn't until the Renaissance that the drug began to saturate most parts of Europe. This development was due largely to a pharmacological breakthrough by the formidable Swiss physician, Bombastus von Hohenheim (1493–1541), better known as Paracelsus. His great feat was to produce a tincture of opium by mixing the drug with alcohol. He named it laudanum and it amounted to the beginning not merely of sedation on a mass scale, but the development of what we now know as pharmacology: 'the search for specific drugs in the treatment of specific diseases.'[36] Successive generations of physicians toyed with Paracelsus' prototype – adding to it sherry and spices – and by the seventeenth century laudanum was regarded as the indispensable tool of medicine. It was the aspirin/Valium of its day, used both to kill pain and sedate. It was considered the answer to diarrhoea, coughs, menstrual cramps and the discomfort of colicky and teething babies.

If Paracelsus invented pharmacology, then its modern era was launched in 1805 when the German apothecary Frederick Sertürner isolated morphine from opium. This separation of what was known as the 'active principle' from its parent was also rightly recognised as a brilliant feat; it allowed for the first time the administration of near exact doses. What was curiously missed by Sertürner and those who fêted him was the danger of addiction posed by a drug that was ten times more potent than opium – which was by now known to cause dependence. Indeed, by 1825 morphine was being marketed as a cure for opium addiction. That there could be problems from the unguarded use of the new drug didn't click even after the hypodermic syringe came into popular use around 1850. In a strange reversal of today's piece of folk whimsy which says you can't get a heroin habit by smoking, only by injecting, it was then believed you couldn't get a morphine habit by injecting, only by smoking. The majority of physicians still were not aware of the consequences of rampant morphine prescribing even after the American Civil War ended in 1866 and some 45,000 soldiers came home, dependent on their fixes.

In England too 'morphinomania' had taken hold – and in the smartest of circles. The author of one 1887 report described how some society women possessed a 'regular arsenal of little injecting instruments . . . Ladies belonging to the most elegant classes of society go so far as to show their good taste in the jewels which they order to conceal a little syringe and artistically made bottles, which are destined to hold the solution which enchants them. At the theatre, in society, they slip away for a moment, or even watch for a favourable opportunity of pretending to play with these trinkets, while giving themselves an injection of morphia . . .'[37]

There was, of course, a corps of progressive physicians who did recognise the problems of morphine addiction, but almost every attempt to correct the situation failed. For a while cocaine was pushed as the answer – users simply switched to leaning on the newer drug, or on both at the same time. The idea that addiction could be knocked flat by administering a more powerful substance continued with the invention of heroin in 1874. Named from the German word *heroisch* meaning heroic or powerful, it was three to four times more potent than its predecessor, and was marketed as a safe, non-addictive substitute for morphine.

A conspiracy theorist might begin to wonder when we consider that it was a German physician who developed laudanum, a German apothecary who isolated morphine, and the Bayer Company in Germany which began commercial production of heroin in 1898. It was also in Germany during World War II that methadone was invented as a 'safe' substitute for heroin. Methadone, we now know, can hold a person by the throat every bit as determinedly as heroin and causes more protracted withdrawal.

Birth of the Junkie

If the abuse of drugs is an inescapable feature of human culture, we don't have to ask: 'When did abuse start?' The answer is easy: 'At the beginning.' Opium was being taken to excess in ancient Greece, and it is clear that more than a decent amount of laudanum was used almost as soon as it was introduced to Britain. But there was no clear distinction between medical and recreational users until the second half of the nineteenth century when doctors and pharmacists began co-opting the sole dispensing rights to opium and its derivatives. Before this, the various preparations (pills, powders, lozenges, wines, tinctures, enemas, etc.) were on sale from several kinds of locations. These included corner grocers, market stalls, and public houses, as well as chemist shops. The new monopoly arrangement not only served the professional interests of doctors and druggists – giving them access to a large pool of fee-paying 'patients' – it signalled the beginnings of the 'medical context'. And that meant anything falling outside was necessarily deviant. As the availability of all psychoactive drugs became more and more severely controlled, with possession rather than just sales restricted, so the junkie and his culture was forged.

Alcohol apart, worries about immoderate drug use in the early part of the nineteenth century centred mainly on what was called 'opium eating'. In fact it was the drinking of tinctures. Panic waves are reputed to have been caused by the 1821 publication of Thomas de Quincey's *Confessions of an English Opium Eater* wherein the essayist writes of the terrors of an addiction gained at Oxford while trying to manage the pain of neuralgia. 'I have struggled against this fascinating enthralment with a religious zeal, and have, at length, accomplished what I never yet heard attributed to any other man – have untwisted, almost to its final links, the accursed chain which fettered me.'

De Quincey let it be known that he had plenty of company among the illustrious classes when it came to opium eating, although he fell short of naming names. It took 150 years and the discovery of a druggist's ledger in a Scottish attic before the handsome habit of the writer Sir Walter Scott was discovered. Between 1823 and 1825, said the records, Scott and his wife had been supplied with 22 quarts (5.5 gallons) of laudanum and 18 dozen opium lozenges and pills.[38] Other literary figures whose output was coloured by their opium experiences included Coleridge, Byron, Shelley, Keats, and Elizabeth Barrett Browning.

The working classes were a bigger concern. De Quincey describes demand, by the 1820s, as being 'immense' in London and spreading beyond.[39] He tells of hearing from several Manchester cotton manufacturers that opium eating was rapidly becoming a habit among the workforce, so much so that 'on a Saturday afternoon the counters of the druggists were strewed with pills of one, two or three grains in preparation for the known demand of the evening. The immediate occasion of this practise was the lowness of wages, which at that time would not allow them to indulge in ale or spirits.'

Reports of such usage aren't especially plentiful but they repeatedly emerge from deepest working-class districts where the factories and ports were located – and also areas like the Fens where women took heartily to the habit. The social fabric of Imperial England, it seemed to the authorities, was under stress.

The fears took on a different shade with the discovery of opium smoking among England's Chinese population. In 1861, according to the historian Virginia Berridge, there were an estimated 167 Chinese people living in the entire country.[40] They lived principally in the Limehouse district in London's East End, and initially had been employed as sailors by that supreme opium pedlar, the East India Company. By 1881 there were still just 665 Chinese, but in those two decades the British public had been alerted to the menace the immigrés and their despicable habit posed. Berridge cites[41] an 1868 article in *London Society Magazine*, among the first descriptions of domestic opium smoking. The account reports on a man called Chi Ki and his English wife who kept open house for smokers. The 'den' is described as 'mean and miserable', but not a threatening place. When Charles Dickens got hold of the theme for his unfinished *Mystery of Edwin Drood* (1870), there is an injection of macabre evil – and it was this note which sounded with increasing resonance all through the last years of the century.

A London County Council inspector notes of his visit to one den in 1904: 'Oriental cunning and cruelty . . . was hallmarked on every countenance. Until my visit to the Asiatic Sailors' Home, I had always considered some of the Jewish inhabitants of Whitechapel to be the worst type of humanity I had ever seen.'[42] The LCC tried to put a stop to opium smoking by licensing all seamen's lodging houses. Where the drug was discovered the licence would be removed, and with it the proprietor's livelihood. But the measure failed because of ambiguity over what was a 'seaman', what was a 'lodging house', and the deftness shown by the Chinese in throwing off the inspectors. The search for the 'wretched den' was in any case a hopeless task, for rather than taking place in a specially commissioned pit, smoking, as Berridge notes, was simply something that went on for relaxation in what was akin to a Chinese social club, usually poorly furnished, but no more so than a local pub. However, it didn't matter that serious investigators repeatedly came away from these places without evidence of depravity; the public at large wasn't going to be deprived. It was a time of widespread anti-immigrant sentiment – most of it directed at Jews – but with enough venom left over for other foreigners. Egged on by increasingly lurid newspaper and fictional accounts, the anti-opium, anti-Chinese movement grew.

The American Experience

Precisely the same drift, but on a grander scale, had been taking place in the US. In contrast to the pocketful of Chinese who trickled into Britain during the nineteenth century, from

1850 onwards America received scores of thousands. They came with the specific purpose of working the mines and fields of the west so that they could save a hatful of money and return home. But the passage over encumbered most of them with debts; the cost of food and lodgings were more barriers to saving and few were able to make that triumphal homecoming.[43] The Chinese who remained in America became perpetual transients. They were obliged to keep separate from 'decent' society, setting up homes in the dingiest red-light districts where they added opium smoking to the domestic vices of gambling, drinking, and prostitution.

'The opium den,' write Terry Parssinen, 'became something of a "rogue's" paradise . . . where thieves, pimps, prostitutes and saloon keepers would enjoy conversation and relax over a few pipes in the wee hours of the morning, knowing that the informal code prohibited violence or robbery within the den.'[44]

The smoking went on in relative peace until, in the mid-1870s, one of those cyclical depressions hit the US economy, and the Chinese switched from being a vital source of labour to an aggravating surplus. Irrespective of the economic downturn, this was a time of major transformations throughout American life, with immigration from all parts of Europe as well as Asia. Many of the newcomers, unwilling to do farm work, began crowding into the fast-expanding cities which began exhibiting many of today's urban problems.[45]

The changes seemed to threaten the core of American identity, especially the dominant position of a Protestant, North European group that had controlled the affairs of the nation throughout the Civil War.[46]

Inevitably aliens began getting more carefully scrutinised – not least the oriental opium fiends. Newspaper stories spoke of the seduction of young whites as part of a Chinese-led global slave trade. As with all panics the stories weren't entirely divorced from fact: there were indeed daring young whites smoking in Chinatown, and there was involvement in prostitution by some Chinese, but it was some jump from there into the deep and fantastical waters that led to America's first anti-narcotic laws. In 1875 San Francisco was the first town to pass an ordinance prohibiting opium smoking. Over the next forty years twenty-seven more states followed suit, but smoking still increased until the mid-1890s when annual importation of crude opium levelled off at around half a million pounds.

This isn't to suggest that the taste for drugs was thus dispelled. With the heat on opium young men and boys of the inner-city slums simply switched to drugs that were cheaper, didn't smell, and could be more easily hidden. That meant heroin and morphine, and to a lesser extent cocaine. By 1930 the old-style therapeutic addict was on the way out. In his/her place came the dangerous street-wise runt.

Modern Use and Controls

The international process of organised controls can be traced back to a series of meetings between 1909 and 1914 which established the framework for narcotics legislation worldwide. The first symposium was held in Shanghai and, at the instigation of the Americans, focused on opiate use in the Far East. Britain was cool on this initiative, not necessarily (as American commentators have suggested) because of her trading interests in the area, but because she was suspicious of America's gung-ho internationalism. She preferred the one-to-one approach and had already established by these means an Anglo-Chinese agreement that limited opium traffic. Also, Britain suspected the US of being more concerned with promoting her own influence in the Far East than in doing good for humanity.

By the time the first of three Hague Conferences came round in 1911, Britain's position was less ambivalent. Alarmed at increased drug smuggling to her Asian colonies, she demanded that the meetings look not just at opium smuggling to the Far East, but at morphine and cocaine too in terms of a worldwide system of control. The Americans agreed, but the Germans, who had their own special cocaine manufacturing interests, threw a proviso into the works: there was no point in the convention pledging itself to fair play, the Germans argued, unless a sufficient number of nations agreed to join in the game with them. So while the framework could be sorted out there could be no commitment until there were thirty-five signatories. This was how the situation was left at the outbreak of the First World War.

For the British authorities the war period brought home just how vulnerable the political health of the nation could be to uncontrolled drug use. In 1916 the Army enacted Regulation 40B of the Defence of the Realm Act (DORA 40B), making it an offence for anyone to supply cocaine or any other drug to a member of the armed forces unless ordered by a doctor through a written prescription which had to be signed, dated and marked 'not to be repeated'. Although this was an unprecedentedly stiff measure, it didn't tackle the general volume of domestic traffic and didn't apply itself at all to the problems of smuggling to the colonies. The next step for the Home Office was to extend DORA 40B to the entire civilian population who, it was argued, faced no less grave a menace from mood-altering drugs, alcohol included. Drink was taxed, premises supplying it had to be licensed, and hours of opening were limited. The most detailed restrictions under the civilian extension fixed on cocaine, but raw and powdered opium came in for only marginally less stringent controls. The Home Office had also wanted to bring morphine into line, but because of its more thoroughly medical context, was unable to wade through the opposition. Further legislative controls tightened up imports of cocaine and raw opium products by means of a new licensing system. By now the Home Office had positioned itself firmly in the cockpit of drugs policy, a position it has never yielded and is never likely to.

At the same time there were bolder moves being made on the global canvas. The Versailles Peace Treaty of 1918 placed responsibility for international narcotics regulations in the hands of the fledgling League of Nations (later it would pass on to the United Nations). Article 295 of the Versailles Peace Pact proclaimed that, within one year, what had been agreed at The Hague before the war but left unsigned would have to be put into action. The pact made it encumbent on individual nations to introduce their own domestic legislation. Britain responded with the Dangerous Drugs Act 1920 (DDA). In effect, DDA was DORA 40, but widened to draw in other drugs such as medical opium and morphine. A lot of its nitty-gritty was reserved for the regulations that would follow the Act's passage through Parliament. The new Ministry of Health had wanted to impose itself in the formulation of

312

these regulations but was easily beaten back by the Home Office. 'The following four years', notes that diligent historian Virginia Berridge, 'saw consistent Home Office attempts to impose a policy completely penal in direction.'[47] There were moves to ban maintenance prescribing to addicts. There were moves to concoct a blacklist of doctor-addicts that would be circulated to wholesale druggists; and attempts to reach into the finest details of prescribing. In short, complained a Streatham pharmacist, the profession was being 'treated as a dangerous body of criminals.'

The British System

From these tensions came the government-appointed Rolleston Committee, under Sir Humphrey Rolleston, President of the Royal College of Physicians. Set up in 1924 and reporting two years later, the main brief for Rolleston's panel was to decide whether or not physicians should be allowed to prescribe narcotics to addicts. In particular, there was the question of long-term prescribing. For, by this time, it was deemed legitimate medical practice to maintain habitual users on their drug of addiction if other treatments failed and if they could live 'normal and useful lives' when given a regular stable dose but were unable to do so if the supply was cut off.[48] Rolleston's working party conducted a strange, complacent investigation calling no addicts, hearing chiefly medical witnesses, and considering only as an afterthought such lower-class habits as the drinking of Chlorodyne patent medicine. In Rolleston's eyes there was principally one sort of addict: s/he was middle class, middle aged, often from the medical profession, and invariably an abuser of morphine. About five hundred such individuals existed nationwide, and rather than representing a threat they were to be pitied. The recommendations were that the UK turn away from the US penal route by allowing the profession a better grip on the problem. Morphine and heroin should continue to be prescribed – long-term if thought necessary – and confidentiality had to be retained between patient and doctor, with no obligation to notify the Home Office about who was being treated, how and why. In this way, the Home Office got its slapdown and heroin continued to be prescribed in Britain for almost forty years, making the system – the British system – a stark and globally contentious curio. One American commentator described the arrangement as 'the epitome of amoral expediency'. In return, it was said of the US decision to enact a total prohibition of alcohol and opium that, 'Barbarians is not too strong a phrase for people who have such an extraordinary savage idea of stamping out all people who happen to disagree with their views.'[49]

The liberality of Rolleston was taken for granted for years, but it was subsequently realised that in the seeds of those recommendations were the makings of a far grimmer regime. The better-deal-for-addicts policy applied only as long as they remained numerically small and decorously middle class. When a new wave of raggedy-arsed users arrived in the late 1950s, UK drugs policy once more revealed its spikier profile and the medical profession its willingness to operate a system at odds with what 'kindly old' Rolleston envisaged. Now the threat was perceived not merely in terms of personal pathology – the individual struggling against a sickness – but as a challenge to what has more recently been called community safety by a class of user regarded as hedonistic and socially deviant. Instead of confidentiality, all addicts were to be notified to the Home Office. Instead of the one-to-one GP arrangement, addicts were to be redirected to special clinics presided over by psychiatrists, with GPs being stripped of their right to prescribe.

The new clinics

The new clinic system was established in 1968 on the recommendation of another government committee – this time headed by Sir Russell (later Lord) Brain. They resulted from Brain's second report; the first, in 1961, more or less repeated Rolleston's recommendations, completely missing the advent of the new-style street addicts. By 1965 their numbers had grown so markedly that Brain was called out once more to look at what might be done. He believed the main reason for the 1960s addiction problem was the wanton over-prescribing by a coterie of private London doctors. Because there was so much being dispensed, addicts were selling off the surplus to friends, creating more addicts who were in turn over-prescribed, and so on. An apparent answer to this malfunction would have been to penalise the doctors concerned, but by this time the new perception of addiction was well and truly entrenched – one that saw it as literally 'socially infectious'. To prevent its spread a total defence network had to be established. This would be done by restricting the right to prescribe heroin and cocaine to a limited number of licensed doctors. They would be psychiatrists, all of them working within a hospital context, and mostly based at new Drug Dependency Units (DDUs). Ordinary GPs would retain the right to prescribe narcotics to non-addicts. But for their addicted patients they could only issue a range of synthetic opioids such as Fortral and methadone. To stamp out duplicate prescribing and keep a check on the number of addicts, a system of 'notification' was introduced.[50] The very term – until now used in the context of lethal, highly infectious diseases – reflected explicitly the new concept of social contagion.[51]

In the new DDUs conflict and confusion were the daily lot as staff sought to act out their social control mandate by means of various coercive 'contracts' with their 'clients'; while the addicts themselves – feeling somewhat disenfranchised and unhappy about their new leper status – refused to play along.[52]

The new addicts

So who were these new addicts that Brain so nearly missed? Many were part of the jazz scene – English and Nigerian musicians and their followers. Later, there came young Americans and Canadians for whom the British system of prescribing was manna. They believed in being cool the way it was imagined the great US jazz players were cool, and heroin, for some, was the necessary apparatus.

A surviving example from that era is Tony R. I met him in the mid-1980s while working on the first edition of this book. He was the child of a couple who worked as butler and servant to some very grand London families. From the earliest age Tony possessed the three most distinctive characteristics that go into the making of a dependent personality: his father was addicted to drink; he constantly looked outside himself for

315

proof of his worth; and he started out, as he puts it, with the 'self-destruct button firing'. The scene he wanted to join from the age of fourteen was the Kingston/Richmond beatniks, comprising jazz clubs and barge parties. He remembers it being peopled with individuals of special talent. There is some justification in such a rose-coloured rear view, since from that corps came the basic components of the British r 'n' b scene of the sixties: Jeff Beck, Jimmy Page, Eric Clapton, Long John Baldry, The Rolling Stones, Graham Bond, etc. Tony's dream was to be a great artist, but he imagined then that it was sufficient merely to disport oneself in the appropriate style for it to happen. He knows this about himself now. He knows much about himself now after a twenty-year drug career during which a great many of his friends perished. That he survived at all is extraordinary. During low times he tried to shoot himself and cut his head off. He has attacked policemen with a meat cleaver, driven a car through a chemist's shop window, and suffered the OD death of his own seventeen-year-old son. He had survived these events and in 1985 was in the business of helping other 'druggies'.

The Richmond scene of his youth never really fully embraced heroin; it took its pleasures from booze, hash, Purple Hearts and speed. Tony got his first smack from a Kingston musician who was being prescribed. Since there was no hangover and no craving he did it again the next weekend. The use of needles started within weeks because, as he puts it, 'I liked the drug, and I always wanted to do things properly.' Plans for college were dumped and instead he got a job as an apprentice name-plate artist. He knew he was hooked, he says, the Monday night he came home from work and, being short of a fix, began sweating and aching as though stricken with malaria. When his mother said, 'You've being doing horse, haven't you? How long?' he wept. She took him to a drug specialist that same night and got a standby prescription. The next day he was registered and twice daily called at the Middlesex Hospital for an injection. This was a cold-hearted way to get fixed, so the next step was to acquire his personal drugs doctor who would allow him to administer himself. The drugs doctor was a gynaecologist, a well-intentioned old man, who gave him Methedrine on the side to jazz up the heroin rush. The gynaecologist thought he was lessening the risk of respiratory collapse by handing out

316

speed at the same time. Such was the old man's generosity that although Tony had developed a voluminous habit he still had surplus drugs to sell off on the Piccadilly exchange.

For a while he enjoyed the darting around – the scoring, swapping, even the Sunday panics when the chemists were closed. Then in 1965 the scene, he reports, changed. A swarm of what he regarded as lower-class, artless gluttons descended on Piccadilly and began consuming with all the refinement of a scoop truck. By the time the new drug dependency clinics were established in 1968 he was ready for them, and to leave behind, if not drugs, then the freak show that went with them. But while on one level the clinics gave him the stability to get and hold down a job for ten years as an addict, on another level they caused a greater hunger in his life by replacing his preferred heroin with the tedium of methadone.

His dissatisfaction with the drug meant periodically returning to do some trading in Piccadilly. He made a connection with local Chinese drug traders, who by this time could see the value of supplying smack-starved white kids. They used him as a courier, carrying packages from the East End docks to Chinatown. His reward was a portion of the drugs.

Corpses cropped up regularly on his daily rounds. Because he cared so little for himself they meant little to him. When encountering a body in the Piccadilly toilets, his first instinct was to go through the pockets to see what drugs were left, and if somebody died in his own place he would consider it a supreme inconvenience – what with the police and all. Dimly recognising what he'd come to, he attempted to quit heroin through hospital detoxification. He tried fifteen or twenty times before finally stopping in 1979, whereupon the most drastic problems of his life began. Although he had left junk behind, he had substituted it with tranquillisers and, more critically, alcohol. His travails between 1979 and 1983 when he finally cleaned up entirely with the help of Narcotics Anonymous are almost farcically grim. The drink took him into the gutter. He went on time-looping benders lasting for weeks. He became a park-bench 'dosser'. It destroyed his pancreas. Eventually he found himself in a mental hospital where he tried to hang himself. He tried to kill policemen, ambulance men, anyone in uniform. He found religion. He shot himself in the head, jumped off Lambeth Bridge, slashed

317

his wrists. He couldn't die and he couldn't live. Then after one particularly savage episode, he was deposited in St Bernard's mental hospital where a doctor told him the only way to tell how 'mad' he was would be to come off everything – booze, tranks, magic mushrooms, the lot. 'It was the first time anyone had ever said this to me in my life.' The idea that addiction cuts across the whole spectrum of drugs was a revelation.

Coming off alcohol was excruciating and in a sense he substituted once more, but this time it was with a fellowship of co-addicts. In 1985, he was still attending Narcotics Anonymous meetings several times a week and was furthering the fellowship's growth by encouraging the setting-up of new local chapters.

Tony's love affair with drugs is as old or new as the turning of the moon. His father had it. His own son had it and perished at an early age. It took hold of a young woman whom we'll call Dilys. She was part of that later sixties generation that Tony accuses of dirtying the West End scene. Dilys, however, was not an artless dimwit but the bright child of a middle-class North London couple. She didn't spell it out, but there was a sense of her having got too much crushing attention as a child, which left her emotionally enfeebled.

'I had what a lot of addicts start out with – low confidence and emotional immaturity. There is this inability to stand up for yourself and accept responsibility. Instead you run to someone else to look after you, or you run to drugs to sort of block everything out. In the end the drugs become an excuse in themselves for not sorting yourself out. I was smoking dope first of all, but got rather bored with that. At university I got hooked on speed because I found it gave me a lot of confidence. I cut myself off the first time because I felt bad about using so much – you know, the moods I got into and the way it isolated me from other people. My friends didn't like me taking it. I then spent a year being very depressed so I got back on because I always felt I had more confidence and ability when I was using speed.'

But the zip soon warped. She became frantic, paranoid, malnourished. The boy she married was simply someone to flaunt at her family: his problems were bigger than her's. Until the breakdown of her marriage she'd always had an aversion to jacking up heroin or any other drug because the

318

image of the junkie appalled her. She still wanted to 'work, not die.' But now on her own with a young child to care for she moved from coke and speed to shooting up smack. The low point came when she took herself down to Piccadilly for a couple of weeks to run in blurred circles with the rest. She remembers a lot of the kids living in squats or in bad hotels around the main stations. A large number were dabbling in burglary and they could be seen selling the proceeds on the street; anything from an LP to their parents' furniture. Most of the traffic centred on pharmaceuticals of the upper/downer variety.

'I suppose, basically, I had finally had enough of messing up my life and I was lucky enough to get a social worker I could trust. She put me on to Phoenix House [rehabilitation centre] which I was shit scared about going to. Phoenix was hard. It was really hard to face up to things and change. But I stuck it out when I felt like leaving because I knew I had nothing to go out to.' After Phoenix she worked for a few months in film and advertising jobs to test herself away from the drugs world. But she found that world 'very impersonal and very shitty. I just couldn't relate to people who cared only about their own trips, their cars and mortgages. There's so much isolation with people not really caring about one another.'

As so often happens with recovered addicts, she went on to work in the field of drugs rehabilitation herself. 'I find people panic,' she says, 'because they've gone to a rehab house and they still can't stop, and they think to themselves, "*God, what is there left?*" They don't realise it's they themselves who have to stop using.'

The third wave

Just as Dilys's generation copied and overtook Tony R's, a sequence of events occurred in the mid-1970s that sucked in fresh waves of users. This was partly to do with availability, partly with the increasingly dismal state of the country. Every age is a troubled one, but the period beginning with the recession of the late 1970s found the UK being thrown into an historical lurch equivalent to the late-eighteenth-century transition from ruralism to industrialism, and where that earlier transitional period was accompanied by one of the most sordid and protracted drinking binges in our history, heroin – according to most commentators of the day – seemed to be *the* drug we were taking with us into the post-industrial microchip epoch. I say 'seemed' because it is too easy to overrate heroin in a society where there is a far more voluminous traffic in other 'hard' drugs such as alcohol and the benzodiazepines – two substances whose 'collateral damage' (family tensions, mental and physical illness, violence, economic loss) is everywhere evident.

Industrial/social change and the unemployment and uncertainty which go with it were at the root of the early 1980s 'working-class epidemic' – tied, of course, to easy accessibility. But fashion also played its part. The discovery by a generation of US and British musicians that cocaine-sniffing could keep them awake after gigs and give them an inflated sense of their talents led to the habit becoming more universally popular. From sniffing coke it is but a short step to sniffing other white-powder drugs such as amphetamine – which was suddenly available everywhere as sulphate. The move to heroin was always going to be more difficult because of the resoundingly poor image the drug had carried since the 1920s. But the bad imagery, paradoxically, was the thing that ultimately appealed. In the mid-1970s, to be rebelliously cool was to be ideally positioned. Rolling Stone Keith Richard was one who embodied these attitudes, and there was many a Richard clone – writing for the *hippest* music weeklies for instance – ready to proselytise on his and the drug's behalf.

A working-class 'epidemic'

While rock stars and their camp followers were sniffing heroin there was no particular panic, but when the drug was taken up by working-class youth then the alarm bells did start clanging. First signs of the epidemic were announced by a couple of researchers at Glasgow University who published a report, 'The Rapid Increase In Heroin Addiction', in 1981.[53]

They pointed to a 388 per cent rise in new clinic cases in six months, plus a quantum leap in pharmacy break-ins. Glasgow, they chimed ominously, was beginning to look like New York. Fifteen- and sixteen-year-olds from the slab concrete estates were jacking up a range of painkilling solutions, many of them foully adulterated. Where they once got ground-up Victory V lozenges cut with their brown Iranian H, they were now

320

getting talcum powder or strychnine with the new whiter stuff. Because of the increased rewards old-fashioned villains had become involved and were practising old-fashioned blood and extortion methods. One man's hands were broken with a baseball bat because he allegedly owed £15. He was later stabbed to death; a now familiar story. The town's drugs squad chief, Charlie Rogers, told me things weren't in fact as hysterically bad as they were painted, and that in comparison to alcohol abuse the heroin problem scarcely existed at all. But some way across town from police chief Charlie's, at a community project I agreed not to name because the people I spoke to there didn't want it dragged through the media gutter any more, there was another perception of drugs, police, and the cankerous, hard-faced system they are asked to defend. Among the area's sixteen–twenty-five-year-olds, I was told, the jobless rate was 75 per cent. Heroin had shown up in force in 1981 and now everything was being tried. Bel Air hairspray was being injected between toes, Beechams powders were diluted and then injected, as was a curious cocktail of methadone and pulped travel sickness pills. There was open dealing in pubs with stolen goods being humped in and out. Prostitution among young girls was increasing. Guns were turning up to enforce sectional interests and there had been so much thieving from Provident (loan) collectors that they no longer made the rounds. Credit was therefore drying up. It was a disease, they said, that spread more deprivation and more crime. 'None of the kids here has any political views,' said the project's leader. 'Nothing. And they don't care because they see no future. That's why it doesn't matter to them what the drugs do – whether they're left with a limp or a hump. And we can't do anything about it, not until they're ready. Then we can give them support.'

I found a similar picture in Manchester, except here the drug was being smoked from foil – Chasing the Dragon – rather than injected. The scene was much more furtive. A young man called Norman took me on a tour of the city's Hulme district. He was himself an addict, just out of a psychiatric hospital where he'd undergone detoxification.

We walked together through Hulme's Bullring, a notorious complex of arcing council blocks that have since been demolished. 'Over there', he said, pointing to a low-rise maisonette, 'are the shooting galleries [where addicts get together and inject, usually from the same works]. I think the council likes to keep them all together. At night the kids come out on the concrete open space and you can hear them smashing their cider bottles. No one else comes out. Funny thing is this used to be a smart area. There's the Henry Royce pub, named after the Rolls-Royce man. On that same site was a Rolls workshop, Rolls-Royce, think of it. And now look!'

But it wasn't just the scuzzier areas of Manchester which were suffering the heroin blitz. Smart areas such as Salford were also affected.

'In our street we've got just one manual worker,' a Salford fire chief and drugs councillor told me at the end of 1984. 'And yet heroin's as easy to come by here as tobacco. A lot of them are getting into it because of the "dare thing". On another level this is one of the areas where you've got a heavy student population, so it's cash. If you're using and dealing a little you've got money. No problems.' The other factor he pointed to was local youth having rejected the old-style recreational pursuit of getting tanked up on booze on a Saturday night. Heroin seemed to them more sublime and sophisticated.

'It's easy to slip into the drug scene,' said the fire chief finally, 'because it relieves the tensions and agonies of mind and makes them relax. My youngest lad can stop bloody well looking for work now. I'm a local councillor and I can't help him.'

Other areas that caught the media's attention early in the 1980s as heroin black spots were Bermondsey and Rotherhithe in South London. Stories began circulating of pushers rolling up in Porsches and young teens racing out of the tower blocks to greet them like it was ice-cream time. The kids didn't even know what they were taking, so the story went: they called it *scag* as though it were another substance. And even when they knew it was heroin, they believed that by smoking it from foil they couldn't get addicted. This alleged ignorance of young users was sometimes borne out, but most often not. Many knew the score precisely but believed addiction would never happen to them, or they used the inherent dangers of junk-smoking as a mark of their personal mettle. Elsewhere in the country, injecting rather than smoking was the preferred mode among the new generation of users.

322

The fixation on the new working-class metropolitan 'junkies' came to dissipate slightly by the end of 1984 as evidence continued to mount of the drug being used in all parts of the UK and by every social type. Whether in Brighton or Chester or those little postcard towns of Wiltshire (where much fixing was going on) there seemed no heroin-free zone remaining – except, curiously, Northern Ireland where, I was told on a visit, the IRA were keeping it out.[54]

By 1986 heroin was assumed to be everywhere and where it was not this was a cause for headlines; for instance the double-decker in the *Southern Evening Echo*, dated 7 March, which declared incredulously, 'Drugs Misuse Not Major Problem', a reference to the findings of a nine-month study of the Southampton area by a local health and social services team.

A case for treatment

Stopping the spread of the heroin contagion was the first objective of the clinics when they opened in 1968. But, within a few years, the senior clinicians themselves were discontented with their social-control function. They had begun by being fairly loose in their prescribing habits (offering injectable methadone on long-term scripts; even heroin) – this so that their junkie clients would keep coming back and the nation, theoretically, would be spared the growth of a new American-style black market dominated by organised crime. But, by the early 1970s, the clinic authorities decided that responsible practice meant moving to non-injectables and – rather than maintenance prescribing – to fairly rapid withdrawal scripts; the new first objective being to get people to quit, and fast. The reality was that many users entered into a series of back-to-back withdrawals, which did nothing to improve their chances of stabilising their drug intake, let alone eliminating substances from their lives.

The new policy lurch failed to expand the appeal of the clinics. But fortunately for the drugged, as well as for the drug-free, there already existed a network (in England at least) of drop-in street agencies and other support groups which were able to take up some of the stress. A number of these bodies had been around since the hippy 1960s, most of them supported by voluntary (i.e. insecure) funding. It was thanks to their street experience and flexible attitudes that the 'epidemic' heroin use of the 1970s and early 1980s caused less harm than it might have done.

By 1983, urged on by its expert advisory committee, the government had let loose what it called the Central Funding Initiative,[55] a rolling programme which, between 1983 and 1990, made available £17.5 million to expand existing English treatment services and to build new ones.[56] Rather than unchecked expansion, the plan was to lace together the various disparate elements – the street agencies, self-help groups, GPs, hospital services, live-in rehabilitation houses – and to establish 'community drug teams' in each district. This new emphasis on co-ordinated 'community provision' somewhat undercut the authority of the consultant psychiatrists who until now had operated virtually unchallenged from their clinic fortresses. In fact, evidence as to the continuing failure of the clinic system was already piling up. Several surveys revealed that a majority of users were unable to hack a regime often involving several weeks' delay for an appointment, which demanded daily pick-up of drugs, compulsory psychotherapy, and made it almost impossible for patients to work or go on holiday (a litany of complaints persisting to this day). A study of a particularly stark case was published in the *British Medical Journal* (BMJ) in April 1986.[57] It found that of sixty drug users referred on to a clinic for help, thirty-seven abandoned the two-week detoxification programme after a few days and only four of the remainder stayed heroin-free after their treatment. The authors – who included the clinic's own consultant psychiatrist – thought the results 'cast doubt' on the value of the clinic service offered at all 106 locations throughout the UK.

Call in the GPs

The first of a series of overtures were now made to GPs in an attempt to persuade them that junkies really weren't such awful people and that they, the general practitioners, belonged 'in the forefront'[58] of the battle against drugs. This was despite the implicit message which had been directed at those same GPs since the advent of the clinics – to the effect that they were far too inexpert and corruptible to be trusted with addicts (a conclusion of the Brain Committee, reached on the basis of the behaviour of a handful of irresponsible London doctors). Following Brain, confidence among family doctors, not unexpectedly, waned. And, without training or other encouragement, the attitude of the practitioners themselves hardened towards the addicts. They came to see them as unmanageable, undeserving even of primary health care, something automatically to be referred on to the experts at the clinics. But by the end of 1987, with the clinics failing to deliver, a re-evaluation was needed on all sides.

According to the advisor on drug misuse to the chief medical officer,[59] 'The old image of drug abusers being difficult and troublesome patients is simply not true as many come from respectable middle-class backgrounds and hold down good jobs. Like it or not GPs need a better understanding of drug problems.'

How confusing, then, that so soon after this placatory message went out, the government should begin a new round in its anti-heroin advertising campaign, delivering up the same old images of users as prostitutes, vomiting down toilets, stealing Mum's housekeeping.

The struggle to enlist and retain the support of GPs – whom addicts themselves generally prefer dealing with – continues through to today. Success, when it does come (as, for instance, in Edinburgh, Birmingham, Liverpool, East London), requires strategic support from an experienced specialist agency. GPs want to know that if they do take on addicts they won't be the only player in town and, thereby, subject to a 'junkie stampede'. They also usually want to be able to concentrate on primary health care and leave the difficult technical questions about the size and duration of a script to those who claim to know better.

Aids

It had long since become the habit to marginalise the junkie figure, to have him/her conveniently vanish at society's periphery. If the early-1980s heroin boom made that more difficult (a lot of the new users looked uncomfortably like 'ordinary' people, the product of 'ordinary' parents) then the advent of AIDS made it imperative to draw them back from the margins and inculcate in them good social habits. By the mid-1980s the link between unsterile injecting equipment and

325

the transmission of this lethal, no-cure disease had become universally apparent. There would be no more cant and simplistic moralising. The health of the whole nation was at stake – which was why the Conservative government of Margaret Thatcher, morally rigorous in its rhetoric but ultimately deeply pragmatic, chose to adopt some of the most innovative anti-AIDS measures to be found anywhere in the world. For so long as AIDS was seen to be a gay plague or the haemophiliacs' curse, official action was torpid and restrained. With the arrival of the infected, injecting drug user, a clearer pathway was seen through to the heterosexual moral majority, and suddenly the posters and media ads were composed in plainspeak: 'It takes only one prick to give you AIDS'.

Free syringes

In 1986, a handful of experimental syringe exchange schemes (new works for old) were started by street agencies in Peterborough, Kingston-upon-Thames, Dundee, Sheffield, and Liverpool. Within a year, fifteen government-sanctioned projects were established throughout the country and subjected to some close scrutiny. The logic behind the schemes was simple. The habit of sharing needles was leading to the rapid transmission of what had been identified as the AIDS virus. Sharing might be in part a product of comradely instincts and/or novice users receiving hands-on instruction from older acquaintances, but mostly it was because needles were in restricted supply. Increase the availability and you decrease the infection rate.

The data collated since indicate that sharing *is* reduced when clean equipment is made available, although users still lack the 'social skills' to say no to a dominant fellow injector who might be the person who actually scored the drugs, or might be an easily offended live-in partner who could, nonetheless, be sleeping with or sharing works with someone else. It has also become plain that not everyone understands that 'sharing' also applies to spoons, filters, water, as well as to practices known as backloading, frontloading, and halving. This is where a pair of syringes are 'docked' together so as to share out drugs accurately.[60]

The argument against easy access to free syringes is that

326

they legitimise not just the consumption of controlled substances but their ingestion via the most dangerous route. How could any government justify, on the one hand, imprisoning people for using prohibited drugs, while simultaneously supplying them with the works for their administration? The answer is: it cannot. Nor could the clinic system, by now directed in the main towards rapid detoxification and abstinence, be squared with the free needles arrangements. The exigencies of AIDS control had exposed contradictions in the British system which had been present for sixty years, ever since a 'liberal' Sir Humphrey Rolleston delivered his findings to government.

The client is king

The crack in the logic of the home-grown system was no better exposed than in a 1988 report by the government's main outside expert body on drugs. Entitled 'AIDS and Drugs Misuse Part 1', it contained a passage that would be much quoted: 'HIV is a greater danger to individual and public health than drug misuse. Accordingly, we believe that services which aim to minimise HIV risk behaviour by all available means should take precedence in development plans.'[61] To this end they urged an extension to the syringe swap schemes (within three years there were 200 of them, distributing some 4 million syringes each year). There had to be a loosening up of substitute prescribing. Clinics, in general, had to make themselves more friendly and cut down on waiting times. *All* GPs needed to be drafted in to provide care and advice for 'misusers'. And there had to be a network of 'community-based' services in each health district which would provide advice and help, not just on drugs and HIV, but on housing, jobs, legal questions, and primary health care.

The relevant specialists should make themselves available. For all services the priority was to attract and keep 'misusers', many of whom had never made contact with any agency and were deeply mistrustful. To achieve this, the customer – namely the 'misusers' – had to be provided, in effect, with what s/he wanted. The location of each service needed to be close to the user population and, if necessary, adopt a mobile role. Opening hours were to be tailored to the users' needs, including, perhaps, evening opening, since addicts were often late risers. The community-based schemes, in particular, had to be 'practical, non-judgmental and informal'.

Free condoms and syringes should be provided, or the user directed to them. Nor was commitment to abstinence necessary. There was to be a whole 'hierarchy of goals' to which users might aspire, during which prescribing could take place. These started with the cessation of equipment sharing, moved on to quitting the syringe altogether, then a decrease in the amount consumed, and, finally, abstinence.

In broad terms the government swallowed whole the Advisory Council recommendations (though failed to provide the funds all this extra activity required), and there followed a further period of service expansion, including a proliferation of 'outreach' programmes (drug workers, equipped with condoms, syringes and expert information, hunting down drug takers in their natural habitats), as well as the establishment of some twenty Home Office 'local drug prevention teams' – a kind of SWAT control effort designed to sharpen the indigenous response and keep in check any possible contagion.

As the (financially stressed) treatment effort grew, so did drug consumption and, it would seem, associated problems of health, community cohesion, and crime. The old debate about whether drugs were a symptom or a cause was earnestly revived. In the second half of the 1980s, during the sham economic boom, there were those who argued that problem drug-taking by the poor/unemployed was invariably a product of boredom, despair, and resentment at the injustice of an unequal society; whereas when the the rich consumed compulsively it was because their lives were so empty and purposeless. The counter-argument was that drug-taking was a matter of personal discipline. People made choices. Blaming outside circumstances was escapist and an insult to those, of whatever social caste, who said no.

A series of substance panics followed, with the 1980s climaxing in a spasm of terror over the Rave scene and the amount of Ecstasy and other drugs being swallowed by the young at their frenetic parties and dance clubs. Then came crack – Yardies, gunfights, monstrous habits precipitating such *un-English* violence. Calculations were done suggesting that, by 1994, drug use fuelled around half of all property crime in the country (about £2 billion out of £4 billion).[62]

Police chiefs and politicians – left and right – lined up to concede defeat in the War on Drugs and to call for, at the least, cannabis to be decriminalised so that those who used it, and nothing else, could be kept apart from the uglier end of the trade.

A new line on AIDS

Suddenly, the years of expanding service provision (whose 'outcomes' had never been systematically quantified) came to an end. With local authorities now controlling much of the cash under new 'community care' arrangements, the squeeze was put on. Residential rehabilitation houses lost their relatively secure funding and local authority drug educators were remaindered. Not only was the country in the midst of a long, deep recession with all the consequent strains this placed on the public purse, but AIDS – the scourge that unleashed so much of the spending – was being critically re-assessed.

In the mid-1980s a heterosexual epidemic seemed imminent. The view six or seven years later was that the original warnings had been over-cooked. Rather than a million cases of HIV infection predicted for the mid-1990s by the Royal College of Nursing, the actual figure was probably fewer than 30,000, with AIDS fatalities during the previous ten years totalling some 5,600. And while the number of heterosexual AIDS cases was steadily increasing, the vast majority still involved gay men and injecting drug users.[63] It was further argued that a sizeable proportion of the heterosexual transmission cases came about through anal intercourse.

The complaint that went with this data evaluation was in two parts: a) too much money was being spent on AIDS – some £26 million each year on 'raising awareness' as part of an overall annual budget of around £200 million[64] (this was said to be more than any disease in the history of medicine); b) if 'ordinary, decent' people were not at risk – only *junkies* and *queers* – why was the nation troubling itself? (This complaint was usually made behind a cupped hand but came through clearly enough.)

There was even the argument, referred to elsewhere in this chapter, that HIV was not the cause of the cluster of diseases and malignancies known collectively as AIDS, and that the whole HIV bandwagon was bogus science – lucrative for drug companies and recipients of research funds, but lethal for those afflicted with the condition who weren't getting help of a relevant kind.

Dissident AIDS voices

My own view is that it is right to be sceptical about an HIV industry that is marked by profiteering and corporate squabbling among the companies making anti-viral 'remedies' and vaccines. As I write these lines, large-scale vaccine field trials are being prepared for Uganda, Thailand, and Brazil. This is despite major safety worries, including evidence that supposedly safe HIV vaccines can mutate back into virulent form.[65] Nor is there evidence that the vaccines – made from part of the HIV virus itself – actually work.[66] Animal trials, as always, have produced confusion. Small pilot studies among humans have ended with members of the study groups becoming HIV-infected (not the fault of the vaccine, the researchers were quick to claim).[67] In not too many years we will no doubt be witnessing mass AIDS vaccination programmes in the UK. But anyone becoming sick as a result of their vaccination will find it an arduous business producing evidence that the vaccine itself harmed them. Not only does the disease incubate for years, but it could always be said that the disease reached them through some other route.

There are other, associated concerns. Western pundits like to point the finger at Africans and/or monkeys as the source of the AIDS epidemic. But there are a number of theories – aired by qualified individuals in the scientific press itself – suggesting that AIDS could have had its genesis in a series of reckless cancer experiments on animals carried out during the 1970s, or in earlier vaccine programmes against polio, directed by Western researchers at populations in central Africa.[68] True or not, there is now a respectable body of opinion arguing that the 'solution' to AIDS does not lie in a new round of scientific adventurism – schemes that involve injecting untested disease products into populations that are highly vulnerable to the triumphalist claims of science.

330

Treatment for sale

Returning to where we were, we can see that the re-evaluation of AIDS, combined with the deep recession of the late 1980s/early 1990s and the arrival of an even more terrifying mind-altering substance – crack cocaine – effectively dislodged heroin from the front page and made it easier for a Conservative government to do what it instinctively does best: turn towards market forces to resolve whatever the 'heroin problem' might be. From April 1993 – following the earlier passage of the landmark NHS and Community Care Act – drug treatment was operating in the context of an 'internal market', with some in the role of 'purchasers' (local and health authorities) and others called service 'providers' (those supplying the actual treatment). It was to be a buyers' market from now on and the providers were going to have to punt their wares amid stiffening competition. Even consultant psychiatrists, who formerly sat at the top of the drug treatment heap, were now mere providers, and suddenly subordinate to health authority managers with money to spend. Throughout the field, there was more nervousness and uncertainty than anyone could remember. And added to the providers' problems was the launching of a series of 'outcome' studies (notably by the Department of Health)[69] designed to measure the effectiveness of what they'd been doing all these years.

No surrender

Yet more change was heralded in October 1994, with the announcement of a new multi-department government strategy.[70] The War on Drugs, the launch document insisted, *could* be won. There'd be no surrender to the decriminalisation lobby. Police, educators, Customs officials, health and drug agency workers needed to draw together and apply themselves with resolute intelligence. Anti-drugs education for the young had been rediscovered and there were to be more accessible treatment options. While law enforcement was to be de-emphasised, it would still take most of the cash; and there were to be some especially fierce measures aimed at drug use in prisons – this amongst a population which, for a decade past, had already shown itself to be in a seething, riotous mood.

Perhaps what was most clearly evident by the mid-1990s was that we were looking at yet another redefinition of the 'drugs problem'. In the 1950s, and before, it had been seen as a question of individual pathology (the 'disease model'). By the 1960s, there was the concept of social contagion (a core of users spreading hedonism and subversive lifestyles). Through much of the 1970s and early 1980s the focus was again on the individual and getting him/her to quit. At the high-water mark of the AIDS scare, around 1986–88, there was an attempt to pamper and reel users in. Whatever they wanted they'd get; just don't infect the rest of us. Then came funding cuts and a fresh perception of AIDS as a disease from which the majority were, supposedly, safe. The 'good times' for addicts were over.

The brand-new concept of the drug problem (circa 1994/95) was 'community safety' – a notion tied up in fear of crime and how to lick it. 'Hard' drug use was no longer about disease or dissolute, heretical young people. It was about theft and violence. From now on government policy, however ineptly, would be directed at its eradication.

Smack in the nineties

But this was lofty stuff. How did the junk scene look from ground level? In 1994, I went 'sight-seeing' in several UK cities and towns; talked to users and dealers, police officers, desperate parents, and would-be healers. The essential story hadn't changed that much from ten years earlier when I had also been trekking the country as part of the research for the first edition of this book. Heroin, it seemed, still filled a vacuum in purposeless lives. It was a kick and an escape. It was business. It set users apart, kept them busy hustling.

On the Isle of Dogs in East London's Docklands, twenty-something junkies from the local estates were doing night-time kamikaze raids on the vast new neighbouring glass and steel office blocks. They were coming out with desktop computers and related gear – the 1990s equivalent of the once-prized video player for an ambitious young thief. They sold them uptown for next to nothing, blowing their takings on injectable smack. The Isle of Dogs was where the British National Party had, temporarily, installed a local authority councillor in 1993/94; an area which had seen twenty years of decline following the run-down of the dock industries; had seen over-crowding, lack of affordable housing, accelerating crime, growing racial intolerance, then – to rub their noses in it – a land-grab of choice riverside sites by city businesses which, in a literal sense, proceeded to wire and fence themselves off from the common indigenous *volk*. Was this an excuse to thieve and fill up on junk?

I was told the story of a young island man who woke up from a heroin overdose while on the way to hospital. He came to with a raging appetite for more drugs, burst out of the moving ambulance, and scrambled off in the direction of his dealer.

Outside Colchester in Essex, I talked with a group of young speed and heroin injectors, part of a sizeable clique who lived on the same not-so-run-down estate. They hinted at the intrigues that passed between them: the gossip and double-dealing. But there was also, they declared, some kind of honour among local junkies. They resisted the idea, as one of them put it, that 'drug use was a manifestation of problems in life. When it comes to it, I like doing drugs.'

They also tried to convince me that so-called 'heroin deaths' were nearly always something different. They gave as an example the case of a local young man, dosed up on junk, who died behind the wheel of his vehicle in a car park. The actual cause of death was hypothermia. Another local case concerned the man who mixed too much heroin and alcohol and overdosed. It was, they insisted, the drink element which killed him. 'A lot of people who do die shouldn't,' it was said. 'People abandon them. They panic.'

These arguments weren't without logic. But they were also, it seemed to me, fairly technical. Yes, heroin is often a mere contributory factor in injury and death. And the drug, when sitting wrapped in a drawer, can't hurt anyone. But it wasn't made for that. Heroin, whatever else might be said about it, is a powerful means to some other end.

In Leith, near Edinburgh, I was talking to an inspired woman – June Taylor – who runs a support service for local street prostitutes (sex workers is now the preferred term) when a couple of eleven-year-old boys she knew paid a visit. The amount they knew about drugs was frightening. Both regarded Ecstasy and speed as the most dangerous of all substances, probably because they'd heard so much about them from their older brothers. They told how they'd recently slipped over on some abandoned condoms near their play area, and described the case of two local girls – aged eight and six – who, having found a discarded syringe on the stairs of a tenement block, took turns in jagging it into their arms. They'd seen it done on TV, or perhaps they were copying some real-life example.

The boys also knew something about crack and AIDS, but not half so much as a man called Jim I spoke to at an exemplary drug agency in South London, known as the Stockwell Project. Jim was one of Stockwell's clients. He had AIDS.

'If I can beat this bastard,' he said with breezy stoicism, 'I'll beat it. If I cannae beat it, then God rest my soul.'

His health had gone up and down since first being diagnosed as HIV-positive in 1983. But his 'full-blown AIDS' developed in early 1993, after parting from a woman with whom he'd lived for four years. The trauma of the split, he was convinced, broke his health. He'd since suffered shingles, four bouts of pneumonia, Bell's palsy – which caused the left side of his face to collapse – and loss of clumps of head hair, revealing, as he put it, the eerily pulsating veins beneath.

He was now feeling better, as a result of following a regime he claimed was diametrically opposed to that which his medics had advised. 'I walk everywhere very fast. I do squats at night, arm-pulls and swings twice a week, compound vitamins, raw garlic, loads of salad, hardly any meat, and I love peanut butter. I also do lots of dope because that makes me want to eat. It opens my stomach up.'

He remained something of a beanpole of a man, thirty-one years old, fair-haired, with the left side of his face still faintly drooping and palsied. Jim is someone we are supposed to regard with contempt. He got infected through the needle, an illness brought upon himself by his own 'degenerate' activities. But who was to judge? He tells his life story of early bumps and falls and you recognise in it echoes of the stories of other drug-fixated individuals you've met along the way.

He was born in a run-down satellite town of Edinburgh. Dad was a partially blind alcoholic whom the women in the family beat up in front of Jim on at least one occasion. One sister also used to 'batter' Jim. The other one, he says, sexually abused him. He was shy and withdrawn as a young child but by the age of eleven was smoking and thieving and, three years after that, breaking into shops and pubs. Thirty months in a special school for 'difficult' youth taught him what he didn't already know about car crime, dope-smoking, and glue-sniffing. He escaped aged sixteen and had never held a straight job since.

Most of his life has been spent in prison, although he'd been out for three years when we met, his longest period yet. Along the way he picked up a heroin and crack habit. 'Heroin I love and hate. It's such a lovely drug, which is why I hate it. It takes all your worries away. Your senses are numbed. Everything's numbed in your body. You feel like a walking zombie and that's what you look like too.'

Jim might have succeeded in numbing himself with his once-favourite drug (he'd quit by the time we met) but he was someone, you sense, who'd always remained more than half-alive to the world and the kind of pain it can dole out.

Getting it Here

The images that prevail are of opium *armies*, heroin *empires*, drug *warlords*, ruthless *enforcers*. But notwithstanding these Hollywoodised images, the opium-heroin trade is, in its essentials, like any other lucrative global agro-business.[71] It has its winners and losers (the producer-peasants being bottom of the pile) and, along most of the manufacturing/distribution chain, the key actors involved are entirely legitimate business people – shopkeepers, restaurant owners, bank managers, commodity brokers, even key movers in religious and social organisations.

But, of course, these individuals cannot operate unrestrained in a free-enterprise capitalist paradise. As one astute observer of the South-East Asia scene has noted, 'There are political-military actors who loosely and fluidly control the physical space in which the production area and communication networks are situated.'[72] These controlling forces can be divided into two broad categories: the first being the soldiers, Customs officials, police and such like who serve under the flag of internationally recognised states such as Thailand, Burma, China and Laos. The second are the locally based men commanding armed units who fight, or claim to fight, for various dissident causes.

'These political-military actors are not only the "regulators" of the [heroin market] but its facilitators as well and, in many cases, partners of the various commercial-economic actors,' says Chao-Tzang Yawnghe of Canada's University of British Columbia.[73]

In return for their facilitating role, taxes and 'tributes' are extracted. In other words, heroin is plain *business*; one that is no more ruthless or hypocritical than many other global enterprises.

Among the more ludicrous manifestations of narcotics punditry are the solemn efforts to chart the routes drugs take on their way from poppy grower to consumer. Typical was a world map reproduced by the *Financial Times* in November 1993 purporting to show the 'main trade routes' but which was so cluttered with arrowed lines and 'bullets' the message it transmitted was that everything was simultaneously going everywhere.

What does seem clear is that the main source of UK heroin continues to be the Golden Crescent countries of South-West Asia (Pakistan, Afghanistan, Iran). Aside from that commonly accepted fact, there is little agreement among the 'experts'. Some see the trade in terms of a carve-up between *organised* crime syndicates (the Mafia, the Camorra, the Triads, the Turkish clans, motorcycle groups, etc). Others prefer a looser scenario: a confluence of *disorganised*, mostly middle-ranking enterprises which co-operate across ethnic lines when it suits them.

It would seem that the most important supply line of heroin to Western Europe continues – at the time of writing – to be the 'Balkan Route', despite it having branched eastward during the early 1990s to avoid the conflagration in the former Yugoslavia. The worst case scenario painted by one group of experts[74] was that 'drug traffickers and elements of organised crime will secure an economic stranglehold on central Europe and Russia, which will result in a flood of drugs entering Western Europe. The relaxed border controls between central and Western Europe and the abolition of internal frontiers within the EC [following the implementation of] the Single Market can only facilitate trafficking.'

An oft-stated view is that organisations from India and

Pakistan have traditionally dominated the UK heroin market. British smack, according to the head of the Dutch narcotics bureau[75] – a man with a good transcontinental vantage point – originates in the 'tribal areas' of Pakistan where it is controlled by a small number of wholesale traders. Each of these traders has his fixed circle of buyers and financiers, who form small groups of a 'fluid' composition. It is these groups which smuggle the heroin to Europe, delivering it to legally resident Pakistani customers. The customers deliver to dealers down the scale, with the greater portion of profits being repatriated back to Pakistan.

But this same Dutch narcotics chief believed that Turkish groups – who play a key role along the Balkan route – were attempting to claim a more solid share of the UK trade.

Help

Some people think they want help with their 'drug problem' but they don't. They've simply found themselves in legal or job problems; or their family is giving them a hard time. There can be no 'cure' for a drug problem that exists only in other people's minds. So the first step is to ask and truthfully answer the question: is my drug use troubling *me*? If so, what is my goal: to cut back and stabilise, to use healthier drugs (e.g. prescribed pharmaceutical stock), or to quit altogether?

Your local drugs advice/information service might help you answer this question, although you could quickly find yourself sucked into a round of counselling before you can take stock. Such counselling varies from having a chit-chat with 'some sad old dear' once a week[76] to multiple weekly sessions with a high-powered psychotherapist. In between, there is the inspired semi-amateur, as well as the artless, the pompous and the hopeless. Counselling is intended to be a non-judgmental process, whereby the 'clients' are helped to see through the clutter of their lives and bring about change. But what kind of change?

For many users, counselling sessions are a mere obstacle on the way to getting a decent methadone script. Depending on where you are in the country and the clinical fashion of the moment, you'll be able to get some kind of script to hold you together.

People choose different methods in their attempt to quit. Some go for an out-patient detoxification, whereby their street opioid is replaced with methadone which is then reduced down in dose to zero. Your GP might offer you this service or s/he'll refer you on to the local Drug Dependency Clinic or Community Drug Team. Service provision is a luck-of-the-draw business, depending on where you live.

Others go into hospital to have themselves purged – although there are few specialist detoxification units in the UK; what's usually on offer is a place in a general psychiatric ward in which four or five beds have been set aside for drug and alcohol problems. Such a programme is often reserved for people using more than one drug, some of which it would be dangerous to withdraw from unsupervised. In-patient detox is usually rapid, perhaps supplemented with sleeping pills or involving the use of the powerful opioid antagonist naltrexone. Some like the fact that, on naltrexone, they can sleep through much of the withdrawal. But beware of side effects, including nausea, vomiting, gut pain, diarrhoea, tearfulness, and prolonged sleep disruption.

Quitting from home

Many people choose to quit from a home base. This is probably the soundest option providing drugs such as barbiturates and tranquillisers are not being used at the same time and there are no other major health complications. Overcoming physical dependence is relatively straightforward even when undertaken abruptly. The peak of withdrawal usually occurs between two and three days after the last dose and normally involves fever, aching limbs, sweating, restlessness, fairly merciless insomnia, violent yawning, spasms, cramps, and twitches throughout the body. The telling struggle comes when the euphoria at having quit is followed by feelings of alienation and anxiety. These feelings will also pass. If an attempt to come off is made and fails, don't despair. It will have been a lesson for next time. However, a rapid succession of flops can injure confidence so it's best to think seriously: why am I trying to go drug-free? And what will I do afterwards?

If, having answered these puzzlers, the decision is still to make the break, it might be worth considering this four-point plan devised by a West London drugs counselling agency:

1. Cut down your daily dose to the minimum possible and resist taking just a little bit more just this one last time. It's difficult, so don't rush.
2. Find somewhere warm, safe and comfortable. You'll need a bed, fresh air and extras like books, records, etc. You'll be able to concentrate on these after a few days. Eat well. Cope with the fever as you'd deal with an ordinary bout of 'flu – cool baths, cool liquids.
3. If you're working take at least two weeks off, but no more than four or you'll mope. Some people go on holiday, but returning to an unresolved home situation can be worse than staying put.
4. Try to enlist the help of a friend to encourage and check up on you. But *stay away* from other users.

Afterwards it's good policy to remain drug-free for six months even if abstinence isn't the final objective. And it's important once in the clear to watch out for excessive booze or tranquilliser use. Many a 'recovering' opiate addict does a surreptitious switch, all the while believing s/he has licked the Big One. Tranquillisers and alcohol are just as difficult to quit.

Help from family and friends

Whatever resolve an addict might muster, s/he can always benefit from family or friends. But these people first need help themselves to understand the problem before engaging it. The same drug agency that gave the four-point quitting plan sketches these basic principles for friends of the addict:

1. Don't panic. Arm yourself with the legal, medical and pharmacological facts.
2. Don't assume the worst. Most drug use is casual, temporary, and leads to no serious problems.
3. Recognise that you might be unable to take on the 'case' yourself. You just might be part of the problem.
4. Recognise that addicts can't be beaten into recovery.

They must be willing partners in the process. If you
help is rejected, don't get miffed. They might come t
you another time.

5. Recognise the problem might not relate to a specific drug
but be part of what the professionals call 'poly drug use'

6. By way of general tips: don't interrogate; calmly acknowl
edge your friend's fears instead of dismissing them o
over-reacting. Resist pressure such as 'I'll die if yo
don't give me money.' Treat each request separately
and if you're to help, only give cash for food and othe
necessities.

Residential services

For a guide to residential 'rehabs', see Apprendix II. A
fuller description is contained in the *Rehab Handbook*, a
plain-English pocket volume, available from the Institut
for the Study of Drug Dependence. At the time of writing
residential services were undergoing a re-appraisal under th
new community care arrangements. Effectively, it mean
length of treatment was often being cut – to meet budgetary
rather than therapeutic needs, so the complaint went.

While there are some excellent rehabs on offer, wha
is sometimes evaded in respectable rehab guides is the
severity of some of the regimes – the kind of psychologica
punishment they can hand out to residents in the name o
personality restructuring. Ex-residents talk of being crushe
and humiliated in confrontational sessions. A combination o
poorly trained staff and lack of independent control an
monitoring has been a problem. It should also be said tha
some ex-residents talk glowingly of their rehab experiences.
They will testify that before their stop-over, eternal misery
beckoned.

Help on AIDS

Mainliners is an agency billing itself as 'working with an
for people affected by drugs, HIV and Hepatitis C.' Their
first-class monthly journal debates these issues, giving space
to users and their experiences as well as to 'alternative
views on HIV, AIDS, and controversial medical therapies
such as AZT (with its problems of toxicity). It also explores

the health benefits of a wholesome diet, exercise, stress control, acupuncture, herbal medicines and so on. (Mainliners, 205 Stockwell Road, London SW9 9SL. Adviceline: Tel. 071–737 3141.)

Other help

For more details on what's available – including self-help groups – see Appendix II.

Notes

1 'Peter McDermott's Guide to the Depressant Drugs', Lifeline, Manchester, 1993.

2 *British National Formulary*, British Medical Association and Royal Pharmaceutical Society of Great Britain, March 1994, p. 178.

3 The most authoritative pro-methadone argument is found in an Australian book: Jeff Ward *et al.*, *Key Issues in Methadone Treatment*, New South Wales University Press, 1992.

4 Andrew Preston, *The Methadone Handbook 2nd Edition*, Community Alcohol and Drugs Advisory Service, Dorchester, 1993, p. 5.

5 Ibid.

6 Ibid, p. 8.

7 McDermott, op. cit., p. 4.

8 This is according to Eric Simon, professor of psychiatry and pharmacology at New York University Medical Center, writing in *Substance Abuse: A comprehensive textbook* (Williams & Wilkins, Baltimore, 1992, p. 196). Simon claims the word is his own invention.

9 Ibid.

10 An idea recited, but not necessarily believed, in a *New Scientist* article, 'Prisoners of Pleasure', by David Concar and Rosie Mestel, 1 October 1994, p. 30.

11 Ibid.

12 Ibid.

13 Ibid.

14 K. Nyberg *et al.*, 'Obstetric medication versus residential area as perinatal risk factors for subsequent adult drug addiction in offspring', in *Paediat Perinatal Epidemiol*, 7, 1993, p. 23.

15 R. Lingeman, *Drugs from A–Z*, McGraw Hill, New York, 1974, p. 104.

16 See *What Works*, an excellent little pocket volume on how to inject safely, published by the Exeter Drugs Project.

17 Not just needles and syringes, but water, spoons, filters.

18 Sarah Layzell, *Staying Safe: HIV and Drug Use*, Standing Conference on Drug Abuse, London, 1993, p. 6.

19 Most notably Professor Peter Duesberg, an American microbiologist and specialist in retroviruses, of which HIV is a prominent example. Duesberg argues that it is chiefly the increased use of drugs (licit and illicit) which is the trigger for the catastrophic breakdown in the body's defences against disease. He has paid for heretical utterances by being stripped of much of his research funding and by being pilloried in sections of both the lay and medical/scientific press.

342

20 Layzell, op. cit., p. 9.
21 Locating whole or even bits of virus in the bloodstream is often both technically difficult and expensive. Therefore many disease diagnoses are made on the basis of the presence of antibodies to the virus in question. The antibodies are produced by the body's immune system as a response to the invasion by a foreign pathogen (bug).
22 Tom Waller, '60 per cent of injectors may be infected with Hepatitis C', in *Druglink*, ISDD, November/December 1994, p. 5.
23 Much of this health-related material comes from Factsheet No. 7, published by *Druglink*, and from *Staying Safe: HIV and Drug Use* (SCODA, op. cit.).
24 Waller, op. cit.
25 Hugh Perry and D. Wright, letter to *Druglink*, November/December 1993, p. 18.
26 *British National Formulary*, op. cit., p. 325.
27 Waller, op. cit.
28 'Calls to ban killer drug methadone', in *The Big Issue*, 24 March 1994, p. 4.
29 Ibid. Untangling Home Office drug-related mortality figures can be a problem. Under a category called 'deaths with underlying cause described as drug dependence or non-dependent abuse of drugs', a figure is given for 'morphine type' drugs (155 in 1992) with no breakdown to show heroin versus methadone. But under the 'poisoning' category we find 82 deaths attributed to heroin and 147 to methadone.
30 *British National Formulary*, op. cit., p. 177.
31 *Drug Notes: Heroin*, ISDD, 1992, p. 5.
32 The ISDD produces some useful digests on drugs and pregnancy – in particular there's its two-part fact sheet and a more detailed booklet, *Drugs, Pregnancy and Childcare: A Guide for Professionals*.
33 In W. Dunlop and A. A. Calder (eds), *High Risk Pregnancy*, Butterworth, London, 1992, p. 267.
34 Mary Hepburn, 'Drug use in pregnancy', in the *British Journal of Hospital Medicine*, Vol. 49, No. 1, 1993, p. 51.
35 Brian Inglis, *The Forbidden Game*, Hodder & Stoughton, London, 1975, p. 73.
36 'Paracelse', *Encyclopaedia Universalis*, Vol. 12.
37 In Charles Medawar, *Power and Dependence*, Social Audit, 1992, p. 31. Medawar's is a diligent and enlightening account of the history of painkilling and sedating drugs – from opium to benzodiazepines and beyond.
38 Ibid, p. 28.
39 Ibid, p. 29.
40 Virginia Berridge, 'East End opium dens and narcotic use in

Britain', in the *London Journal*, Vol. 4, No. 1, 1978, p. 3.

41 Ibid, p. 4.
42 Ibid, p. 14.
43 Terry Parssinen, *Secret Passions, Secret Remedies: Narcotic Drugs in British Society 1920–1930*, Manchester University Press, 1981, p. 212.
44 Ibid, p. 213.
45 David Musto, 'Historical perspectives on alcohol and drug abuse', in *Substance Abuse: A comprehensive textbook*, op. cit., p. 2.
46 Ibid.
47 Virginia Berridge, 'Drugs and social policy: the establishment of drug control in Britain, 1900–1930', in the *British Journal of Addiction*, Vol. 79, No. 1, 1984, p. 23.
48 Richard Hartnoll, 'Going the whole way', in the *International Journal of Drug Policy*, Vol. 4, No. 1, 1993.
49 John Marks, letter to *The Lancet*, 22 June 1985.
50 Confidentiality is built into the notification system. It is not designed with a view to monitoring the activities of individual addicts. Worries persist, however, that the police in some areas could in theory breach the system via their powers to inspect the prescribing records of chemists.
51 While the thriving street trade in amphetamines was recognised, as was so-called 'polydrug abuse' (users trying a range of substances), Brain confined his treatment recommendations to heroin. For historical and career reasons it suited the treatment establishment to focus on heroin and ignore the much larger phenomenon of stimulant 'abuse'. These luminaries knew more about heroin and had a method of treatment – useful or not. Stimulants were more of a puzzle. Come the cocaine/crack 'epidemic' starting in the late 1980s, those seeking help were left largely high and dry.
52 See Rachel Lart, 'Changing images of the addict and addiction', in the *International Journal on Drug Policy*, Vol. 3, No. 3, 1992, p. 119. 'Leper status' is my phrase, not hers.
53 J. Ditton and K. Speirits, 'The rapid increase of heroin addiction in Glasgow during 1981, background paper, Department of Sociology, Glasgow University, 1981.
54 Even by 1994 there was still very little heroin use in Northern Ireland (only 70 people were registered as dependent users) and 'virtually no injecting', according to local consultant psychiatrist Diane Patterson. The reasons, she claimed, were the strength of community and family life; the security situation (which made it difficult to bring drugs in and ship them around); and the unwavering refusal of medics in the province to prescribe either

heroin or methadone, except in 'controlled clinical conditions'. Patterson's remarks were reported in *Druglink*, July 1994, p. 4.

55 The initiative was in response to the 1982 *Treatment and Rehabilitation* report by the government's own Advisory Council on the Misuse of Drugs.

56 Scotland got no such help and was to pay the price throughout the 1980s and early 1990s in terms of huge numbers of overdose deaths and some of the highest HIV infection rates in the world.

57 Roy Robertson *et al*, 'Use of psychiatric drug treatment services by heroin users from general practice', in the *British Medical Journal*, Vol. 292, 12 April 1986, p. 997.

58 Phrase of the then Health Minister, Ray Whitney.

59 This was Dr John Strang, quoted in a *Doctor* magazine interview that coincided with a new video training package for doctors backed by the then Department of Health and Social Security.

60 Neil Hunt *et al.*, 'You say sharing, I say . . .', in *Druglink*, July/August 1994, p. 10.

61 'AIDS and Drug Misuse, Part I', report by the Advisory Council on the Misuse of Drugs, Department of Health and Social Security, HMSO, London, 1988.

62 This was according to Labour Party calculations. They were based on an estimated 22,819 addicts needing nearly £30,000 a year to finance a gram a day heroin habit, and that stolen goods can only be sold at one-third of their actual value. While drug-related property crime is a serious business, these calculations were unreliable. Not all money for drugs is acquired through theft. Users often fund themselves by work and dealing. Nor do they have an unwavering consumption level. Many get state methadone, or they'll quit from time to time – voluntarily or as a result of spells in jail or hospital.

63 Data from Angela Neustatter, 'AIDS – the biggest hype of the century?', in *Living*, June 1994, p. 24; and from Communicable Disease Report, Vol. 3, Supplement 1, PHLS Communicable Disease Surveillance Centre, London, June 1993.

64 Neustatter, op. cit.

65 '*Safe* AIDS vaccine mutates into virus', in the *Independent*, 15 September 1994, p. 8.

66 No one will know whether the vaccines will work or not, according to a *New Scientist* report (22 October 1994, p. 10) until the trials take place. Recipients would be warned that 'the vaccines are experimental and not finished products'.

67 'AIDS vaccine suffers setback in US', in the *British Medical Journal*, 11 June 1994, p. 1527.

68 For an outline of these theories, see my own 'Monkey Business' article in the *Independent Magazine*, 19 September 1992, p.

24; also, for the argument against immunisations in general, 'Vaccination: The hidden facts', also by this author, in the *Evening Standard Magazine*, September 1991, p. 74.

69 Due to report in early 1996.

70 *Tackling Drugs Together*, a consultation document on a strategy for England 1995–98, HMSO, October 1994.

71 Chao-Tzang Yawnghe, 'The political economy of the opium trade: implications for the Shan state', in the *Journal of Contemporary Asia*, Vol. 23, No. 3, 1993, p. 306. An illuminating and highly recommended paper.

72 Ibid.

73 Ibid.

74 Valerie Seward, 'Combating drugs trafficking and abuse: the challenge to Europe', a report based on Wilton Park conference 385, 7–11 September 1992, HMSO, London.

75 Jan van Doorn, 'Drug trafficking networks in Europe', in the *European Journal on Criminal Policy and Research*, Vol. 1, No. 2, p. 96.

76 See McDermott's *Guide to Drug Treatment* and his *Do-It-Yourself Detox* (Lifeline, Manchester), both of them wryly witty, comic-book format manuals, authored by someone who's been there.

POPPERS

What are they?

Poppers and *rush* are the street names for a range of inhalants belonging to a group of chemicals known as alkyl nitrites. Variously formulated as amyl, propyl, and butyl nitrite, they are highly volatile and flammable liquids, yellowish in colour, smelling sweet and fruity when fresh and of old socks when stale. Their reputation as a mighty enhancer of the sex act has made them especially big in gay circles but, more recently, they've found favour among young 'straights' on the dance scene.

Only amyl nitrite has a history of medical application. Discovered in 1857, ten years later it was being used for the treatment of the pain from angina. The relief came through the drug's ability to open up the vessels delivering blood to the heart. The format it came in was a small glass capsule known as a vitrellae, which was enclosed by cotton wool. The vitrellae was crushed with a pop between thumb and forefinger and the vapour inhaled. It is this popping noise which gives the recreational nitrites their best-known street name, even though the products used for purposes other than medical do no such thing: they come in little Tipp-Ex-sized bottles with screw or plug tops.

Most poppers on sale in the UK are US imports of propyl nitrite and carry nudge-nudge brand names such as Rock Hard, Heart On, Bolt, Ram TNT, Climax and (less suggestively) Liquid Gold. Since they are not recognised as medical products, neither their possession nor sale is illegal (as of October 1994). Outlets include sex shops, clubs, and pubs.

Purity

Any move to stamp on existing nitrite supplies would inevitably lead to the production of less pure 'bathtub' poppers – a phenomenon already witnessed in some gay neighbourhoods in the States where legal pressure against the drug has been ratcheted up since 1969. Even the purity of currently sanctioned stock can only be guessed at. There is little news of up-to-date samplings but a 1981 investigation into various brands, carried out by the Stanford Medical Laboratories in California, found them to contain kerosene, hydrochloric acid, and sulphur dioxide, among other impurities.[1]

Sensations

Depending on location and expectation the experience will differ. Used on the dance floor they are said to deliver a shaft of dizzy, giggly, disconnected energy that lasts just a couple of minutes. They are frequently used alongside Ecstasy and even Vicks nasal spray to enhance the rush. In lovemaking, poppers can lower inhibitions, relax the body, and prolong – in the mind at least – orgasm, so that it seems to stretch for minutes, though, in fact, while poppers might excite the senses, they can easily dull the organs. Poppers' ability to relax the anal sphincter muscle make them popular with gay men who wish to practise anal sex without obstruction.

The down effects include flushed face, headaches, weakness, nausea, coughing, and cold sweats.

Tolerance

After continual use for two or three weeks, tolerance develops to the drugs' psychoactive effects – i.e. they no longer bring on a high. An equivalent period of abstinence will probably restore sensitivity.

Dependence

The nitrites can encourage psychological dependence. Symptoms of physical addiction – with traumatic withdrawal problems – have not so far been widely reported.

Medical Effects

Skin rashes and irritation of the throat and eyes occur in some users, especially where there is contact with the liquid, as distinct from the vapours. Crusty lesions to the skin around the nose, lips, face, penis, and scrotum have also been reported.[2]

Nitrites' physiological effects include a fall in blood pressure and a reflex increase in heart rate to maintain the flow of blood to vital organs. As a result, people with blood pressure disorders, or heart problems, should be wary of using the drug.

Another of their features is to cause healthy haemoglobin (an important red pigment in the blood formed from a protein and an iron compound)) to convert into an abnormal, malfunctioning version called methaemoglobin. If levels of methaemoglobin rise too high (a condition known as methaemoglobinaemia) the result can be breathlessness and headache, with the tongue and lips turning blue.[3] If levels carry on rising the symptoms start resembling those of severe anaemia: massive haemorrhaging, blood vessel collapse, coma, and death. Sufferers of anaemia should, therefore, also be wary about using poppers.

Reported fatalities

Six of thirteen cases of nitrite-linked methaemoglobinaemia cited in the medical literature resulted in death, although all but one had swallowed rather than simply inhaled the nitrites, and the other victim already had heart/circulatory problems.[4] The difficulty of attributing death to nitrites, even when they are being used at the point of expiry, was highlighted in a 1992 paper published in the *Journal of Medicine, Science and Law*.[5] Two deaths were described – both having previously been blamed on the drug, even though other factors clouded the issue. Case one was a sixty-year-old man who collapsed in the street and was dead on arrival at hospital. Natural causes was the coroner's initial judgment. A second autopsy was carried out when it was discovered that the man's bank cash card had been used several times since his death, suggesting that he could have been the victim of a theft. Because of the levels of methaemoglobin discovered in his blood and an amount of nitrite in his stomach, cause of death was newly attributed to amyl nitrite. Yet this second autopsy also revealed that he had heart disease, that he had been drinking, that there were areas of mild bruising to the face and multiple deep bruising to the upper limbs and the trunk.

Case two was a thirty-one-year-old man found dead on his sofa-bed by his flat-mate. The deceased, well known as favouring bondage sex, had been dallying on his last night with a nineteen-year-old youth, who later testified that the older man had wanted poppers poured on to a cloth and the cloth secured around his nose. He also asked to be trussed up with a leather strap running from his neck to both wrists. Various sexual acts followed including the insertion of dildos. The post mortem found a swollen and congested brain and a wide-open anal orifice that was covered with 'fissures and lacerations'. Death, as we have seen, was officially blamed on the amyl nitrite, and yet the author of the aforementioned report was not convinced: '. . . death could not be definitely attributed to amyl nitrite, as it could have been precipitated [by] or even totally attributed to either reflex cardiac stimulation by the leather strap around the neck or the forceful dilation of the anal sphincter by the dildos.' In other words, the bondage games – with or without amyl nitrite – could have been the killer.

The Milligan affair

A 'nitrite-related' fatality that inspired a frenzy of media coverage was that of Tory MP Stephen Milligan, whose body was found, in February 1994, sprawled on a kitchen table. Binding his feet was electrical flex that was also pulled around his neck. Except for stockings and suspenders and a plastic bin-liner tied loosely over his head, Milligan was naked. In his mouth was a half-chewed quarter of orange. In his bloodstream was amyl nitrite. The coroner was equivocal about the cause of death. Most 'expert opinion' believed Milligan died from suffocation while practising 'autoerotic asphyxiation', a self-imposed partial strangulation designed to heighten orgasm. It seems that the use of nitrites was part of the erotic kit.

The AIDS connection

The darkest shadow cast over the nitrites is the alleged part they play in causing Kaposi's sarcoma (KS), a malignant tissue disease that occurs frequently in gay men with AIDS. In the early days of the AIDS epidemic, some argued that nitrites had to be implicated because the data showed that practically every time KS turned up there was a history of nitrite use. But as more data piled in and the original figures were freshly analysed, the causal link between nitrites and KS/AIDS looked less and less certain.[6] That remains the picture.

Those who argue that nitrite sniffing does lead to KS suggest the following two-step 'mechanism': as poppers are metabolised (broken down) by the body some of the resulting by-products end up being carcinogenic (capable of causing a cancer); also, nitrites themselves depress the immune system, leaving the user vulnerable to the (so-far unidentified) disease agent that is assumed to be responsible for KS.[7] Other people might ingest the KS 'disease agent' but they are immunologically strong enough to fight it off.

An obvious argument against the nitrites-are-to-blame hypothesis is that the drug is just one of a multitude of toxic, immune-suppressing, cancer-causing substances that people (particularly those in certain risk groups) are subjected to in their daily lives, and that to fix obsessively on nitrites betrays a peculiar narrowness of vision. Other formidable immunological 'insults' come from antibiotics, immunisations, the whole array of licit and illicit drugs, X-rays, vehicle pollution, toxic residues in meat, residues from the chemicals that are sprayed on to crops, as well as the radioactive and chemical waste that is pumped from factories and nuclear plants into the air and waterways.

Toxic shock

Such 'insults' readily pile up in particular individuals. Take the case, for instance, of a gay male who, over a period of years, contracts a variety of named and unnamed infections of the urogenital tract, the throat, and elsewhere. To counteract them, he is given a series of (immune-depressing) antibiotics and other powerful drugs and vaccines. As the number and regularity of the symptoms mount, so more drugs are prescribed. He is probably already using (immune-depressing) street drugs and is unlikely to be eating properly. If his number is called, he will suffer a complete immune collapse leading to a more dramatic sequence of opportunistic infections and other maladies which, collectively, are diagnosed as AIDS.

HIV will probably be implicated because AIDS is rarely diagnosed these days if HIV antibodies are not present – no matter if the clinical symptoms in an HIV-free individual add up to a classic AIDS case. Even so, there have been several reports of non-HIV cases of AIDS.

Returning to nitrites: that gay KS sufferers tend to have a history of nitrite use is hardly astonishing. Poppers have been ubiquitous on the gay scene since the 1970s. Then again, many heavy nitrite users have had no problem with KS.

'Rimming' and Kaposi's sarcoma

The conjunction of sex, gays, AIDS, and nitrites has been thoroughly researched in recent years, with most investigators pointing to nitrites being associated with 'casual', multi-partner sex, often without the use of condoms.[8] This feature is usually interpreted to mean that nitrites incline people to go high-risk, but it is just as easy to turn the formulation on its head and argue that people inclined to such high-risk adventures are also the type to use copious amounts of nitrites.

A sex-linked theory that achieved some prominence in medical circles during 1992 was summarised in the title of a paper published in *The Lancet*.[9] It was called 'Risk of Kaposi's sarcoma and sexual practices associated with faecal contact in homosexual or bisexual men with AIDS'.

The sexual and other habits of sixty-five gay and bisexual

London men with AIDS were examined, in particular to establish the prevalence of a sex act known as 'rimming'. This is where the mouth and tongue make contact with the anal ring of a partner (and, inevitably, with traces of his excrement). The investigators were looking, especially, for '*insertive* rimming', which presumably entails deeper tongue contact.

While 18 per cent of the men with KS said they had never indulged in insertive rimming, among those who had, the incidence of KS rose the more that rimming was practised. It was found in 50 per cent of men who rimmed less than once a month, but in 75 per cent of those who performed at least once a week.

'The men with Kaposi's sarcoma also tended to be more sexually active,' noted the authors, 'and were more likely to engage in other sexual activities that entailed contact with faeces [such as unprotected anal penetration and 'fist fucking'] than were the men who had other features of AIDS only.'

As to poppers: these 'were not related to Kaposi's sarcoma risk, after taking into account whether the subjects had practised insertive rimming.'

But, of course, as soon as one hypothesis looks like it might grow wings and fly, up jumps another expert with a bundle of data that proves exactly the opposite. A month after publication in *The Lancet* of the faecal-contact report, a letter appeared in the same journal from an Australian team saying that their own studies – and others like them – revealed that whereas the number of men with AIDS in whom KS developed had dramatically fallen, there had been no corresponding decrease in the numbers practising insertive rimming.[10] What price, in other words, the connection between KS and bum-kissing?

Rips and scrapes

Finally, while groovers on the male gay scene are mostly resentful about the targeting of nitrites – for many of them it is their drug of first choice – worries do persist in those circles. It is now generally recognised that poppers, along with most other drugs, do depress the immune system. There is also some acceptance of the idea that use of nitrites might not only encourage the abandonment of normal restraints but that, by relaxing the sphincter muscle, they make vigorous anal sex so trouble-free that the result could be extra rips and scraping of tissue which could more easily open the way to infection.

Patterns of use

In showbiz circles amyl nitrite was popular in the 1950s. A decade later it became celebrated in US gay circles, a development the government acted upon in 1969 when the drug was restricted to prescription-only sales. The manufacturers switched to butyl nitrite, a close chemical relative with moderately less potent effects. To avoid tangling with the authorities, the butyls were marketed under the feeble subterfuge of being 'air fresheners'. 'Remove cap,' ran a typical set of instructions, 'leave in vacated room for half an hour. Return to an outstandingly fragrant atmosphere.' By the early 1970s they were, according to a campaign document written by two gay American activists, 'an accepted, even obligatory part of the gay male lifestyle in some cities. . . . At gay discos, men shuffle around on the dance floor, zombie-like, holding popper bottles under their noses . . . Ordinarily rational men become hysterical when it is suggested that the nitrite inhalants are harmful to the health and may play a role in causing AIDS. Since poppers have become necessary for them to function sexually, giving up poppers would seem, at least in the beginning, like giving up sex itself.'[11]

Neither were they impressed by the manufacturers' room-deodoriser deceit: 'Heroin [might as well] be sold as a mosquito-bite remedy ("for external use only"). Live hand grenades could be sold as "paperweights".'

The UK broadly followed the pattern of use in the US, lagging perhaps two or three years behind: first there was their appearance on the gay scene then, by about 1982, among straights in places like Leeds, West Yorkshire, and Manchester, where they were sold over the counter in pubs, clubs, and sex shops.

Today, their appeal lies in their cheapness (about £5 for a bottle that lasts all night), their legality and easy availability.

Gay clubgoers in places like London and Brighton, especially younger ones, seem as keen as ever to pop a bottle. The young, post-rave dance crowd have also taken to them. One Manchester report suggested that more than 20 per cent of the city's school students have tried the drugs. A survey of older Scottish youth produced figures of between 5 and 10 per cent.[12]

But while nitrites have acquired some cachet among both straight and gay youth, in some circles popper 'goons' are considered about as urbane as sniffers of butane gas. One twenty-two-year-old North London man told me: 'You're not going to see it in any of the smarter clubs or at any half-decent party. It's pretty naff, pongy stuff, used by kids because it's cheap and easy to get hold of and because they don't know any better.'

The Law

By 1978 the American butyl business was estimated to be worth $50 million a year. Less than a decade later, the turnover had perhaps tripled.[13] When, in 1988, Congress banned 'air freshening' butyl nitrite, the manufacturers once more jumped sideways and started churning out propyl nitrite. A US ban of every kind of alkyl nitrite was threatened during 1991 but, so far, hasn't come to pass.

The legal status of nitrites in the UK is equally uncertain. Amyl nitrite is still not controlled under the Misuse of Drugs Act as a substance of abuse but there are controls placed on it under the Medicines Act. Pharmacists may sell it for the treatment of angina (although its use for that illness has been superseded by longer-acting preparations). As to whether or not a prescription is needed, even the legal and medical experts seem unclear.[14]

There appear to be no effective sanctions against the sale or possession of the other nitrites, nor against someone brewing up their own stock from chemicals bought on the open market.

Notes

1 J. Lauritsen and H. Wilson, *Death Rush: Poppers & Aids*, Pagan Press, 1986, p. 6.
2 H. Haverkos and L. Dougherty, 'Health hazards of nitrite inhalants', in the *American Journal of Medicine*, 84 (3, Part 1), 1988, pp. 479–82.
3 'Drug notes: Poppers', ISDD, 1994.
4 Ibid.
5 E. R. Sarvesvaran *et al.*, op. cit. 'Amyl nitrite related deaths, *Journal of Medicine, Science and Law*, Case Reports 267, 1992.
6 J. Vandenbroucke and V. Pardoel, 'An autopsy of epidemiologic methods: The case of poppers in the early epidemic of the acquired immunodeficiency syndrome (AIDS)', in the *American Journal of Epidemiology*, Vol. 129 (3), 1989, pp. 455–7.
7 As outlined in 'Nitrite inhalants: Promising and discouraging news', editorial in the *British Journal of Addiction*, 84, 1989, pp. 121–3.
8 An example being J. Dudley and R. Kaslow, 'Recreational drug use and sexual behaviour change in a cohort of homosexual men', in *AIDS*, 4 (8), 1990, pp. 759–65.
9 V. Beral *et al.*, 'Risk of Kaposi's sarcoma and sexual practices associated with faecal contact in homosexual or bisexual men with AIDS', in *The Lancet*, Vol. 339, 14 March 1992, pp. 632–5.
10 J. Elford *et al.*, 'Kaposi's sarcoma and insertive rimming', in *The Lancet*, Vol. 339, 11 April 1992, p. 938.
11 Lauritsen and Wilson, op. cit., p. 5.
12 Ibid.
13 Ibid, p. 6.
14 ISDD, op. cit.

SOLVENTS

Intro

The origins of sniffing for pleasure are rooted in the eighteenth and nineteenth centuries, when the fashion for using nitrous oxide, ether and the more dangerous chloroform became widespread. But sniffing among a whole spectrum of youth is very much a product of the modern age. More than one hundred commercially available products are now used to obtain lift-off. They include lighter fuel, glues, rubber cement, typewriter correction fluid, nail polish remover, magic markers, petrol, paint and paint thinners, cleaning fluids, aerosols, fire extinguishers and even the 'volatile' contents of decorative table lamps.

In the early 1980s, before heroin arrived in a big way to jolt opinion-formers, what was then known as 'glue sniffing' provoked the majority of all drug-scare headlines. More than half the 3,500 press cuttings collated in 1983 by the Institute for the Study of Drug Dependence related to sniffing. In those days the habit was closely identified with two perilously anti-establishment youth tribes – skinheads and punks – and so it was little wonder polite society recoiled from this volatile mix.

But the years pass and the rhetoric runs cold. More young people than ever are dying from the sniffing habit (two or three every week). Yet Parliament hasn't stirred on the subject in years and the press has picked up and discarded at least half a dozen other killer substances since then.

Why do young people sniff? Availability is one answer. Mum's aerosol hairspray will often be the first 'drug' product a young person has access to. It's also fun to experiment. Adults tell them the whole thing's miserable and they're likely to die if they take the stuff. But they know plenty of kids who tried it and had a real good laugh.

Another reason is that something like a can of butane lighter fuel is comparatively cheap, it's clean, and it doesn't stink too much. You can't get busted for being in possession, and the 'trip' is strong and quick. It gets you hallucinating like LSD but doesn't go on for hours like LSD.

Yet these young people will know that no kudos attaches to the sniffing habit, not even from their peers. It hasn't done so since the earliest days of punk, when the most elegant justification for glue-sniffing was that it was an ironic comment on gross materialism. The scene these days seems unrelievedly squalid, with surveys indicating that it is inner-city working-class runt-culture that most enthusiastically takes to the fumes. Sniffing killed four times as many young people from the lowest social class as from the highest between 1981 and 1990[1]. And when we look overseas, a similar pattern is apparent.

Among the estimated 100 million street children worldwide, volatile-substance-sniffing is widely practised. It's done to stay alert to possible violence, to bring on sleep, to dull physical and emotional pain, or as a substitute for food.[2] The products selected are the cheapest and most readily available: glues in shoemaking areas; solvents where there is nearby industry. In Uganda, street children gulp the fumes of aviation fuel and petrol. In Guatemala, as many as nine out of ten rough-sleeping youngsters are thought to be dependent on paint thinner and cheap glue. A South African survey of a group of their own young homeless showed high levels of brain damage, with the 'subjects' unable properly to think, speak, remember things, or physically co-ordinate their movements.[3]

Volatile substance use – given its association with poverty and alienation – is a political matter, requiring political remedies. But it is also personal. Not all the deaths and injuries are of children living in sewers. First-time experimenters from stable homes also come to grief. Thirty-eight per cent of those who died from sniffing in the UK during 1991 had never tried it before.[4]

What all would-be sniffers require is credible information from sources they can trust. They should be informed of the most and least dangerous substances and practices. The information might not dissuade them from using, even

358

long-term, but their chances of coming through unscathed will be improved.

What are they?

Anything that gives off an intoxicating vapour is a candidate for sniffing, no matter what other unappetising chemicals and solid particles the product might contain. Generally speaking, there are two kinds of ingredients that meet the sniffability test – solvents and propellant gases. A useful all-inclusive term for both these is volatile substances. This signals that they readily evaporate at room temperature and, in so doing, give off a 'sniffable' vapour. One more clarification: the fumes are not so much sniffed as inhaled through the mouth and nose.

What we are talking about, then, is the inhalation of volatile substances that occur in a vast array of products used in the home, by commercial businesses, and by industry.

Solvents

The solvents of interest are volatile hydrocarbons (chemical compounds of hydrogen and carbon) that derive largely from the oil industry, but also from coal and fermented vegetable matter. Industry is keen on this family of chemicals since, along with other substances, it can deploy them in products that would otherwise solidify in their containers. The job of a solvent is to keep the product dissolved until it is spread, poured, or squirted, and then to evaporate from the product quickly without trace. It is this volatility which gives the hydrocarbons their intoxicating effect. But as well as keeping products such as glue and paint in a liquid state, solvents are used to liquefy materials once they have gone solid. An example is nail varnish remover – a solvent that dissolves nail lacquer for its easy removal.

Propellants

These are pressurised liquid gases used to propel the advertised product (hairspray, paint, etc.) from the can. Butane is most often used these days. The other main category is the halogenated hydrocarbons, otherwise known as chlorofluorocarbons – the infamous CFCs, whose destructive impact on the ozone layer (which protects earthly life from cancer-causing ultraviolet radiation) led to a search for alternatives.

The products

Contact adhesives and other glues

Once easily the most sniffed of all volatile substances (VSs), adhesive products are now less openly available to young sniffers as a result of a 1985 legislative clampdown.[5] But they are still widely used, with Evostik being a particular favourite. They seem to be among the least intrinsically hazardous of the VSs, partly because just the vapour rather than the whole item is consumed, partly because the vapour drifts off the semi-solid glue rather than being rammed down into the lungs as is the case with pressurised gases, and also because they contain fairly simple hydrocarbons – notably toluene – as opposed to the unassimilable, ozone-destroying chlorofluorocarbons (CFCs) found in aerosols. Another solvent generally borne by the adhesives is commercial hexane, containing variable amounts of n-hexane, which is known to be harmful.[6] Altogether, thirteen of the 122 sudden sniffing deaths recorded in 1991 (the last figures available at the time of going to press) were linked to contact adhesives.

The usual method of use is to put a blob of glue in the bottom of, say, a freezer bag, crisp packet, or the flimsy bags available at supermarket check-outs, and then deeply inhale the fumes half a dozen to twenty times; known as *huffing*. Some warm the bag and pump it up and down to vaporise the solvent more speedily. It is often a group activity with the bag, like a cannabis joint, being passed from mouth to mouth. More serious sniffers, in their search for a denser hit, will enclose themselves in a vaporous atmosphere by placing a glue-laden plastic bag or blanket over their heads. Both these enclosure methods are hazardous since the user is cut off from fresh air and if (as is quite possible) s/he passes out while continuing to draw in the vapours s/he might well asphyxiate.

Nail polish and nail polish remover

Like the glues, these are generally considered to be less powerfully toxic than some other sniffed items. Their principal solvents are acetone, amyl acetate, and ethyl acetate, and they are typically used by brushing a cuff or other material with the substance and inhaling from close quarters. Inevitably, they are more popular among girls, who will have a legitimate reason to buy and possess such items.

Rubber solutions (for fitting carpets)

These contain toluene, commercial hexane, and 1,1,1-trichloroethane. The products would be sniffed straight from the container.

Petrol

Petrol-sniffing was the pastime that preceded the glue and aerosol fads in the US, and was especially noted among minorities such as Mexicans, and the native peoples of America and Australia. It seems never really to have taken off here, which is as well since UK petrol, unlike the US product, still often contains tetraethyl lead, a particularly toxic substance for children. Its main solvent is benzene, mixed with other hydrocarbons. Rarely used indoors, petrol is instead sniffed straight from the car or bike tank. It can also be poured on to a rag and inhaled.

Dyes (for shoes, etc.)

Sniffed straight from the container or poured on to a rag and inhaled, dyes usually contain acetone, commercial hexane, and other less volatile hydrocarbon solvents. They seem to be rarely used.

Gas lighter fuel

At the time of writing, this was the most popular of the volatile substances and also the most lethal – accounting for forty of the 122 sudden sniffing deaths logged in 1991.[7] Made up of liquid butane and virtually nothing else, the appeal of lighter fuel is that it is 'clean' (no paint, no fly spray), virtually odour-free, and it leaves no stain. The most straightforward method of use is simply to uncap the canister, clench the nozzle between the teeth, and squirt the chilly butane gas down the throat. Being packed under pressure, it acts as its own propellant. The gas might also be squirted into a plastic bag, from which the fumes are then inhaled. This is safer than taking it straight down the throat.

Although it is packaged like one, lighter fuel is not strictly an aerosol. It has no diffuser incorporated into its release nozzle which, in products such as deodorants, produces a misty spray. When the lighter refill nozzle is pressed it releases a powerful cold liquid stream which, upon contact with the atmosphere, turns into a gas.

Aerosol products

In this category are perfumes, deodorants, anti-perspirants, cleaning agents, paint sprays, hair lacquers, pain-relief sprays, fly-killers, damp start and de-icer. All contain three principal elements: the advertised product; a solvent to keep it from solidifying; and pressurised liquid gases to propel it from the can. The solvent could be a number of substances: water (starch products); alcohol (hairspray or perfume); or kerosene (insect sprays). The main buzz factor is the propellant gas, which will probably be butane, pentane, or a CFC.

The problem with sniffing aerosols is that it is difficult to inhale the propellant gas fumes without also consuming sprayed particles of paint, lacquer, or whatever the principal ingredient might be. Users will try filtering out 'impurities' by spraying the product into a balloon, hoping the concentrates will stick to the sides, or by spraying on to a cloth and then inhaling. For those seeking an intense dose – no matter what solids they might ingest along the way – plastic bags are placed or even tied over the head; or sniffing of the unfiltered spray is conducted under a blanket. The method free from all trickery is simply to spray into the atmosphere and suck.

The more gas in a can and the less solid matter, the more appealing to sniffers a product will be. High on their lists are pain-relief sprays and anti-perspirants. The aerosols were linked to 22 per cent of the sudden deaths in 1991.

Aerosols made their first appearance on the US market in the 1950s, but not until October 1967 did the 'abuse' issue come alive when the Du Pont Corporation produced a statement acknowledging at least seven deaths caused by glass-chilling products that were supposed to be used for prettifying cocktail glasses. The Federal Trade Commission ordered that in future all such products should carry a 'Death May Result From . . .' warning, and journalists took up the theme with campaigns offering details on how and what could be sniffed. Educational programmes were developed by trade associations and literature distributed to schools. By March 1972 some three hundred deaths had been recorded, and though the glass-chillers were by now withdrawn, the variety of aerosols being inhaled had increased and so had the fatalities. It was the experience of the US authorities which led to the British government adopting its cool approach; avoiding printed warnings and gauche educational assaults. The concern then, and still today, is that such moves trigger interest in substances where none existed.

Cleaning agents

This category includes domestic and industrial cleaning agents, degreasing materials, plaster remover (e.g. Zoff), and, above all, typewriter correction fluids such as Tipp-Ex. The vapours derive from trichloroethylene, trichloroethane, other chlorinated aliphatic hydrocarbons, and methylene chloride.

At the time of writing, Tipp-Ex was perhaps tying with glue as the second most popular of all the volatiles after butane lighter fuel – easy to shoplift, simple to use even in the classroom (a few drops dabbed on a sleeve and, with the chin resting in the palm, the fumes are sniffed). The German manufacturers of Tipp-Ex responded to concerns in 1990 by introducing a new water-based correction fluid. But the original trichloroethane-based version is still doing good business.

Typewriter correction thinners were linked to eleven of the 122 sudden sniffing deaths in 1991.

Fire extinguishers

The traditional method is to decant the liquid into an empty beer can or plastic bag and inhale the fumes; or a piece of material or cotton wool might be soaked and the vapours sucked. They contain an unfriendly solvent called bromochlorodiflouromethane.

Young sniffers often steal the extinguishers from rail or bus stations. At the March 1990 inquest of a twelve-year-old Peckham, South London boy, the London Central Bus Company revealed that 365 extinguishers had been stolen from its depot in just five months.[8] In December of the same year, a Poole, Dorset inquest heard from the local bus company how 170 of its devices had been stolen or vandalised in seven months. The hearing was into the death, from a heart attack, of a sixteen-year-old boy who had been sniffing from a stolen extinguisher. Of the 122 sniffing deaths in 1991, six were attributed to fire extinguishers.

In the above-listed products certain gases, chemicals and solids have been identified as the key psychoactive (mood-altering) constituents. And yet much of what else goes into these products remains a commercial secret. There are any amount of additives to improve consistency and flavourings to entertain the nose, and these might also be absorbed by the sniffer, whatever the filtering precautions. The effect on the body of simple hydrocarbons such as toluene is still not really known. The impact of these unspecified materials is a correspondingly bigger mystery.

Sensations

The inhaled vapours are absorbed through the lungs and pass rapidly through the blood to the brain. They act on the central nervous system, sometimes as a stimulant but generally as a depressant, putting a clamp on that part of the brain (the cortex) which is believed to 'check' primitive instincts. The result is what the professionals call 'disinhibition'. General body functions like breathing and heart rate are depressed and there is a 'stoned' feeling lasting from a few minutes to half an hour. Headaches, sickness and dizziness are not uncommon, particularly for novices. The majority of users will stop at this point. Continued or deep inhalation causes disorientation, drowsiness, numbness, and perhaps unconsciousness – much like the effects of medical anaesthetics. Recovery is usually quick, but complications arise if the source of the vapour is not removed or after the person has blacked out. Typically, this would occur if the person is alone and sniffing with his/her head in a bag or under blankets. Despite all kinds of scary possibilities, most sniffing bouts do not end in grief.

The experience is said to be much like that of being drunk and, as any drinker knows, having a few can produce results as varied as euphoria, aggression, deep melancholy, the giggles, and raised libido. The key factors are the user's mental state: how is s/he feeling? What has been eaten? Is s/he alone or in a group, and does that company inspire an elevation or depression in mood?

Hallucinations

Hallucinations are never attributed to alcohol, except by some heavy/chronic drinkers, yet they are often experienced by sniffers of all kinds of volatile substances. Some (pain-relief sprays, typewriter correction fluids) are held to be especially potent triggers to the imagination, leading to a variety of visual and auditory imaginings. Users talk of shooting stars, babbling cartoon characters, angelic music, and witches. Power delusions are also commonly reported, such as being able to fly, to turn stone into liquid, pass through brick walls, even travel to other worlds. A group, sniffing together, seem capable of experiencing jointly the very same images – which they then collectively control.

Inevitably, the 'cases' most intensively studied are those who are most easily on tap – namely, people who come forward for medical treatment or are in trouble with the law. The experiences of such individuals are almost certain to be more downbeat than those of typical users but they can still be revealing. A group of forty-three youngsters –

lighter fuel and glue regulars – gave in-depth interviews to a research team for a 1987 paper published in the *British Journal of Psychiatry*.[9] Eighteen arrived by way of the Leeds Addiction Research Unit, the rest were from special units for young offenders run by the then Department of Health and Social Security.

Most had been using for more than a year and nearly half every day. Clear differences emerged between the glue and 'gas' trips. Glue caused slowed-down, fragmented speech and thinking. Gas produced the opposite effects. 'It's as if you're really brainy,' said one respondent. All reported what the researchers called 'illusionary misinterpretations': trees coming alive, gravestones changing into orange aliens. 'Tactile hallucinations' were also common: *I could feel knives sticking in my legs . . . a long, greasy, slimy worm was trying to climb out of my throat.*

Stories of witches and graves opening up and things coming out of them were common, as were tales of spaceships and little green men. One boy went back in time and was given chase by Romans in leather armour who wanted to capture him for the slave trade. What the researchers called 'delusional ideas' were most common among the toluene group. Two were convinced they were dead during a sniffing session. One thought he had changed into his best friend. Another decided the Devil was operating the world from an underground city where UFOs were buried. Some of the delusional ideas turned out to be nearly lethal. A girl who thought she could swim but couldn't jumped into a lake and had to be rescued. Others reported jumping out of trees and from the windows of buildings, under the impression that they could fly. None was seriously hurt, although one broke an ankle.

For all of these young people, sniffing was associated with positive expectations and, initially at least, 'elation of mood and pleasant perceptual change.' But the continued use of volatiles was often associated with a release of internal conflicts and, in particular, 'unresolved feelings about death and their parents.'

Most individuals will know the difference between a VS dream and reality. The danger arises when they become so intoxicated that they are no longer bothered or are unable to take cues from their bodily reactions. Among the sniffing deaths on record is a boy who drowned in a canal watched lethargically by his stoned friends. He simply bobbed out of sight. Another was a boy who plunged from a high-rise flat after crawling out on to an unguarded ledge that under normal circumstances he presumably would not have gone near. It is because of such accidents that young users must be discouraged from sniffing in potentially dangerous places.

Patterns of Use

Considering the number of annual volatile substance deaths of young people, the whole area is remarkably under-researched in terms of knowing who's taking what, why, and the kind of long-term impact the habit is having on users who don't die. Scientific as well as media interest peaked during the early 1980s and was already tailing off before the end of the decade. Perhaps what the 'glue story' lacked was a foreign enemy upon whom the blame could conveniently settle – the equivalent of a South American coke bandit. The producers in this instance are top-ranked industrial concerns, while the dealers are high-street retailers from whom we buy our newspapers and electric kettles. To remove all temptation from potential sniffers would mean reformulating or even jettisoning literally hundreds of favourite consumer products – the hairsprays, fly-killers, fire extinguishers, rubber cements. A less stressful option was to keep a low profile: say little and do less. And this was what was done.

From the information available, various assumptions can be made about the nature of the volatiles habit. Studies from the late 1980s indicate that between 4–8 per cent of secondary-school pupils have sniffed something or other.[10] But there is considerable variation across the country, with Scotland and the north of England judged to have high consumption rates and East Anglia amongst the lowest. A two-part survey of 776 school pupils from Manchester and Merseyside, conducted in 1991 and again a year later, found that around one in eight had sampled 'solvents' by the time they were sixteen. (This was against a background showing that nearly half had tried something illegal.) The Department of Health tried offering some solace when, in a 1992 guide to parents, it avowed that most who try sniffing 'will only experiment; they won't sniff for very long.'[11]

The London-based Institute for the Study of Drug Dependence estimates that about a tenth of those who start sniffing wish to carry on. They'll do so for perhaps a few months, usually sniffing in groups. Only a small proportion of these individuals will continue long-term.[12]

More boys than girls report having tried sniffing and the attrition rate for boys is also very much higher (among fifteen- to nineteen-year-olds, almost ten times more males than females per million died from sniffing in 1991). The peak experimenting age is probably around thirteen or fourteen, and even the government will admit that there is more use in the deprived inner-city areas.[13]

Sniffing Alone

A distinction can be made between the solitary and the group sniffer. Apart from any conclusions to be drawn about the psychological health of a persistent solitary user, the chances of coming to grief are increased. A study that examined 140 UK sniffing deaths between 1971 and 1981[14] found that most occurred alone, at home, with the age group most at risk being the fifteen- to sixteen-year-olds.

Getting Hooked

Tolerance

A novice glue user is likely to be satisfied with a single experimental blob that will keep him or her buzzing for up to half an hour. The level of subsequent use, if there is to be any, is entirely variable. Those who become regular users will generally require increasing amounts to achieve the same high and might find themselves in a spiralling pattern of use in which scarcely credible amounts of volatiles are consumed: perhaps five or six cans of butane lighter fuel a day or twenty-five tubes of model aeroplane glue.

Addiction/dependence

A psychological dependence can develop for any mood-altering substance, volatile solvents included, especially if their use has served to mask some deep-set problems. A physical dependence can also arise, although on the scale of such things (barbiturates and alcohol being in the high, danger zone) it is usually comparatively mild. Distinct withdrawal symptoms occur in perhaps 50 or 60 per cent of such users. Typical features will be sleep disturbance, irritability, shakiness, sweating, fleeting illusions, and nausea. Less often there will be stomach cramps, lower chest pain, and facial tics.[15]

Health

Sudden deaths

While there is plenty of debate in medical circles about the long-term effects of volatiles on the brain, liver, kidneys, and blood system, one clear-cut phenomenon is what are known as 'sudden sniffing deaths': an individual inhales a volatile product and his/her heart or respiratory system fails. S/he will possibly choke on vomit, or the liver and kidneys will pack up. Many of the sudden deaths in the UK have been due to asphyxiation caused by plastic bags over the head, or to the use of other paraphernalia such as tubes.

Also common in recent years have been fatalities resulting from the freezing effect of butane gas when it's sprayed directly against the back of the throat. It is cold enough to freeze the larynx and cause the lungs to fill with fluid – an experience akin to drowning.

Inhaling butane, and other propellant gases, can also cause a fatal cardiac arrhythmia. This is where the heart is thrown into severely abnormal rhythms. The presence of the gas makes the heart more than usually sensitive to the 'fight or flight' hormone, adrenalin. When a user is under stress (from, for instance, being chased) the release of adrenalin into the system can prove too much.

Volatile substance deaths have been monitored since 1971

by St George's Hospital Medical School in London. In that first year, two fatalities were recorded. For 1991, 122 were logged. The total for the whole twenty-year period was 1,239, with an average annual rise of around 5.5 per cent.

At first, glue was the major product involved. But as the legal and media pressure bore down on the adhesives, so other products began figuring more centrally in sudden deaths – notably aerosols and gas fuels. In 1983 gas killed nineteen people. Five years later the tally was fifty-three. The equivalent aerosol figures are thirteen and forty-six. Proportionately, gas fuel deaths decreased slightly between 1989 and 1991, but they were still killing more people than all the other volatiles.

The 'mechanism' of death also tells an interesting story. The St George's team specifies five routes to oblivion: direct toxic effects of the substance(s) concerned, inhalation of vomit, suffocation from a plastic bag, trauma (including hanging, drowing, and falling), and other/not known.

Throughout the twenty-year period, direct toxic effects have been given as the reason for roughly half the annual deaths. Inhalation of vomit and trauma have also carried off a fairly constant proportion of people – about 13 and 12 per cent respectively. The biggest change has been in the numbers dying each year after sticking a plastic bag over their heads. For the first ten years the average was nearly 23 per cent of the total. The 1991 figure was just 7.4 per cent – evidence that this harm-minimisation message, at least, was getting through.

Among the most disturbing bits of data to come from the St George's study is the high number who die the very first time they try sniffing: in 1991, 38 per cent of the total.

Long-term effects

This is an extremely complicated area, not least because a large number of different products are used, often containing several volatile substances, each of which interact unpredictably. Additionally, the products are peppered with additives, not all of them listed, as well as solid matter. Another difficulty is establishing what happens to a 'normal' cross-section of recreational sniffers over a period of time, since much of the information on adverse effects comes from industrial studies where the exposure of workers has typically been to *low* concentrations. Or else it has come from laboratory experiments on animals which – apart from being a cruel use of fellow creatures – cannot be trusted either. While a mouse can demonstrably suffer when abused in a laboratory, his/her body chemistry is not the same as a human being's; nor is it the same as a monkey's, a cat's, a dog's, or any of the other animals used for these poisoning 'procedures'. Each will respond differently to the same chemical insult, to the point where some animals will actually thrive on chemicals that kill other species.[16] For this reason, the data gleaned from such experiments will mislead rather than illuminate.

The main argument among researchers centres on how long the damaging effects of certain volatiles last, with some insisting that the problems quickly reverse themselves and others reporting that (especially with use over several years) the result can be permanent damage to the brain, nerves, liver, kidney, muscles, stomach, and intestines.[17]

One leading researcher in the field has concluded that 'the risk of developing any impairment due to solvent abuse is small. Where it does occur there may be factors such as lack of oxygen, or individual susceptibility which might act singly or in combination, making it impossible to predict who might be at risk.[18]

Benzene (found in petrol), and trichloroethylene and trichlorethane (found in typewriter correction fluid), have been fingered as the substances most likely to cause kidney and liver damage.[19] Another product found in petrol – tetraethyl lead – is identified as a likely source of brain impairment.[20]

In a recent report from Austria, a researcher said that she 'sometimes' saw a range of long-lasting problems caused by volatile substances which included epilepsy, lack of muscle co-ordination (especially linked to toluene), brain degradation, and congenital malformations in babies born to sniffing mothers.[21]

A British research team speculated that the reason why there were comparatively few reports of damage to vital organs was because 'in a young and otherwise healthy population, any chronic organ toxicity arising from [volatile substance use] has to be gross in order to become clinically apparent.'[22] The evidence they'd looked at led them to believe that toluene, trichloroethylene and trichlorethane 'can cause permanent damage to the kidney, liver, heart and lung in certain volatile substance users.'

Where brain damage is found in young sniffers, there is 'reasonably good evidence', according to another team, that intellectual performance will suffer. They went on to suggest that even where no physical damage is apparent, sniffers usually perform worse in IQ tests than abstainers.[23] But attributing these low scores to the volatiles themselves is another matter. A 1989 survey of 160 London school pupils – half of whom had sampled the fumes – found that while the sniffers performed 'significantly less well' in tests of vocabulary and verbal intelligence, once social background was accounted for, the differences were 'no longer significant'.[24]

Heart

As has already been indicated, the use of various volatile substances can cause arrythmia – an irregular heartbeat pattern. This condition can lead to heart failure if, while sniffing – or shortly after – the user becomes stressed emotionally or physically. The advice for sniffers must be 'don't tear off in a panic if you're found out', and for those who catch young people in the act, 'don't give chase'.

Pregnancy

Since all the volatiles are capable of passing through the placental barrier and entering the bloodstream of the foetus, there is an – as yet unquantifiable – risk of the developing child being damaged. See the cocaine chapter for general comments on drugs and pregnancy.

Identifying a User

A sniffer without guile will signal use in fairly obvious ways. The odour may cling to clothes, there may be freezer bags, milk bottles, crisp packets, plastic bread bags and other paraphernalia lying around in strange places, possibly with chunks of hardened glue in them. If dry-cleaning fluids are being used there may be curious fade-stains on sleeves and lapels; or spill-marks on bedclothes, window ledges, carpets. There will be physical signs too. A number of them are typical of the teenage years, so beware of making rash assumptions. The most common will be cold-sore-type spots around the mouth and nose, cracked lips, a cough, runny nose, watery eyes, a pallid, tired look – reminiscent of the symptoms of a stubborn cold. There may be weight loss together with listlessness. These symptoms will invariably clear up once sniffing stops, probably in a week to ten days.

The law

Inhaling volatile substances is not, in itself, illegal. Nor is it an offence to purchase or possess the products concerned (although since the 'sniffing epidemic' started there have been many irate demands for a ban on all suspect items).

Recognising that total prohibition is an impossibility, the government enacted a piece of legislation in the mid-1980s directed at dissuading shopkeepers from supplying young people with the means to get out of their heads. The Intoxicating Substances Supply Act 1985 – applying to England and Wales – makes it an offence to supply or offer to supply a person under the age of eighteen with substances where traders know or have reasonable cause to believe that the product concerned will be used for intoxication. Maximum penalties include a six-month prison term and/or a fine of £2000.

In practice, the law is a sleeper, with fewer than a dozen prosecutions a year. The problem seems to be obtaining proof that the retailer knew a product would be sniffed; few are so careless these days as to offer up 'sniffing kits' with plastic bags and the like.

The law has, in any case, done nothing to reduce the death-rate from volatiles and has probably served to increase it by directing young users away from the now-more-difficult-to-obtain adhesives and on to lighter refills and aerosols, products that are intrinsically more hazardous.

'Where substances such as adhesives have been removed from the shelves and are harder to buy,' noted one drug worker who is experienced in the ways of volatile sniffing, 'substances such as aerosols and gas refills still remain easy to buy. And for places where shops restrict sale of even aerosols, shoplifting remains an effective way of obtaining substances. Hence legislation designed to protect young people from the social, health and crime risks associated with volatile use can force young people to steal a less safe product as a result.'[25]

Scotland has been ahead of the rest of the UK on several fronts: they had the first publicised 'glue epidemic'; the first specialised clinic; the first successful prosecution of a glue-kit pedlar; and the first piece of anti-volatile substance legislation (enacted 1983) called the Solvent Abuse (Scotland) Act. While not expressly banning sniffing, it added the practice to the list of conditions whereby a child might be referred to the 'Reporter'. This person then decides whether to inform the parents, ask social services to 'take a look', or pass the child on to the Children's Panel which has the power to place him/her in residential or non-residential care. The numbers of referrals was in the 500 to 600 region for the first three years, since when the practice has tailed off. Very few youngsters are nowadays reported to Children's Panels simply for volatile substance sniffing.[26]

Other Controls

Arresting sniffers for being 'drunk' in public is a possible option but there is little official enthusiasm for embarking on a course that would likely catch thousands of youngsters in the criminal net, particularly if they are committing no separate 'outrage' such as thieving or assault, for which laws already exist. And yet because there is an amount of public distress at the very sight of young people with their faces in crisp packets, swaying and giggling, various laws have been turned against sniffers. Generally, an arrest will be for obstruction, public nuisance, criminal damage, and a range of similar offences. Local bye-laws have also been dusted off, such as in Neath where a sixteen-year-old girl pleaded guilty to contravening a local statute making it an offence to 'cause annoyance or commit a nuisance to public decency or propriety'.

Though sniffing has been ruled not to cause 'drunkenness', volatile substances are included in the provisions of the Road Traffic Act, making it an offence to be in charge of a motor vehicle while 'unfit to drive through drink or drugs'.

Other policy options

In the early 1980s, the nation was entranced by the glue-sniffing epidemic. A decade later opinion-formers and legislators were bored, even though, by now, two or three young people were dying every week. In the House of Commons not a word was uttered on the subject between December 1988 and May 1994. The silence was broken by David Hanson, former director of the campaign group Re–Solv, who, after reeling out the dread statistics, called for more money, better co-ordination between different government departments, and a good dose of preventive education for all those who labour 'at the interface with young people'. Such people included retailers of the products themselves, the police, youth workers, and doctors. All needed to 'know about the causes, the symptoms and the remedies, so as to help ensure that young people do not get involved in the first place,' said Hanson.

What Hanson's message omitted was the serious conflict of interest between the key political and moneyed interests. While the Department of Education was prepared to go the 'harm minimisation' route and even put out a reasonably intelligent and useful booklet for parents,[27] the Home Office was fearful of the political consequences of not talking Rambo-tough. Business had another agenda. In 1991, British manufacturers put 45,000 tonnes of butane into aerosol products, 90 per cent of which was consumed on home soil. The cigarette lighter and refill business is also of some consequence with around 15 million items sold annually.[28]

The chairman of the Association of British Lighter Manufacturers declared that he had no idea young people were snorting butane refills until just a couple of months before a special November 1992 seminar on 'volatile substance misuse' at which he was a participant.

Not so the managing director of one of the largest refill businesses, Keene World Marketing of Buckinghamshire. Geoffrey Keene told *New Scientist* magazine that he had known about sniffing since 1988 but blamed media hype for much of the problem. 'Britain, the US, Canada and Australia all have media which responds to these sorts of hairy stories. The publicity then tends to breed it.'[29]

Other than making deep adjustments to the political and social status quo calculated to improve the mass of young people's prospects, and other than educational sorties that warn and inform, there are various sniffing-control options to be considered. Most, however, come with drawbacks. Here are the main ones:

Ban all sales of recognised volatiles to under-16s. Apart from being unfair to legitimate young consumers, the sniffer will always find an alternative – probably one that's more dangerous. Or s/he will shoplift what s/he wants or nick it from under the sink at home.

Use an 'aversive', foul-smelling additive to make the products uninhalable. Again, pity the ordinary consumer. Every single item capable of being sniffed would have to be so doctored, and finding a suitable aversive substance is in any case extremely difficult. The Ministry of Defence's chemical defence establishment at Porton Down worked on it for some time and failed. The substance must be potent, yet it cannot be flammable, cause allergies, or in any way be dangerous to the majority of purchasers.

Put clear warning signs on the sniffable items. This will amount to a 'sniffer's guide'.

Given the above drawbacks, it is little wonder that there is scarcely any support for such controls, whether from the 'caring agencies', the government, police, or industry.

Help

It is not helpful to pounce on young experimentalists in a panic, much better to talk calmly with them, discover what and how much they're using and by what method. Set before them the risks; even if they don't quit they might at least be steered towards safer habits. Try to find out whether the sniffing is for 'fun', to relieve teenage boredom, or whether it masks deeper problems. Sniffing that goes on

376

for more than six to nine months and which is done without friends and/or gluttonously will signal something other than recreational use. Then, clearly, the underlying problem has to be unfolded, and a commitment drawn from the user to quit the habit. How this commitment is achieved will vary, but one of the big obstacles will be a failure to see that alternatives to the habit can possibly exist. Most experienced counsellors recommend old-fashioned healthy pursuits to take the place of the volatiles. All the while self-confidence should be boosted in readiness for the awkward road of volatile substance 'deprivation' lying ahead. A few years ago, a remarkably sensible document was produced by Manchester drugs expert Rowdy Yates.[30] It was designed for professional counsellors but could equally aid parents and friends of compulsive sniffers. Among his recommendations:

- Avoid dwelling on the particulars of volatiles and their effects since 'this can often reinforce the self-image that the process is attempting to change.'
- Avoid getting into 'yes you are – no I'm not' arguments about when the last sniff was had and what it was. 'Better to acknowledge this is a difficult area and move on to the problems which lie behind the denial – fear, inadequacy, lack of self-respect.' A more honest relationship will develop.
- Though there'll be a long-term target (to quit or cut down to a manageable level), also have a series of short-term objectives – no matter that they are slight. These can be celebrated when reached.
- Avoid depicting small lapses as grave failures. Rather, 'use the experience to develop new strategies to overcome particular difficulties and situations.'

Some habits, clearly, are going to be beyond the wit of the user and his/her family and friends. Experienced help will be needed. See Appendix II.

Damage limitation

Fashionably called 'harm reduction' in treatment circles, this is a strategy for limiting the negative impact of drugs. It recognises that not everyone will be able to or even be interested in quitting – not according to someone else's timetable, anyway. For volatile substance users (and those concerned for them) there are several practical steps that can be taken to reduce their risk of dying, coming to serious grief, or harming others.

1. It should be recognised that aerosols and butane gas are more intrinsically dangerous than glue and other toluene-based adhesives.
2. If aerosols and butane are to be used, it's much safer first to spray the solution into a plastic bag and inhale from that. Butane lighter fuel fired directly into the throat is especially risky because of its freezing effect.
3. The use of booze or other drugs with solvents brings extra risks.
4. If a bag is to be used, choose a small one. Never place a bag over the head. It can cause asphyxiation.
5. It is better to use with others than alone in case a medical emergency occurs. (Not that this amounts to a suggestion to go on a recruiting drive.)
6. If you do sniff alone, be wary of doing so in a confined space – such as under a blanket – where no air circulates. If you pass out and the fumes are still coming at you (e.g. from an open bag or pot of glue) you could lapse into fatal coma or choke to death.
7. Volatile substances are generally flammable – they easily catch fire and might actually explode. Naked flames or even a cigarette might trigger an inferno that could engulf someone who is already surrounded by volatile vapours.[31]
8. When heating solid products such as polishes and dyes in order to release their volatile fumes, remember that the risk of explosion, followed by the spraying of large amounts of hot liquid over those in the vicinity, is high.[32]
9. In an effort to escape detection, sniffers often hang out in dangerous places, made more so once they are under the influence and into a drowsy, hallucinatory, paranoid, delusional state. High-risk locations include railway embankments, the sides of roads, rooftops, the branches of trees, canals, and river banks.
10. To repeat a tip given earlier: if you're caught sniffing,

don't run off in a panic. And if you're the one who encounters a sniffer, don't give chase or over-stress him/her. It could lead to cardiac arrest.

11. When approaching a sniffer, bear in mind that paranoia and anxiety might induce them to act violently. Approach calmly, offering reassurance.
12. Persistent solitary sniffing is usually a tip that the use is problematic.
13. Try not to panic if your child is sniffing.
14. Don't be discouraged if the quitting/cutting back isn't instant or if there are lapses. A 'cure' requires understanding that there are healthy and satisfying alternatives to the fumes.

Notes

1 A. Esmail *et al.*, 'Death from volatile substance abuse in those under 18 years', in *Archives of Diseases in Childhood*, 69, 1993, pp. 356–60.

2 Re-Solv *Newsletter*, June/July 1994, p. 2.

3 P. Jansen *et al.*, 'Glue Sniffing: A description of social, psychological and neuropsychological factors in a group of South African "street children"', in *S. Afr. Tydskr Sielle*, 20 (3), 1990, p. 150.

4 '1991 Mortality Figures', factsheet published by Re-Solv, Stone, Staffs.

5 The Intoxicating Substances Supply Act, 1985. This was supposed to have restricted the sale of all sniffable products. But, because of the simplistic equation in the public mind between sniffing and glue, and because it is logistically simpler to target just one kind of product, aerosols, lighter fuel, and other items have not received the same attention.

6 'Solvents: drug notes', ISDD, London, 1993, p. 7.

7 '1991 Mortality Figures', op. cit.

8 'Teenagers sniff deadly fire extinguisher gas', in the *Sunday Independent*, 16 December 1990.

9 A. C. Evans and D. Raistrick, 'Phenomenology of intoxication with toluene-based adhesives and butane gas', in the *British Journal of Psychiatry*, 150, June 1987, p. 769.

10 'Solvents: drug notes', op. cit., p. 3.

11 'Solvents, a parents' guide', Department of Health, February 1992, p. 4.

12 'Solvents, drug notes', op. cit., p. 3.

13 'Solvents, a parents' guide', op. cit., p. 5.

14 H. R. Anderson *et al.*, 'An investigation of 140 deaths associated with volatile substance abuse in the UK (1971–1981)', in *Human Toxicology*, Vol, 1, pp. 207–21.

15 Evans and Raistrick, op. cit., p. 772.

16 For example, rabbits can eat deadly nightshade with impunity, though it can kill humans. Penicillin is highly toxic in guinea pigs but is widely used in human medicine. Morphine depresses the central nervous system of humans, rats and dogs, but stimulates cats, goats, and horses. Coumarin (a food flavouring) produces liver damage in the rat and dog but not in the baboon.

17 For instance, see 'Solvents: drug notes', op. cit., p. 8; Simon Wills, 'Volatile substance abuse', in the *Pharmaceutical Journal*, 250 (6730), 20 March 1993, p. 381.

18 In 'Solvents: drug notes', op. cit., p. 8.

19 Kevin Flemen, 'Volatile Substance Use: A basic briefing', The Hungerford Project, London, 1993, p. 23.

20 'Solvents: drug notes', op. cit., p. 8.
21 Re-Solv *Newsletter*, February/March 1994, p. 2.
22 R. Marjot and A. A. McLeod, 'Chronic non-neurological toxicity and volatile substance abuse', in *Human Toxicology*, 8 (4), 1989, pp. 301–6.
23 O. Chadwick and H. Anderson, 'Neuropsychological consequences of volatile substance abuse: a review', in *Human Toxicology*, 8 (4), 1989, p. 307.
24 O. Chadwick *et al.*, 'Neuropsychological consequences of volatile substance abuse: a population-based study of secondary school pupils', in the *British Medical Journal*, Vol. 298, 24 June 1989, p. 1679.
25 Flemen, op. cit., p. 29.
26 'Solvents: drug notes', op. cit., p. 4.
27 'Solvents, a parents' guide', op. cit.
28 Justin Russell, 'Fuel of the forgotten deaths', in *New Scientist*, 6 February 1993, pp. 21–3.
29 Ibid.
30 Rowdy Yates, 'Sniffing for Pleasure', Lifeline Project, Manchester.
31 Flemen, op. cit., p. 24.
32 Ibid.

STEROIDS

Intro

The founder of a city-centre drugs agency in Nottingham, about to lecture some eight- to fourteen-year-old youth club members, tells me: 'I know for a fact that most of the questions they'll ask tonight will be about steroids. I'm for ever being asked about steroids.' In the Wirral, a community nurse reports that the big question on the lips of the school kids she goes visiting is, 'What drugs can you take, miss, to make you bigger?'

Male youth has always modelled itself on beefcake. But whereas in earlier times they sought to replicate the 'advanced' physiques of a Victor Mature or Charles Atlas, such characters – in our own era of 6ft 4in protein-overloaded fifteen-year-olds – now look manifestly puny. The exemplars these days are TV's all-action Lycra-clad giants, The Gladiators, or the star performers on the World Wrestling Federation circuit.

We won't speculate here as to whether such individuals have ever used anabolic steroids, but what we can be clear about is that the pressure is now on young males to conform to a certain idealised body profile and that a proportion of these male children are deciding that the fast way to get as *big* as their heroes is to take a chemical assist. The evidence is already accumulating that steroids are no longer confined to the sealed world of competing body-builders, strength athletes, and the like, but are close to becoming a mainstream street drug.

A survey by a Dumfries research psychiatrist, published as long ago as 1991, found that nearly one in twenty male students at a Scottish technology college were using the drugs – mostly to 'enhance appearance' rather than for athletic performance.[1] And from Nottingham two years later came news that more than half the 840 injectors using the free needle exchange scheme established by a city-centre drug agency were steroids users.

The barriers are breached. Not only are those chemically-boosted gym regulars (female as well as male) looking less and less like a group apart, but the secret elixirs that they have been consuming since the 1940s are now the property of the common majority.

In this sense, the steroids 'craze' represents the first major innovation in underground drug use of the modern era. The most common pattern of street usage before steroids had been associated with a spectrum of up/down/hallucinatory experiences, at one end of which is recreational fun use and, at the other end, escapism, pain relief, and suicide. What's common to virtually all the drugs discussed in this book is that they are broadly non-efficient, certainly in the long term. Though cocaine provides a lift and heroin puts the pain of the world at a distance, and while there are some mellowing, mind-expanding benefits derived from cannabis and LSD, people do not take these drugs to remodel their lives along more efficient lines. They are used to turn down or hype up reality – from love to suicide.

Anabolic steroids, on the other hand, are aimed at avid self-improvers. They are the perfect accompaniment in an age of perfectibility, an era in which the citizen has been replaced by the consumer who, ironically, is him/herself reduced to a mere commodity by virtue of an increasingly rigorous social and capital marketplace.

To get a buyer, a product must be packaged and presented right. So with those who strain for a more heroic body image; they want to be admired and taken up. Or perhaps we're being too sociological. Steroids are something to try. They are powerful, they are interesting, and the more authority wrings its hands and seeks to banish them, the greater will be their allure.

Given the potentially serious impact on physical and mental health these drugs can present, the time to develop an intelligent strategy in response to their increased use is now.

What are they?

To explain what anabolic steroids are we must first describe testosterone from which they are usually derived and with which they remain structurally related.

Testosterone is the most powerful of a group of naturally occurring male hormones whose job is to prompt the development of a whole range of 'masculine' characteristics. As well as the growth and proper functioning of the male sex organs themselves, testosterone also plays a key role in the 'virilising' process that occurs during male puberty – including the deepening of the voice and the growth of body hair. All these male effects are categorised as androgenic.

But testosterone also has anabolic effects – that is to say it causes general growth in body tissue and, during puberty especially, a rapid increase in muscle mass.

The synthetic anabolic steroids also have a combination of virilising and muscle-building capacities (it has so far proved impossible to produce a product that does one and not the other) and are, thus, more properly called anabolic-androgenic steroids.

The catalogue of medical conditions for which steroids are prescribed is formidable. The list includes persistent anaemia, breast cancer, post-surgical muscle wasting, poor appetite, the loss of 'condition' by terminally ill patients, various blood circulation disorders, slow growth in adolescent males, and as hormone replacement therapy for 'menopausal men'.

Steroids come in several forms:

- Water-soluble. Usually in oral though sometimes injectable form, these are excreted by the body fairly rapidly – in from one to four weeks.
- Oil-based types that are soluble in fat. These are injected into the muscle and absorbed into the fatty tissue. They remain in the body for up to eight months or even longer, making them easier to detect in sporting dope tests.
- They also come in patches, sublingual (under-the-tongue) tabs, capsules, implants and – rarely – as suppositories and sprays.

The majority of steroids on sale 'recreationally' in the UK are counterfeits of genuine pharmaceutical products that may long ago have been discontinued by the drug company concerned. Others are veterinary products (genuine or faked) with horse remedies being especially popular since body-builders look with admiration at a well 'ripped' racing animal and want whatever tonic got him that way.

Mexico, India, Spain, and Canada are often cited as source countries for the recreational products, and while they might approximate the genuine article as suggested by the name on the label they might just as easily contain the likes of vegetable oil, liquid aspirin, or something more malign.

A 1993 survey[2] of body-builders, weight trainers, and other athletes found that the following products were most commonly used. First comes the brand name then, in brackets, its chemical classification:

Dianabol (methandrostenolene); Deca-Durabolin (nandrolone decanoate); Testosterone; Anavar (oxandrolone); Winstrol/Stromba (stanozolol); Primobolin (methenolone); Anadrol (oxymetholone); Equipose (boldenone); Finajet (Trenbolone); Maxibolin (ethylestrenol).

Other performance-enhancing preparations

The use of steroids to improve the way the body looks and performs often leads to the consumption of other powerful preparations, either to maximise the impact of steroids, or to counter their damaging side effects. The following list includes some of the more popular items, together with a selection of unwanted side effects.[3]

Antibiotics. These are used in an effort to prevent or reduce the spread of acne – one of the common side effects of steroids. It is now generally recognised that antibiotics, unless used sparingly, encourage the development of disease organisms against which no drug has any impact.

Anti-estrogen preparations. Used to prevent or control what medics know as gynaecomastia and what serious steroids users refer to as 'bitch tits' or 'BTs' – small breast-like growths that develop under the male nipple. It seems that excess male hormones are converted into the female hormone oestrogen (which is present in small quantities in all males), by a process known as aromatization. In other words, any steroids-assisted attempt to become more of a man means becoming more of a woman too. A commonly used anti-estrogen product is tamoxifen, used for breast cancer treatment and whose common side effects in women include hot flushes and vaginal bleeding and discharge. Less commonly, there are skin rashes, major visual problems, hepatitis, cancer of the womb lining, deep vein blood clots requiring hospitalisation, and life-threatening clots in the lung.[4]

Human Chorionic Gonadotrophin (HCG). Steroids tend to depress the body's natural ability to produce testosterone (The body stops bothering since it's getting so much of the synthetic version pumped into it.) HCG, derived from the urine of pregnant women, is intended to stimulate the testes into recommencing testosterone production. It is generally used just before steroids users go into one of their periodic rests from use, known as an 'off cycle'. The purpose of an 'off-cycle' is to avoid over-saturation.

Clomid. This is a female fertility drug, used for the same reason as HCG.

Human Growth Hormone. HGH is given increasingly to children who are considered to be 'too short'. It promotes growth throughout the body, including that of bones. Some steroids users take HGH hoping for similar effects to those produced by steroids themselves, but they risk developing a condition known as acromegaly. This is where the bones – unable to grow lengthways once maturity is reached – simply thicken. The signs of acromegaly can be seen especially around the skull, skin, face, hands, and feet. Other symptoms are diabetes, impotence, and enlargement of various internal organs.

Diuretics. Their authorised use is for people who have a build-up of fluid in the body related, perhaps, to heart failure or high blood pressure. Diuretics encourage a lot of peeing and, thus, excretion of these unwanted fluids together with the impurities they contain. Steroids users also commonly suffer fluid retention, developing a bloated

look. Apart from disposing of these surplus liquids, diuretic
also speed the elimination of any banned drugs that migh
have been consumed. A third benefit is that they can hel
users meet weight limits applying to their events. Side effect
include impotence, tiredness, skin rashes, thirst, nausea, an
dizziness

Potassium supplements. Apart from sometimes causin
nausea and vomiting, diuretics can lead to the excretion o
important salts – notably potassium, whose loss can caus
muscle weakness and impaired heart muscle function. Potass
ium supplements are intended to counter this outcome. Bu
potassium is itself toxic in excessive doses. For the majorit
of users the question of how much diuretic versus potassiun
should be taken is a matter of guesswork since few will hav
access to relevant laboratory screening of blood circulation
cholesterol levels, kidney and liver functions.

Thyroxine. A naturally occurring hormone prescribed fo
hypothyroidism, a condition whereby the body tissues fai
to get the energy they need. Body-builders and other 'gyn
junkies' sometimes take thyroxine hoping it will increase
their metabolic rate and thereby reduce body fat. Side
effects include heart-beat irregularities, angina, headaches
muscle cramp, diarrhoea, flushing, and sweating. Too mucl
thyroxine can also lead to an irreversible condition known as
exopthalmus, whereby the eyes protrude and bulge.

Corticosteroids. Use of steroids makes possible extra-hard
training, which can cause joint and muscle damage. Corticosteroids are taken to reduce any resulting inflammation. Side
effects, particularly from high-dose prolonged use, can be
serious. They impair the body's natural immunity to infection,
can cause diabetes, muscle wasting, mental disturbances
(including depression and paranoia), brittle bones, and the
suppression of clinical symptoms that may allow diseases
such as septicaemia or tuberculosis to get to an advanced
stage before becoming visible.

Clenbuterol. An anabolic-type drug generally used for
fattening cattle. It became the fad item after earning notoriety
at the 1992 Barcelona Olympics.

388

Thiomucase. Injected into clients at beauty treatment parlours in France and the USA. Some competitive body-builders take it for its supposed 'fat melting' properties. Treatment is painful and potentially dangerous.[5] Creams are also available.

Esiclene. Believed to produce better muscle definition by causing tissue irritation at the site of injection.

Erythropoetin. A synthetic version of a naturally occurring hormone that stimulates the production of red blood cells. Its main medical use is for the treatment of various forms of anaemia. Erythropoetin improves athletic performance in much the way altitude training does – by increasing the oxygen-carrying capacity of the blood. However, the side effects – especially resulting from combined use with diuretics – are potentially fatal. This is because exercise tends to thicken the blood, whose red cell count will already have been increased as a result of erythropoetin's use. Complications can include blood clotting, heart attacks, and strokes.[6]

Amphetamine. Steroids seem to provide the aggression and commitment any athlete needs to undertake a severe training regime. When steroids stop working their magic – as they invariably will – amphetamine, another hard-driving drug, is resorted to. Or it might be used in tandem from the outset.

Effects

The popularity of anabolic steroids with sports people, body-builders, club doormen, police and the like is due mostly to their apparent ability to increase muscle mass and strength. How do they work? Probably in two main ways: by helping the body retain its stores of nitrogen, a basic constituency of protein from which muscle and other tissue is formed; and by blocking the process of protein breakdown (known as the catabolic effect) which occurs during intensive training. Steroids also seem to encourage harder work-outs and reduce the time needed to recover from them – initially, at least.[7]

All these alleged effects are disputed, chiefly by those within the medical profession who oppose the 'sporting' use of steroids. They claim – and have backed their case with various surveys – that any apparent gains from anabolic steroids are due to the drugs' placebo effect: i.e. a person taking them will be encouraged to train harder and thereby develop more bulk. They also argue that extra muscle doesn't necessarily translate into more strength – an argument I've heard from strength athletes (weightlifters, etc.) who view body-builders as nicely packaged puffballs. (Body-builders, in turn, will say of lifters and strongman competitors that they are nothing but 'fat slobs'.

As to the medical trials 'proving' anabolic steroids offer no real gains, these have been criticised on several fronts.[8]

1. Results are usually judged from the consumption of 'therapeutic' doses, whereas athletes are known to take from ten to a hundred times these amounts.
2. Specific exercises are designed to produce gains in specific muscle groups. Those conducting the trials tend to measure things more randomly.
3. For steroids to work they need to be coupled with a high-protein diet. This element has sometimes been missing in trials.
4. Similarly, any gains depend on the user exercising harder than s/he would normally do – the additional effort made possible by the steroids themselves. Some trials have restricted the subjects to their usual regime.

As to the puffball factor, it is now generally accepted that steroids will produce more strength and not just muscle bulk so long as they are combined with intensive training and a high-protein, high-calorie diet.[9]

The rush

Given that the medical profession still hasn't got used to the idea that steroids can inflate the user's physical body, the idea that they might also provide a 'buzz' is considered too weird for serious discussion. But users themselves talk

390

unabashedly of the special feelings they get after injecting or swallowing the drugs. Depending on the kind of person they are, their underlying mood and other factors, the experience will differ. But the kind of terms used are *euphoria . . . fantastic confidence . . . a feeling of enormous power . . . a teeth-gritting rush . . . like you're totally on top of things . . . nothing can hurt me . . . full of yourself . . . randy . . . moody, ready for aggro . . .*

The highest expression of steroid aggro is the so-called 'roid rage', a roaring temper tantrum that has been linked with acts of sadism and murder. Do steroids *cause* such violence in otherwise peace-loving individuals? Or do they merely act as 'disinhibitors', releasing what was already there but for so long repressed? See below for more on this subject.

Health Impact

The question of the damaging health effects of steroids is seriously under-researched. Investigations to date have looked mostly at the 'therapeutic' doses (i.e. quantities much lower than those used by sporting types) given to medical patients suffering conditions such as anaemia. Ethical considerations apparently impinge upon studying, in a controlled way, typical gym users.

But even when a serious effort is made, researchers are up against difficulties peculiar to the steroids scene. There is the enormous variety of 'performance-enhancing' products habitually consumed, the majority of which are fakes and might contain anything. On top of this, users are vague about the doses they take, being unable to talk – as can the average heroin injector – in terms of milli- or micrograms.

Physical

Nonetheless, there is an oft-repeated list of side effects associated with steroids use. It includes stunting of growth for those who've not yet attained full height. In women, they are linked with deepening of the voice, growth of body and facial hair, shrinkage of breast tissue, and enlargement of the clitoris – effects that seem to be irreversible. Menstruation is also affected.

In men they can cause decreased sperm production leading to infertility, as well as shrinking of the testicles and growth of breast tissue ('bitch tits').

In both sexes they often produce acne and, less frequently, disorders of the liver and kidneys, which might result in jaundice, tumours, and cysts. They can elevate the level of blood cholesterol (the 'bad' low-density lipoprotein sort) and raise blood pressure, thereby increasing the chance of heart attack and stroke.

In 1993 a British survey team from the Centre for Research on Drugs and Health Behaviour put this list to the test when it interviewed 110 serious steroids users (97 men, 13 women) and asked what had befallen them as a result of their drug use.[10] Only 17 of the 110 reported no side effects; 12 listed seven problems they believed were caused by steroids.

For both men and women 'holding water' figured most often (62 mentions). For women, menstrual irregularities cropped up just as frequently, with the growth of body hair and voice-deepening following close behind (almost half the respondents). Four reported clitoral enlargement.

More than 50 of the 97 males said their testicles had shrivelled ('testicular atrophy') and nearly as many complained of acne. Also figuring were sleeplessness (about 37), high blood pressure (25), growth of body hair (35), 'bitch tits' (30-plus), tendon injuries (25), nosebleeds (21), more frequent colds (16), loss of hair/baldness (12), lymph node swellings and liver problems (around 5 each). This is not the complete side-effects list.

Sixty-four per cent of the total sample underwent no medical monitoring and so might be missing non-symptomatic conditions that could, ultimately, prove more significant.

Behavioural

Reports of steroids-induced behavioural problems are now plentiful – everything from mild depressions to raging psychotic crack-ups. As always, assigning blame where it belongs is difficult, not least because the category of individual who obsessively weight-trains to inflate his body image might just be the sort to lash out anyway.

Dr Precilla Choi of Nottingham University's psychology department, herself a weight trainer, has researched this area as dutifully as anyone. She reports that paranoid schizophrenia, manic episodes, and major depression following withdrawal have all been found in athletes using anabolic steroids.[11]

She says that users themselves tell of increased feelings of aggression, irritability, suspicion, negativism, feelings of power and anxiety. In studying twenty-one steroid consumers attending a needle exchange clinic in Wales, Choi heard from one man how he'd ripped a door off its hinges and broke it in pieces after losing his temper while ironing a shirt. Another told of smashing a car by kicking it. A third individual got into a 'mad rage' in a pub and started throwing beer glasses around.

Roid Rage

In a 1990 study[12] of a small group of strength athletes – three of whom used steroids and three didn't – one subject told Choi's research team that, while on steroids, he believed 'absolutely nothing could hurt me'. This led him, repeatedly, to step out in front of moving traffic until one day he got knocked down. He also confessed to extreme hostility. 'I followed [a woman] home . . . right to her doorstep and I intended to kill her . . . I grabbed hold of her . . . She dropped to the floor and even though I thought her neck was broken and she was dead I still stamped on her face 'cos I hated her so much . . . I went home and it didn't worry me. I felt no guilt . . . she deserved it.'

Subsequent research by Choi among Boston, Massachusetts gym regulars found that steroids users were, by their own accounts, involved in significantly more fights, verbal aggression and violence towards their partners while actually consuming the drugs compared with when they were in an 'off cycle'.[13] And the aggressiveness, Dr Choi notes, 'is not only limited to those who are aggressive by nature but may extend to previously non-violent individuals.' Examples of apparent 'roid rages' from this Boston study include one subject throwing a brick at his girlfriend, another fracturing several bones in his partner's hand while squeezing it, and a third picking his partner up and 'flinging her across the room'.

While such evidence doesn't settle the question of the existence or otherwise of 'roid rage', it does lead to the conclusion that steroids are, at the least, capable of unleashing long-repressed violent urges in individuals who might otherwise never manifest them. The argument, in fact, is much the same as that over alcohol; some people come home with a bellyful of booze and beat up their spouses. Others get love-stricken.

It's the highly androgenic steroids such as Testoviron, Finajet, Dianabol, and Testosterone Cypionate which seem the most likely triggers of a roid rage, and while these tendencies are likely to subside during off cycles, using them over long periods might generally 'shorten the fuse'.[14]

A UK survey bigger than any that Choi has carried out is the aforementioned Centre for Research on Drugs and Health Behaviour study of 1993[15] which asked 110 steroids users about their psychological states both while they were on and while they were resting from steroids.

Positive sensations easily overshadowed negative ones during 'on cycles', with some 83 per cent reporting feeling 'more powerful' and 51 per cent reporting an increased sex drive. Other benefits included feelings of euphoria, confidence, and a general sense of being 'pleased with myself'.

On the downside were reports of more unintended aggressiveness, impulsiveness, and (less markedly) paranoia and an 'urge to harm others'. But during these on cycles many will have been building up with rigorous training to some kind of contest or performance, and so nerves will inevitably have been frayed.

During off cycles, depression seemed to occur more often, but respondents also said they were better able to relax.

Sex

Many male users talk arrestingly of increased libido, of multiple ejaculations and of erections that won't go away. Given that anabolic steroids are designed to mimic the effects of the natural male sex hormone, testosterone, these stories have a degree of plausibility. But what goes up invariably comes down. While libido can be temporarily raised, it might later be suppressed to vanishing point.

The permanent enlargement of the female clitoris following steroids use might be unwelcome aesthetically, but some women report getting extra sex pleasure as a result of the change.

Dependence

One mark of the addiction/dependence potential of any drug is what happens when you quit taking it. Too much pain often induces further use for the relief it brings. There seems to be no evidence of steroid use leading to major physical trauma upon withdrawal of the sort that can be caused by alcohol or barbiturates. There are scattered reports[16] of fatigue, craving, depression, muscle and joint pains (perhaps from old, forgotten injuries), loss of appetite, restlessness, nausea, chills, and a general malaise. But such symptoms are answered to by no more than a (fairly significant) minority of users.[17]

Another mark of addiction potential is the amount of repeatable pleasure to be had from a substance. That so many steroids users talk of being imbued with transcendent power and confidence is a clue to the kind of psychological grip the drugs can exert.

The joy of steroids was starkly described in a 1989 American paper by Dr Paul Goldstein, an astute observer of the scene.[18] One dumb-bell addict told him: ' . . . this stuff gives you a new level of aggression and power that you can't achieve on your own by thinking it out any more. You just can't. You try! Like you're lifting a dumb-bell and you give up. But you go to the gym when you're on that stuff and everything is going good, and your levels are real built up high . . . You take that weight, 40 pounds heavier, and you do it. Screaming! Crazy joy! Ecstasy! It's like having an orgasm. It's better. You don't have any idea what it's like . . . it's total orgasm. Oneness. It's like a one-cell creature reproducing itself . . . You just feel so good that you just want to buy 20 bottles more.'

Another user described to Goldstein how steroids-boosted gym work consumed him body and soul. 'You get into the vicious cycle of doing more and more and more, and doing new sophisticated stuff . . . Then once you're on the stuff you feel differently . . . all of a sudden you're making gains . . . and you're strong. And you have no pains like you had before. You're very euphoric. You feel kind of indestructible. And

395

nothing matters. They can steal your car. You know, so what? If you caught the guy you would kill him. But if you didn't, alright, the car's gone. As long as the gym is open . . . Don't steal your food. Don't steal your steroids. But you can take my car, my wife, take anything you want. That's really how you become. And you don't know it. You're in this fog.'

Injection

The majority of steroid users inject – perhaps 80 per cent of them. Injection brings with it the usual hazards of viral and bacterial infection, collapsed veins, and abscesses. Since many consumers are competing athletes and body-builders, they aim to insert the needle in a place that won't leave tell-tale marks. A favoured site is the gluteus medius muscle in the buttocks (a region concealed by trunks or shorts). This means getting a friend to do the jabbing, a favour that's likely to be reciprocated, perhaps with the same works. The question of whether much sharing goes on produces different answers. When asked direct questions about sharing, most steroid users will shake their head, but engage them in more detailed discussion about their injecting practices and as many as three-quarters will admit to having shared equipment at some time.[19]

Once shy of such places, steroids users now resort mostly to the needle exchanges for their clean works – the establishments set up for more traditional street drug users. A second main source of what are known in the gym world as pumps and pins are their own steroids dealers. But while access to clean works doesn't seem to be a major problem, there is still a startling amount of ignorance about how and where to inject safely. Nerve damage and large fibroid growths are common, as is the assumption that it is necessary to draw blood when injecting.

History

The consumption of performance-boosting substances is at least as old as the Olympic Games of ancient Greece, during which time sheep's testicles were part of the doping regimen. In the modern era, the canal swimmers of Amsterdam and nineteenth-century racing cyclists are among the sporting types who've used various items for extra propulsion. Participants in six-day cycle races during 1879 were alleged to have prepared variously with caffeine, sugar cubes dipped in ether, alcohol cordials, and nitroglycerine (favoured by sprinters). In 1886, a British cyclist died from using an ephedrine-based drug which he'd taken to mask fatigue and remove the natural bodily restraints intended to protect against over exertion.[20]

Anabolic steroids were being used by athletes as early as the 1940s, though probably sparingly. By the 1950s the range of synthetic steroids increased and so did the uptake. By the 1960s/early 1970s the drug companies, according to one old hand, 'realised there was a hell of a market here for the stuff. So they threw some dollars into research . . . Now they are using anabolics that work so fast, they are so powerful . . . I don't think the body has caught up with the dosage or the science of it all . . . Twenty years from now you're going to see a whole bunch of people dying. But you are going to have to wait twenty years.'[21]

By 1968, according to US Senate Committee testimony by Olympic hammer-throw gold medallist Harold Connelly, 'it was not unusual to see athletes with their own medical kits, practically a doctor's, in which they would have syringes and all their various drugs. I know any number of athletes on the '68 Olympic team who had so much scar tissue and so many puncture holes on their backsides that it was difficult to find a fresh spot to give them a new shot.'[22]

By the 1980s, Olympic dope cheats were making big news. A record fourteen competitors were thrown out of the 1984 contest. Three years later, following a two-year investigation, the US federal grand jury handed down a 110-count indictment charging thirty-four persons with steroids trafficking, among them British 1972 silver medal sprint hero David Jenkins. Jenkins was later sentenced to seven years' jail, to be followed by five years' probation and a $75,000 fine for his lead role in a steroid-smuggling operation that encompassed a production plant in Tijuana, Mexico and distributors throughout Europe and the US.[23]

Around the time of Jenkins's arrest the total US black-market trade was estimated by federal law enforcement officials to be worth around $500 million a year with every sign of continuing rapid growth.

As to who and how many were using, a 1984 report based on confidential surveys and the testimony of coaches and former users suggested that 80–100 per cent of top American body-builders, weightlifters, and field athletes made use of steroids.[24] But the drugs were also powerfully attractive to those unconnected with top-drawer sporting circles. A 1988 survey found that 6.6 per cent of a national sample of high-school males reported using anabolic steroids.[25] A series of other less formal student surveys produced even more dramatic results: 65 per cent of pupils in a 1986 Miami high-school poll knew someone who was taking steroids; 38 per cent of high-school football players surveyed in Portland, Oregon during 1988 knew where to score.

Bulging muscles were in. They were the passport to a lucrative athletic scholarship and to that dream girl in the micro bikini. A Philadelphia physical therapist who worked with athletes stated: 'People think the cocaine issue is big. It's not as big as anabolic steroids. Among kids it's epidemic.'

'We face a lot of problems,' echoed the executive secretary of the Florida High School Activities Association, 'but we feel the number-one concern is steroids.'[26]

The UK scene

Here in the UK similar patterns were observed, although they were slower to surface and the numbers involved were more modest. In western Scotland in 1987 and in the West Glamorgan area of Wales in 1992, surveys of gym users found that, respectively, around 20 and 39 per cent were taking steroids.

More telling was a survey published in January 1991 by Dumfries clinical research psychiatrist, Dr Douglas Williamson, which found that nearly one in twenty male students at a Scottish technology college were using the drugs – mostly to 'enhance appearance' rather than for athletic performance.[27] Williamson believed the figures could be extrapolated for the UK as a whole, which meant that the drugs 'may represent a public health problem that ranks after only alcohol, tobacco and cannabis use.'

From Nottingham – a big gym town, locale for several major

body-building contests – came more eye-catching figures. By 1993 the city's main centrally located drugs agency, Drug Dependents Anonymous, had a total of 840 injectors participating in its free needle exchange scheme designed to limit the spread of HIV. Of this total, fully 500 – or more than half – were steroids users.

In Mid Glamorgan and Northampton special steroid-specific services were being set up, and in Liverpool an innovative project called Drugs and Sport Information Service was established. Its director and sole full-time worker was Pat Lenehan, former psychiatric and general nurse. The Lenehan objective was to penetrate the closed jock culture of the gym and, thereafter, persuade users that steroids are not simply 'an aid to digestion', as one local gym-owner disingenuously described them to me, but a drug whose imprudent use can have potentially catastrophic effects. 'Harm minimisation' and information about non-drug alternatives was the name of Lenehan's low-key game.

'What is required', he avowed, 'is a response separate from other drug services because these guys don't consider themselves drug addicts in the usual sense of the word. These guys are often massive, very fit and very knowledgeable about what they're using.'

Sherry Lambert, who was running a telephone sales company in Preston, Lancashire when I spoke to her in 1993, got a measure of the steroids phenomenon after going public on her steroid-using boyfriend in the woman's magazine *Take a Break*. The 1990 article detailed his metamorphosis from 'lovely person to monster', describing how he used to break up the household furniture, punch holes in windows, and make impossible sexual demands – that's prior to his sex drive shrivelling altogether. At the end of the piece, Ms Lambert announced the formation of the Steroid Abusers' Wives Association. 'Several hundred' women immediately joined up, she told me, many of them with horror stories of their own.

Liverpool's Pat Lenehan identified three features that are likely to aid the continued expansion of the underground steroids market:

1. **The sex angle**. Stories of multiple ejaculations and erections that won't quit appeal to not a few young

399

males, even though such superhuman feats are distinctly time-limited.

2. **Making the hard cases harder**. Surviving 'on the street' can be tough. What harm can a little extra muscle do? While anabolic steroids cannot build muscle from the comfort of an armchair (strenuous exercise is required) the gains the drugs make possible inevitably exceed, and by some distance, what can be achieved naturally.

3. **For vanity's sake**. Several muscle-heads I spoke to confessed to pathological levels of narcissism – or what might be called a reverse anorexia. The mirror becomes their lover (and every wall of every gym is lined with them) as they stare ceaselessly at their bulging images. 'You watch your legs coming out, your chest building up and your back getting bigger,' a nineteen-year-old Merseyside youth told me, 'and it's very attracting. It's like you become addicted by your own ego.'

Users and dealers

Nineteen-year-old Merseysider Jerry Vale[28] lived until his early teens in southern California where his major hobbies were boxing and hanging out on the golden beaches of Santa Monica and Venice. He was a thin boy, though well enough muscled. But he'd look around and see nothing but bleach-haired giants for whom life seemed a breeze. And he'd go to the movies and swoon before screen images of big Arnie Schwarzenegger, Western culture's most fabulously grotesque creation of the moment.

'I found that these big guys in the States they had all the girls. They looked good and seemed to feel good about themselves in that they were very, very positive.'

He bought a stack of muscle mags and, after ordering a set of weights from a catalogue, started training at home in the garage five nights a week. An older friend with experience of top body-building competitions introduced him to proper work-out routines and to training in the gym. It was in the gym that steroids came his way. In six months he gained two and a half stone, mostly of muscle, which took his weight to around fifteen stone. Emotionally, there was a switch too. Listening to him, in spring 1993, describing the violent rages that beset him, the fidgeting and facial itching that generally prefigured each episode, I was unable to suppress thoughts of Dr Jekyll/Mr Hyde and the demon potion that transformed the one into the other. Too extreme a notion, of course. More sober minds would say that steroids cannot make a person act in a way that is foreign to his nature and that there are, in any case, far more potent and pervasive triggers to violence than steroids: alcohol, for instance. But Vale himself believed the contrary – that without the steroids his bouts of aggression would never have occurred, no matter the circumstances.

Most of his victims had been moderately lippy customers at the Liverpool city-centre club where he worked as a doorman three nights a week. For the price of a wisecrack, one received a broken nose. 'I've been warned constantly by the owner of the club that I have to calm my temper down,' he said. 'I've bashed heck out of people just because they were giving me cheek.'

He was a grey-skinned, high-shouldered youth with thick, short black hair and open nostrils. His mother, with whom he lived alone, appeared to be terrified of him. 'There was an incident the other day,' he said, 'where I couldn't find my deodorant and I went absolutely mad and wrecked my bedroom. Mum understands but she doesn't have much to say in the matter. She just has to put up with it, although I do try to stay in my room if I'm in a bad mood.'

At first he consumed steroids only in their tablet form and found not only that his libido dramatically waxed and waned, but that he was 'prone to lying in bed for days, too tired, sick and exhausted to move.'

His body ultimately adjusted, after which he included regular intramuscular injection as part of a steroids regime that usually involved six weeks on the drug (the 'on cycle') and six weeks off. The problems worsened. As well as rage episodes he developed a large swelling on the side of his neck which was refusing to go away; it's at its worst soon after each jab. There were also frequent nosebleeds. 'I wake up in the night', he complained, 'with my pillow soaked in blood.'

Pat Lenehan of the Drugs and Sport Information Service was hoping to get Vale to see a GP, and also – at the very least – consume his steroids more sensibly. Vale seemed to want to comply but was talking only of 'stopping for a period if told to by a doctor.'

Until that time, his 'doctoring' had been done by other

doormen at the club where he worked. It was they, he suggests, who coaxed him into starting in the first place, teasing him about his comparative lack of bulk and his youth. When the serious side effects started he went for advice to an established underground steroids dealer, a thirty-six-year-old redundant builder whom we shall call Martin Lake and who was himself something of a gym junkie. I met both men in Lake's flat, located on the second floor of a dishevelled low-rise council block a couple of miles from the city centre. The interior, with its glass and steel furniture, its black leather three-piece, was immaculate.

Late believed that virtually all Vale's side effects resulted from the bad, in fact malicious, advice he got from his nightclub colleagues. They misled him about what sort of steroids to take and in what quantities. But even for the well-informed, Lake admitted, safe use can be a problem, given that perhaps 95 per cent of steroids products on the gym circuit are counterfeits of the 'licit' prescription items. The stocks themselves are thought to originate in countries such as India, Canada and, especially, Mexico, where – roid legend has it – a phony company called International Pharmaceuticals set up shop during the mid-1980s, allegedly with a $1 million stake from former Panamanian leader General Manuel Noriega. The plant was closed down by the Mexican authorities two years later but vast quantities of IP products, all of them convincingly packaged, were still sloshing around gyms throughout Europe and the US. Lake showed me some samples.

It was because he mistrusted what he was himself being dealt as a consumer that Lake took to dealing. He says he researched the field as best he could, checking out his main suppliers. He dealt for about a year but then became so unsatisfied with stock quality that he withdrew from both selling and consuming. 'There is just too much crap around,' he told me.

Until the early 1990s, steroids dealing is reputed to have been a gentlemanly affair, conducted for the mutual convenience of users rather than for pure profit. Gym habitués are not intrinsically violent individuals, I was repeatedly told; their pursuit provides a disciplined framework for whatever aggression they might harbour. 'But today,' said Lake, 'the whole thing is a lot more heavy and complex.' The big dealers were invariably gym-connected but also had other interests such as sportswear and training equipment. A major order placed with one of these men, he said, can be met within twenty-four hours, using runners and portable phones. Sometimes things get unpleasant. Lake had twice been threatened for helping steroids consumers identify counterfeit products. And he knew of two small-scale traffickers whose vehicles were set on fire by more prominent players upon whose territory they were allegedly encroaching.

Lake didn't suggest that the scene was anything like as violently competitive as mainstream drug-dealing can be. There are, for the moment, enough customers to go around. But he did sense an amount of marking-out of territory, and was especially troubled by the appearance of increasing numbers of amphetamine and cannabis dealers. 'At the moment steroids is a separate scene but, given time, it will definitely be a street drug like any other.'

West London steroids dealer Tony Johnson supports the picture sketched by Lake. A 6 ft 4 in seventeen-stone-plus bouncer who was on the brink of competing seriously in body-building contests when we met, Johnson became involved in steroids dealing for the same reason as Lake: he wanted supplies whose quality he could trust for himself and friends. Obtaining stock from his main provider, he said, 'can be as simple as ordering a pizza.' Syringes and needles came by the boxload from friends who worked in chemists. Like Lake, he recognised that there was much 'useless crap' in the system, as well as the beginnings of formidable tensions. The dealer who originally supplied him was driven out of business by 'men from up north' who held a shotgun at his nose. They resented the low prices Johnson's supplier was charging.

'Over the last couple of years [we were talking in spring 1993] it's turned out that a lot of the stuff sold down here is coming from northern dealers. There's apparently a big counterfeiting crew up there who are expanding their operation.'

Also like Lake, he believed that many of the side effects attributed to steroids were invented by a sensation-hungry media that refused to face the truth about the real roots of social violence. The problems that did occur, he said, were invariably caused by ignorance. He offered as an example his friend Freddie Garner, who when they first met was using a steriod called Equipose, designed for racehorses. Equipose was, in fact, one of the most popular products on the gym circuit. But Equipose didn't suit Freddie Garner. On his £200-a-month habit (five times the usual outlay) he was having 'very, very bad fits of anger,' said Johnson, 'punching people on the door at the club he worked at as a bouncer and for no reason at all.'

Garner agreed that his steroids use did get out of hand, despite him having originally turned to them for 'medicinal reasons' as much as for any desire to create a more heroic body aesthetic. He was one of a small but increasing number of hard-core users of 'recreational' substances who were resorting to steroids to restore their depleted physiques. Garner's own weakness had been crack cocaine. In the first five months of 1992 he burnt up £10,000 worth of the drug – money obtained as compensation for a workplace injury. He became emaciated and manic. His wife fled with their four-year-old daughter to a women's refuge, although Garner says he never actually hit her; they are now back together.

'Do you want to know the secret of why people use drugs?' he asked. We were in a shiny municipal gym in Hounslow, West London. As Garner, Tony Johnson, and two other friends worked out, a couple of schoolgirls, aged about fourteen, sat in a corner expertly examining their forms. 'The answer,' said Garner, 'is that they can't bear being by themselves, with themselves.'

He was born in London's Paddington twenty-eight years ago, his father a Nigerian diplomat, his mother a white West German doctor. The race mix, he said, left him confused about his identity, a confusion that was reinforced when he was sent to an all-white boarding school in York which instilled in him 'feelings of inadequacy and self-loathing'. By the age of fifteen, already expelled from school, he was 'out of control, alienated and heavily into heroin'. At age eighteen, he left his family and moved to Brixton where he embarked upon a self-destructive search for black roots. More drugs, petty crime, and conflict with the police followed. Then, while peddling cannabis in Kensington market, he met his wife, Ginny, a 'trendy white uptown girl'. She convinced him of the need for change. But there followed years of 'struggling against habitual patterns of behaviour' – a process from which he had still not fully emerged.

It was through his work as a pool attendant in West London that Garner discovered the attractions of the gym and, inevitably, the short-cuts that steroids offer. He got bigger, took a job as a club doorman, and eventually established his own informal security agency which has helped find work for nine or ten gym buddies – his dealer friend Tony Johnson among them. Garner is an intelligent man, and unsparingly self-critical. He recognises that there is much 'warped over-compensation' in his obsession with body size and estimates that many of his gym friends also have profound insecurities. The immense Tony Johnson, for instance, was once a gangly, skinny child, at the mercy of a tyrannical father.

'This summer will be the last that I'll be using steroids,' Garner told me in 1993. He had recently found Buddhism, a discovery that led him to shear off his dreadlocks so that he might evince, as he put it, a 'quiet, sober self-respect'. Steroids, he contended, *are* a bad deal. Besides leaving him with a mild case of 'bitch tits', he is forced to wonder: 'Would you pump someone you loved full of steroids just to get them big?'

A year after our first conversation he was still on track, by now working with young people, seeking to prevent them falling into the drugs trap.

The Cure

At the time of writing, simple possession and use of anabolic steroids, whether by tablet or injection, is perfectly legal. Suppliers had also been given a virtual free hand until a November 1994 Home Office announcement that, in future, trafficking would be an offence under the control of the Misuse of Drugs Act (MDA). The proposed maximum penalties were a £2,500 fine and three months' imprisonment where the case came before magistrates, or five years in prison and an unlimited fine when heard in crown court.

One police officer who favoured this turning of the screw was Detective Inspector Carol Bristow of the Metropolitan force who, by 1994, had twenty-eight years' experience of drugs, sexual assault, murder, and child abuse cases.

In 1992 she analysed fifteen murder and rape cases from across the country – selected at random by computer – and found that nine involved body-builders, at least three of whom were known steroids users. A dossier presented to her superiors at the Yard produced no response. She is convinced that steroids are not simply 'disinhibitors' but lead men, and sometimes women, into uncharacteristic violence. 'I have no evidence of violent men becoming more violent,' she told me, 'but I do have evidence of pussy cats becoming violent quite suddenly.'

Among the stand-out cases she pointed to is that of John Steed, the M4 rapist, who in 1986 was convicted of killing a prostitute in central London. Steed, the Old Bailey jury heard, was a body-building fanatic and steroids injector. But they also learned that his emotional equilibrium had been tilted years before when, at age five, he watched his mother being violently raped by his father. A second case Bristow cited is that of Christopher Snarski, another body-building steroids obsessive, who was jailed for twelve years in March 1991 after setting fire to the family home in Bracknell, Berkshire, killing his two young daughters. Snarski was said by his defence to have become confused and paranoid as a result of his steroids addiction. But equally disorientating, it would seem, were his £10,000 worth of debts and the two jobs he was holding down which kept him busy from dawn until late at night.

Such contributory circumstances can invariably be found when 'steroids-induced violence' is examined with a little care and caution. Even the apparently meticulous research work of academics like Nottingham University's Precilla Choi (see above), which point to the simple formulation that steroids create or 'invent' violence, requires a sceptical reading. As one Northampton dealer challenged me: 'Compare it with alcohol. Men all over the country get pissed, go home and knock the missus's teeth out, smash the house up. That's a very common occurrence. If a person is law-abiding they won't become suddenly criminal because they've taken some steroids. But with violent people it's very easy to look to something to blame. You get people jumping on the bandwagon in court cases. These husbands, if they're going through problems with the marriage, money problems, problems at work, it's very easy to blame the steroids.'

But DI Carol Bristow has no doubts about the way violence

and steroids go together, nor about the constructive part the MDA can play in suppressing the drugs' use, especially when directed at dealers rather than simple users.

Mike Baker, a fifty-six-year-old former Mr Europe who now runs a gym in Northampton, believes some of his fellow gym-owners bear a large part of the responsibility for the growth of steroids use. 'They don't take a stand against it', he told me, 'because they are profiting financially.' They are either involved in dealing themselves, Baker added, or turn a blind eye to its use in order to ensure that their clientele keep coming through the door. He wanted no repetition of an incident that occurred in 1991 when a once good-natured weight trainer went into a rage over a snapped cable on a piece of work-out equipment. He hurled a heavy block of metal through a window, attacked Baker with a broom handle, and tripped him down the stairs.

Walter O'Malley, a fifty-three-year-old former Mr World who runs a hard-core gym in Warrington, took a less prohibitive view. He refused to say whether or not he uses steroids because 'if I say "no" people wouldn't believe me anyway, what with me reaching such a high standard.' Nor would he erect banning notices in his gym, for this would only serve as 'a rod for my back . . . in that people would think I've got something to hide.'

He believes steroids' side effects are greatly exaggerated. 'After all, anything that makes you strong can't be bad.' He favours their open supply under medical supervision. To prohibit them under the Misuse of Drugs Act, he said, would be to drive them further underground, make them scarcer, more expensive, and encourage more desperate acts by those seeking to buy or sell. In this prognosis O'Malley is supported by most experienced drug agency personnel currently working with users of heroin, cocaine, and the like. Prohibition, they recognise, has failed to staunch the flow of these other drugs and can be said to be a prime incentive to commit theft, property crime, and similar offences.

For men like Pat Lenehan, of Merseyside's Drugs and Sport Information Service, the answer is harm minimisation – the provision of 'non-judgmental' treatment and education directed at stopping people damaging themselves and others. It requires, he says, informing a new client group about alternative ways of reaching maximum performance. The

Home Office is – as I write – considering whether or not to ban simple possession of steroids, having already rejected such a course in 1988. If they do reverse that earlier decision the consequences in the shape of conflict between the police and gym regulars could become quickly apparent. But even if the status quo is maintained, steroids are likely to bag an increasing share of the drug-scare headlines.

Notes

1 D. Williamson, 'Anabolic steroids: Edinburgh's lesser known drug problem', in *Edinburgh Medicine*, No. 65, 1991, p. 6.

2 P. Korkia and G. Stimson, *Anabolic Steroid Use in Great Britain: An exploratory investigation*, The Centre for Research on Drugs and Health Behaviour, London, 1993, p. 79.

3 Most of the details obtained are from the *British National Formulary*, British Medical Association and the Royal Pharmaceutical Society of Great Britain, No. 27, March 1994.

4 Side effects list drawn from 'Recruits to a risky business', in *New Scientist*, 11 June 1994, p. 44; and 'Good health after bad?', in the *Guardian*, 11 May 1994.

5 *New Scientist*, op. cit., p. 80.

6 P. Lenehan, 'Drugs in Sport', paper published by the Drugs & Sport Information Service, Liverpool, 1993.

7 P. Lenehan, factsheet on performance-enhancing drugs, published by the Drugs & Sport Information Service, Liverpool, 1993.

8 See, for instance, Williamson, op. cit.

9 'The Steroid Papers', ISDD, London, 1993, p. 9.

10 Korkia and Stimson, op. cit., p. 89.

11 P. Choi, 'The alarming effects of anabolic steroids', in *The Psychologist*, Vol. 6, No. 6, 1993, pp. 258–60.

12 P. Choi *et al.*, 'High-dose anabolic steroids in strength athletes: Effects upon hostility and aggression', in *Human Psychopharmacology*, Vol. 5, 1990, pp. 349–56.

13 P. Choi and H. Pope, 'Violence towards women and illicit androgenic-anabolic steroid use', in the *Annals of Clinical Psychiatry*, Vol. 6, No. 1, 1994, pp. 21–5.

14 ISDD, op. cit., p. 15.

15 Korkia and Stimson, op. cit., p. 95.

16 Ibid, p. 99.

17 Ibid, p. 99.

18 P. Goldstein, 'Anabolic steroids: An ethnographic approach', report submitted for NIDA Research Analysis and Utilization System meeting on anabolic steroid abuse, March 1989.

19 Korkia and Stimson, op. cit., p. 104.

20 Goldstein, op. cit., p. 6.

21 Ibid, p. 25.

22 A. Hecht, 'Anabolic steroids: Pumping trouble', in *FDA Consumer*, September 1984, pp. 12–15.

23 Korkia and Stimson, op. cit., p. 14; and Goldstein, op. cit., p. 16.

24 P. Choi *et al.*, op. cit., p. 349.

25 W. E. Buckley *et al.*, 'Estimated prevalence of anabolic steroid

use among male high school seniors', in the *Journal of the American Medical Association*, 260 (23), 1988, pp. 3441–5.

26 Goldstein, op. cit., p. 4.
27 Williamson, op. cit., p. 6.
28 The names of users and dealers appearing in this section are pseudonyms.

TOBACCO

Intro

The once-ubiquitous habit of tobacco smoking is running into tough times in the 'mature', health-conscious markets of the industrialised North. In the US, especially, it is under attack from a health lobby inspired by a series of scandals suggesting that the industry has suppressed important health data and manipulated nicotine levels so as to cultivate addiction in its customers.

But in Africa, the Far East, and the former Soviet satellite states of eastern and central Europe there's still plenty of sag to be taken up by the world's leading dealers in the leaf. The game played is a hard one: where financial inducements don't succeed in prising open hitherto closed markets, threats of trade sanctions have been used. And while we in the 'developed' North now require on-pack health warnings and set limits for the amount of tar we'll stomach, no such protection is afforded consumers in these virgin territories.

Are the activities of the tobacco companies, a) evidence of liberty in action, or are they b) the taking of liberties? The answer is a), according to the UK lobby group FOREST (Freedom Organisation for the Right to Enjoy Smoking Tobacco), a right-wing libertarian organisation whose brief is to maintain freedom of choice and counter 'biased allegations' about smoking and health. Despite its money (substantially more than £200,000 a year in 1993), almost wholly deriving from global tobacco businesses whose annual profits can run to several billions of dollars, FOREST positions itself as the friend of the little guy; antidote to a bullying, hectoring health lobby that includes the Department of Health, the Royal College of Physicians, the British Medical Association, sundry MPs, and the campaign group Action on Smoking and Health (ASH).

411

FOREST's chief argument is that its opponents hype up the dangers of smoking while leaving out the good bits such as the 'proven' beneficial effects nicotine has in preventing the likes of Alzheimer's disease, ulcerative colitis, and one or two cancers. Its supporters crunch the health data with panache (though rarely convincingly), but it is when they resort to bellowing rhetoric that they are at their liveliest.

Adolf Hitler is regularly invoked as a 'pioneer of the anti-smoking movement' and, thus, FOREST's opponents are granite-faced 'health fascists . . . a serious danger to us all'. At other times, there is a resort to dripping sentiment. One of its MP supporters declared that '. . . to attack the right to smoke is necessarily to attack the freedoms for which our ancestors fought and suffered. It is also to show contempt for a system of government which – in spite of its admitted faults – has been a model for half the world and is the present hopeless envy of the other half.'[1]

While most of the group's pamphleteers lean heavily towards the free-market right, socialists are also given space when their message fits: 'Smoking is a class issue,' one Terry Liddle has declared.[2] 'Smoking . . . is part and parcel of being working class. For the working-class youth the first cigarette, like the first drink, is both a rebellion against the staid and stolid world of adulthood and a rite of passage from childhood into that world.'

A bigger name than Liddle joined the valiant battle for smokers' rights during 1992. Margaret Thatcher – apparently a non-smoker herself – is reputed to have accepted $1 million from Philip Morris, manufacturers of Marlboro, the world's biggest brand, in return for the use of her 'services and skills' over a three-year period. The health 'fascists', naturally, were outraged, and even Winston Churchill, MP, grandson of the wartime leader whose memory Thatcher reveres, thought it 'very sad indeed when you think of the effort that is put by so many people into cancer prevention and heart disease prevention.'

Aside from Thatcher's support, another useful development for Philip Morris during 1992 was the death of Wayne McLaren, the renegade former model for the company's Marlboro Man series of cigarette ads in which he posed as the rugged, stoic cowboy in the big hat, a guy who reached for a Marlboro whenever the world crowded in apiece. After being diagnosed in 1990 as having lung cancer, McLaren took against the tobacco industry, speaking out at Philip Morris stockholders' meetings and publicly attributing his ailment to thirty years of cigarette smoking.

Crisis in Marlboro country

While the US industry was able to shake off McLaren's complaints, more serious trouble lurked just around the corner. In 1993 came a report from the US government's Environmental Protection Agency which, for the first time, classified 'passive smoke' – the stuff that drifts over from a smoker's cigarette – as a Class A carcinogen: a material presenting a serious cancer risk.[3]

Smoking was banned from more and more public places and a series of uncompromising public health campaigns and media investigations was launched, culminating in an August 1994 ruling by a panel of experts that nicotine was, after all, a true drug of addiction and not a mere 'flavouring', as claimed by the industry.[4] This left the way open for the powerful Food and Drug Administration to regulate tobacco as it does other addictive substances. 'The public thinks of cigarettes as simply blended tobacco rolled in paper,' FDA chief David Kessler told a congressional hearing in April 1994, 'but they are much more than that. Some of today's cigarettes may, in fact, qualify as high-technology nicotine delivery systems that deliver nicotine is precisely calculated quantities – quantities that are more than sufficient to create and sustain addiction.'

The FDA could seek a total ban on tobacco – but this was unlikely given the $48 billion in tax revenues the industry generates every year, and the powerful friends it still has in Congress. If not a total ban, the FDA could press for prohibition on all products with amounts of nicotine above a level judged capable of causing addiction. The problem with this option was readily acknowledged by the FDA itself: it would leave 50 million tobacco addicts hungering for cigarettes that offered a decent hit. A black market would almost certainly emerge to meet their needs.

Business as usual in the UK

The tobacco industry's relationship with the UK government during this same period had been altogether less tumultuous. The industry's complaint for years had been that taxes are too punitive (about 76 per cent of the price of a pack of twenty is tax) and that there were too many restrictions on advertising, sponsorship, and the kind of public places in which people can smoke.

The tax question was now so serious, according to an industry newsletter[5] – especially since the virtual abolition of European Union border controls – that large-scale smuggling into the UK of low-priced continental brands is an inevitability. The average smoker, buying some three hundred packs of cigarettes a year in this country, could save about £300 by buying them in Spain, perhaps on their summer holiday. The consequences of such a trend, it was argued, would be dire not just for UK tobacco manufacturers and retailers but for the Exchequer too, given that lost domestic sales equal lost tax revenues.

And yet, despite such complaints, the industry was not yet in a terminal condition. While sales, by the early 1990s, had stabilised, production costs were down and profits were continuing to rise. It would also appear that the industry still had allies in government. The February 1994 announcement by a Conservative health minister that his department would not enforce a ban on tobacco advertising was described by the Labour opposition as a 'corrupt payoff'[6] for favours rendered during the 1992 general election campaign, when Imperial Tobacco made available to the party billboard poster sites.

An Imperial spokesman later acknowledged that 2,000 poster sites were indeed on tap to the Tories – although the party had been obliged to pay for them – and that 'the reason we were allowing them this opportunity was because they were the only party that stated in their manifesto that they would vote against the proposed EC directive on the banning of tobacco advertising.'

The anti-smoking group ASH said that the no-ban decision – reinforced when Conservative backbenchers subsequently talked out a private member's bill – would cost around 4,400 lives a year, a figure it arrived at by calculating the number of new smokers who would be drawn to the habit and die prematurely as a result of the continued existence of advertising.

But the government and the tobacco companies had their minds on more immediately relevant figures. The priority for both sides has always been to maximise their tobacco-related income. Government does this by continuing to ratchet up tobacco duties – though not at a rate that deters existing smokers faster than new ones can be recruited. A prime method by which new smokers are pulled in is by advertising. The industry (despite its claims that ads merely inforce brand loyalty) understands all this, which is why it considers steadily escalating taxes an acceptable trade-off for continuing to enjoy the right to push its wares in the public marketplace.

What Is it?

Tobacco comes from the dried leaves of the plant genus *Nicotiana*, whose most popular and widely cultivated species, *N. tabacum*, is native in its original state only to the Americas.

Manufactured cigarettes have commanded the dominant portion of total tobacco sales since the turn of the century. In the UK we go for Virginia-type 'blond' mixes which are now beginning to colonise other markets – such as France – where dark oriental flavourings have been traditional. The average mass-produced cigarette will contain from half a dozen to thirty varieties of tobacco. It will also be enlivened by a selection from the 150 or so additives that are permitted under UK law, ranging from dwarf pine-needle oil to geranyl isobutyrate.

Yet despite the flavouring options, the average cigarette today contains just half the quantity of tobacco it had in the 1930s. This, ironically, results from the public's demand for narrower, longer cigarettes capped by ever-lengthening filter tips. It also results from the switch to low-tar brands, a proportion of whose bulk comprises the previously discarded sweepings and stems. The bulk is further inflated by a 'puffing' technique which usually involves injecting freon, a refrigerated gas that vaporises at room temperature. Some of the rest of the mass comes from air, water and steam, which is pumped in to make the leaf 'more pliable'.

The smoke

The smoke that users draw into their lungs and twirl into the atmosphere contains thousands of different chemicals in the form of gases and particles. The particulate phase includes nicotine, benzene, and the stuff known as 'tar'. The gas phase includes carbon monoxide (the main poisonous gas from car exhausts), ammonia and formaldehyde. So far, around sixty of these thousands of chemicals have been identified as known or suspected carcinogens (capable of causing cancer).

Tar

Probably the most important of smoke's constituents is tar, the dark, treacly goo which forms as the smoke cools and condenses. It is this cancer-causing material which carries the flavour, and although it could be eliminated by breeding special plants and by heavy filtering, the result for the smoker would be a gust of flavourless warm air. Tar yields per cigarette have been falling substantially during the last two decades as customers switch to the cleaner smoke of the filter tip. (These now account for 97 per cent of all UK sales.) And tar yields will come down further after 1997 as a result of a European Union diktat that will outlaw anything above 12 mg.

Nicotine

Pure nicotine is one of the most lethal substances known – able to kill within minutes of a few drops being applied to the tongue. In the concentrations found in cigarettes it acts as a mild stimulant, producing small increases in heart rate and blood pressure. Nicotine is usually cited as the reason why smokers continue craving tobacco, although decades of research into brain function and human psychology have failed to explain how and why the drug produces its 'wide spectrum of behavioural effects'.[7]

Nicotine is found only in tobacco plants and is carried into the smoker's body in tiny droplets of tar which get sucked down with the smoke. A typical cigarette delivers about 2 mg of the drug, although less than this reaches the bloodstream, and – from there – the brain. The lethal dose is believed to be about 60 mg when taken in its pure state. The easiest way to consume such levels would be to swallow a dose of the pesticide nicotine sulphate.

Carbon monoxide

Carbon monoxide is an inevitable consequence of the combustion that takes place while smoking. The yield per cigarette depends on how closely packed it is and the kind of paper used. Tighter cigarettes without 'ventilated' filters and which are smoked right down to the butt will deliver more of the car-fume gas. One of its effects is to deplete the oxygen-carrying capacity of blood, leading to an oxygen deficit of as much as 15 per cent.

Other Products

Pipe and cigar tobaccos

Pipe and cigar tobaccos have a higher tar content than cigarettes, but because practised smokers don't generally inhale the fumes they run comparatively less of a health risk. Not so the reformed cigarette smoker who switches to one of the other products and carries on taking the smoke down.

Snuff

Snuff is pounded, flavoured tobacco. It delivers as much nicotine per snort as the typical cigarette, but because there is no fire there is no tar or carbon monoxide.

Non-tobacco smokables

Herbal and other non-tobacco cigarettes are subject to the same laws of combustion as the tobacco sort, and therefore deliver up carbon monoxide and tar. But they contain no nicotine. The same applies to smoked hashish, marijuana, crack, and heroin.

Sensations

The answer to the question why do people want to smoke is no closer to being answered now than when the leaf was first introduced to European society four hundred years ago. Tobacco produces neither euphoria nor stupefaction, and yet smokers return to it over and over with a compulsion that could be said to make many heroin addicts look moderate. It is not only rare for a smoker to miss lighting up every day, it is rare for him/her not to light up ten, fifteen, up to a hundred times daily. (The national average is seventeen for men and fourteen for women – although males and females are fast drawing together.)

What pleasures are forthcoming? In the early 1960s, psychologists tended to talk in terms of 'oral gratification', a concept tied up with early parenting and thwarted sexual urges. Smoking, with its 'appealing' taste and smell and the pretty rings of smoke, was judged to be recompense for some sort of emotional deficit. Today, the scientific fashion is more mechanistic. Genetics, and molecular biology in general, dominate, and so the focus now is on components of brain cells – known as receptors – upon which nicotine is said to act.[8] Laboratory rats, as usual, are the luckless stand-ins for a series of merciless experiments, as scientists try to establish the precise mechanisms leading to nicotine 'addiction'.

The average smoker, in describing the attraction, would resort to more straightforward explanations. There is the hit factor as the smoke is drawn into the lungs. For the novice this experience is burning and exalting, and even though the impact diminishes as the lungs become familiarised, the experience remains an important one for many smokers. Then there is the flavour – nutty and sweet with the darker blends such as Gitane; sappy and bright if it's a Virginian.

Though, pharmacologically speaking, nicotine is a mild stimulant, smokers will describe the cigarette experience

418

in much more versatile terms: it takes you up when you're feeling low, brings you down when you're too fired up; makes you relaxed, friendly, and communicative; gets you going; helps you think; takes your mind off your problems.

These states of being are plainly at odds with each other and yet experimenters with pure nicotine seem to confirm that the drug truly does have this multi-faceted ability. Smaller doses stimulate whereas larger ones depress. But then other tests suggest the upping and downing isn't dose-related, more a matter of personality. Still more tests indicate that nicotine has practically no bearing on how much people smoke. Subjects given injections of the drug carried on smoking at the same rate and in the same manner as though the injections had never happened.[9]

Health Impact

The health argument over smoking goes back in Britain at least to 1604 when James 1 published his spirited tirade *Counterblaste to Tobacco* . . . In modern times the issue was revived by the Royal College of Physicians who, in a 1962 report, linked smoking with lung cancer and implored the government to do something about rising consumption. The public itself responded by momentarily cutting back, but a year later was smoking more than ever. The pattern was duplicated in the US following a report by their own Surgeon General. The masses, it seems, cannot be persuaded from their vices by gore stories alone – and young people are often positively attracted to high-risk activities.

The dramatic reductions of recent years – down between 1974 and 1992 from 45 per cent of the population to 28 per cent – are probably as much to do with an increasingly punitive tax regime as any other factor. But even this relationship is unclear. Surveys show that poorer households not only spend a greater share of their income on tobacco, they spend more in absolute terms than the wealthy; the more people earn the less they smoke.[10]

So what are the smoking hazards? Since that first Royal College report, the news has got no better. According to the government's own statistics, smoking-related diseases cause around 110,000 premature deaths each year in the UK.[11] That's six times as many as the combined total caused by road accidents, suicides, homicides, fire, illicit drug use, and AIDS.

But besides death there is all the misery of smoking-related diseases, the financial cost to the sufferer these cause through lost work, and the drain on the NHS resulting from millions of individuals knowingly injuring themselves.

It is often argued by the freedom-to-smoke lobby that tax receipts from tobacco sales – £8.2 billion during 1993/94 – easily exceed what is spent treating those suffering smoking-related sickness. In other words, there is a net gain for the state. The bill to the NHS is currently around £437 million,[12] but other costs have to be considered. These include the payment of sickness and invalidity benefits to ailing smokers, as well as pensions and social security giros to those the smokers leave behind. Added to this are the 50 million working days said to be lost every year through smoke-induced sickness,[13] plus the human and material costs of between 6,000 and 7,000 fires that result every year from smokers losing track of their combustibles.[14]

The idea that smokers pay their way and, at retirement age, discreetly exit is disputed in passionate terms by a forty-eight-year-old housewife from Matfield in Kent.

'My uncle had his first smoking-related heart attack at forty-five and was a burden to the state until his death at sixty-one, having suffered a multitude of ills related to heart disease and the side effects of all the drugs he needed. My mother-in-law is sixty-nine and has had smoking-related emphysema for over twenty years. She too is costing the state. A good friend's husband, who was a heavy smoker, had a stroke. Not only was he relatively young but she has had the burden and sorrow of living with a man who is a shadow of the man she married. Smoking takes its revenge slowly and costs a great deal in sorrow, pain and money.'

There are four principal ailments with which smoking has been shown to have a causal rather than a coincidental relationship – lung cancer, bronchitis/emphysema, heart disease, and arterial disease.

Lung cancer

Some of the most plausible data linking lung cancer with smoking comes from studying the smoking habits of doctors between 1954 and 1971. The proportion of male physicians smoking cigarettes halved during this period from 43 per cent to 21 per cent, while among all men in England and Wales the number of smokers remained the same. Lung cancer among doctors during the period fell by 25 per cent, whereas in the general population it rose by 26 per cent.[15] It also appears from this same study that the risk of the disease increases in direct proportion to the number of cigarettes smoked. Those who consumed up to fourteen a day were eight times more vulnerable than non-smokers, and twenty-five-a-day-or-more types were twenty-five times more at risk.

Lung cancer has actually started declining among men in recent years. This is due largely to the reduction in smoking and, to a lesser extent, to the low-tar filter cigarettes that have come to dominate the market.

For women, lung cancer is on the increase, and this seems to correlate with a sharp rise after the Second World War in the number of female smokers. If lung cancer deaths among British women keep rising at their present rate, the wrecking power of the disease will overtake that of breast cancer by the year 2010. It already has in Scotland and in some parts of England.

Since lung cancer is seeded many years before the disease appears, quitting smoking will not instantly eliminate risk, but the danger will start decreasing to the point where after ten to fifteen years, according to the American Cancer Society,[16] the ex-smoker whose habit was moderate is only at slightly greater risk than someone who has never smoked.

Emphysema/bronchitis

The new preferred term for these progressively disabling conditions is chronic obstructive lung disease (COLD), which better indicates what's happening. Fundamentally, the air passages to the lungs are being narrowed and damaged and much of the lung tissue itself destroyed. Onset of the disease is gradual and a good deal of harm will probably already have been done by the time the familiar breathlessness becomes

421

disabling. It has been argued that at least 90 per cent of COLD deaths are attributable to smoking,[17] and though the death rate has been decreasing in recent years, the condition still managed to kill nearly 30,000 people in 1992.[18]

Heart diseases

There are two principal manifestations of coronary heart disease – angina and heart attack. Both occur because the arteries carrying blood to the heart muscle become blocked or narrowed, often by deposits of fatty substances – a condition known as atherosclerosis. A heart attack results from the severe blockage of a coronary artery, either by those fatty materials, or by a blood clot. With the heart muscle denied its normal supply of oxygen, part of it dies – as does the patient himself in a quarter of all cases.

The part played by smoking in heart diseases is less clear-cut than for lung cancer. Though the Department of Health has estimated that about a quarter of mortalities are smoking-related, it is evident that other factors play a principal role in this most prevalent of all causes of death. Not least there is lack of exercise, the consumption of too much animal fat (milk and cheese included), obesity, high blood pressure and, to a lesser extent, the hereditary factor. While the 1991 mortality rate of nearly 93,000 men and 78,000 women represents a decline since the 1960s of, respectively, 10 per cent and 2 per cent, the fall in other industrialised countries has been far more dramatic.

Whatever the other contributory factors, middle-aged smokers on fifteen or more cigarettes a day seem to be three times more prone to the disease than their non-smoking counterparts. And at least 80 per cent of heart attacks in men under forty-five are thought to be due to smoking.[19] Women under sixty-five are much less liable to be felled by heart problems than men but they too are being stricken more often.

Researchers usually isolate nicotine and carbon monoxide as smoke's ravening factors as far as the heart is concerned. The first increases the great organ's workload, while the carbon monoxide denies it the normal supply of oxygen. Additionally, smoking tends to make blood stickier and therefore less able to flow through the narrowed arteries and more likely to form a thrombosis or clot.

Arterial disease

Disease of arteries other than in the heart area is also more common in smokers. More than 90 per cent of all individuals with serious arterial disease of the legs are regular smokers.[20] This is a condition that, if unheeded, can lead to gangrene and amputation of the limb.

Other smoking-related diseases

Lung cancer, bronchitis/emphysema, and heart and arterial diseases might be the Big Four smoking risks, but there are several more ailments with which the habit is linked, sometimes, it has to be said, fairly tenuously. These include cancers of the mouth, throat, oesophagus, bladder, pancreas, kidney, and cervix; also asthma and cot deaths. There is, additionally, what the Royal College of Physicians calls a 'well-recognised association' with peptic ulcers in the stomach and duodenum.

Women and smoking

Apart from falling prey more frequently to the 'male diseases' of lung cancer and heart failure, other special hazards face women. Those who take the contraceptive pill and also smoke are ten times more likely than non-smoking pill users to have either a coronary attack, stroke, or blood clot in the leg veins[21] – an effect that is even more marked in women over forty-five.

Women's fertility, their well-being during pregnancy, and the health of their children also seem to be compromised by smoking. An American survey found that, of a group of women studied, fewer of those who smoked were able to conceive, and those who did fall pregnant took longer to do so.[22] Men who smoke are affected too: higher rates of arterial disease limit their ability to mount an erection. And, once the organ does get going, it is likely to produce fewer, more sluggish sperm, which will be less able to reach and penetrate the female egg.[23]

The impact on babies

That babies suffer as a result of their parents' habit is now well documented, although there always remains the problem of separating out other health-damaging factors that coincide with tobacco use. These include the consumption of other drugs (prescribed or scored on the street), pollution, and poor nutrition. The focus is usually on women – 32 per cent of whom, according to a 1991 Gallup poll, continue smoking during pregnancy. But North Carolina researchers, scouring the health records of thousands of children born between 1959 and 1966, claim that the offspring of men who smoked more than twenty cigarettes a day were twice as likely to suffer birth defects, such as hare lip and malfunctioning hearts, as the children of non-smokers. A parallel study found that leukaemia and cancer of the lymph nodes were twice as common among children of men who smoked in the year before their children were born, while brain cancer was 40 per cent more common.[24] Commenting on the findings, leading American biochemist Bruce Ames said: 'I'm already convinced that a good proportion of the birth defects and child cancers are coming from male smokers.' He could detect no such links traceable to women. Ames also warned that the genetically based damage could 'reverberate down the generations', affecting the grandchildren and great-grandchildren of smokers.

Where women and pregnancy are concerned, it is now fairly well established that the various poisons contained in tobacco smoke are able to pass through the placenta into the baby. This can result in smaller, more feeble babies who might continue lagging as they grow older. Tobacco use during pregnancy is also reported to double the risk of spontaneous abortion (miscarriage)[25] and to promote other complications, such as bleeding and premature detachment of the placenta.[26]

Death of the baby at or soon after birth has been shown to happen more often the greater the number of cigarettes smoked by a woman during pregnancy. For those using in excess of twenty a day the risk is more than a third higher than that faced by non-smokers.[27]

However, the news for women – and their children – who quit before the twentieth week of pregnancy is good. Their risk of having a low-weight baby is believed to be similar to that of a non-smoker and they will also be less vulnerable to the other hazards.

Passive smoking

The issue of passive smoking (i.e. the involuntary ingestion of other people's smoke) is the most passionately disputed area in the great tobacco debate. That's because if smokers really are injuring innocent bystanders then the freedom-to-enjoy line promoted by the likes of FOREST begins to unravel. FOREST argues that the data have been given an unfair spin. But, while there is indeed some over-eagerness on the part of the antis, too much evidence has now piled up for anyone to pretend that the use of tobacco is no one's business but that of the smoker.

Young children are the first victims. The Department of Health estimates that, every day, fifty under-fives are admitted to hospital with symptoms of passive smoking.[28] Such children suffer high levels of bronchitis and other respiratory diseases and run an increased risk of cancer later in life. Where both parents smoke, the child is receiving the equivalent of 60 to 150 cigarettes a year into his/her lungs.[29]

For adults consistently subjected to other people's smoke, there is, according to the fourth report of the government's Independent Scientific Committee on Smoking and Health (1988), an extra 10 to 30 per cent chance of contracting lung cancer. This means that 'several hundred' of the 40,000 annual UK lung cancer deaths can be laid at the door of passive smoking.

Dependence

There is only one universally recognised drug in tobacco: nicotine. Being a mild stimulant, it's possible to build a tolerance to its stimulative effects, which would necessitate a bigger and bigger dose, leading, ultimately, to physical dependence. In practice, most people reach a ceiling well below this dependence level and then even out their consumption. The amount they use from then on fluctuates according to their state of being – which is precisely the way they'll use other drugs. When a craving for tobacco does develop, this will generally have a psychological and not a physical basis. And even after years of comparatively heavy smoking, people can still quit on the spot, experiencing few if any of the classic withdrawal symptoms.

One perverse by-product of the obsessional research into nicotine is that the drug is now being dispensed as a smoking 'cure'. As well as the various patches, a leading research scientist is predicting that we shall one day see nicotine-type drugs that mimic the effects of the genuine article but which 'do not share its undesirable effects'.[30] This is a familiar phantom – the safe, non-addictive substitute for a drug whose side effects have at last been officially recognised. The pharmaceutical companies have always chased this particular ghost because it is lucrative to do so. And the licensing authorities are invariably willing to vouch as safe a new product on the basis of unsubstantiated claims because the public will swallow what they are licitly given – until told not to; at which point the item concerned leaches out on to the street where some people will indulge messily and damage themselves in a way the manufacturers and political authorities say couldn't possibly have been anticipated. *Nicotine tablets?* One (unsubstantiated) claim for the drug is that it reduces the chances of succumbing to Alzheimer's disease, a progressively disabling condition leading to dementia. Nicotine tablets probably are on their way and, although the bottle might say they're safe, the ingenuity of the street user, out for the ultimate high kick, will demonstrate otherwise.

Earliest Use

The origins of tobacco smoking can be traced back to the Maya civilisation of Mexico at around 500 AD. This, though, is a modest assumption about tobacco's pedigree. References to the smoking of various plants have been found in the Vedic scriptures of India dating from a couple of thousand years BC, and tobacco is likely to have been one of the selection that was consumed. Commercial trading on an international scale began with the arrival in the 'New World' of European interlopers

426

some four hundred years ago. From Chile to Montreal the native people of the new lands were smoking, chewing, eating the leaves, and drinking the juice of the plant. In the West Indies it was customary for small leaves to be wrapped in larger ones or in a palm leaf, the prototype of the modern cigar. In Mexico they were sniffing through tubes made of tortoise shell and silver. Further north the pipe was traditional, sometimes made of marble, sometimes of lobster claw.

The Portuguese, as masters of international commerce before the rise of the Dutch and English, were the first to cultivate the plant outside the Americas and did most to convert the rest of the world. But its arrival in England – around 1565 – was probably by means of French or Flemish sailors acting at the behest of English herbalists. For the first couple of decades it was used here strictly medicinally – for purging 'superfluous fleame and other gross humours', as one contemporary account had it. Then, in 1586, a great cache of the stuff was brought back to England from the West Indies and, on the instructions of Sir Walter Raleigh, was surveyed and written up.[31] It was thanks in large measure to Raleigh's patronage that smoking became a social ritual and that, increasingly, tobacco was sold from specialist shops. By the 1600s public houses were also in on the action, as were grocers, drapers, chandlers, and goldsmiths. Virginia in what is now the USA was the source, and the colony soon became the world's tobacco capital with every open space in the township employed for the growing of the leaf.

Other American colonies followed and cultivation started in every part of the world. Though some regions gave the plant a frigid welcome, the Portuguese hit lucky in what was to become Malawi and Zimbabwe, while the Dutch were equally successful in Indonesia where the soil and climate were ideal for producing the thick, juicy leaves that go into cigar manufacture.

As Europeans became more engrossed in the trade, so the medicinal claims for the leaf grew ever more fulsome. 'There can be do doubt', according to a Dr Johannes Vittich,[32] 'that tobacco can cleanse all impurities and disperse every gross and viscous humour, as we find by daily experience. It cures cancer of the breast, open and eating sores, scabs and scratches, however poisonous and septic, goitre, broken

427

limbs, erysipelas, and many other things. It will heal wounds in the arms, legs and other members of the body, of however long standing.'

Among the converts were the faculty of Eton College, who obliged their boy students to smoke a pipeful every morning to keep them healthy. Penalty for disobedience was a flogging.

When it came to smoking for pleasure, this – in early-seventeenth-century England – was essentially a pastime for the wealthy, given that it demanded expensive metal pipes and other bits of apparatus. Later, the introduction of clay and wood pipes meant that the lower orders could join in, and yet groups like the London dandies still devised means of setting themselves apart. The fashionable kit required a case of expensive clays, an ivory or metal box to hold the weed, ember tongs to convey a heated coal to light the pipe, a metal stopper to compress the tobacco into the bowl, a pick with which to clear said bowl, a knife to shred the tobacco, and a small scoop in which the tobacco could be dried.[33] Patented methods were devised for in/exhaling the smoke, with names such as the *Gulpe*, the *Whiffe*, and, perhaps most excitingly, the *Cuban Ebolition*, whereby smoke was expelled from the nostrils. The new habit clearly vexed members of the clergy. King James, too, was not pleased, although his *Counterblaste To Tobacco* was apparently aimed as much at his political enemy Raleigh as the new drug. He followed his tirade by raising the import duty on tobacco by 4,000 per cent and, subsequently, by establishing a royal import monopoly – not the first or the last time sovereign and political powers have profited handsomely from what they claim to find morally obnoxious.

But James's lunge at the smoke habit was modest compared with what was going on elsewhere. In Switzerland smoking could mean the pillory, in Persia suffocation by smoke, in Turkey having a pipe-stem thrust through the nose, in China decapitation, and in Russia flogging, castration, slitting of the lips, or exile to Siberia.

By the end of the seventeenth century, snuff had jumped up to steal the limelight from pipe smoking, a position it held until the early nineteenth century. Snuffing involved paraphernalia and etiquette even more extraordinary than that for smoking. A gentleman was known by his snuff; he laid it down as he would a cellar of wine. That ladies also took to snuffing is illustrated by the will of one Mrs Margaret Thompson whose coffin in 1776 was filled with unwashed snuff handkerchiefs and her body borne by the six greatest snuff-takers in the parish. Inevitably the habit spread to the lower orders, whereupon the product became more and more adulterated with coal or powdered glass, and was ultimately jettisoned from smart circles. *Hints on Etiquette*, published in 1835, called snuffing 'an idle, dirty habit practised by stupid people in the unavailing endeavour to clear their stolid intellect.' By this time cigars were drawing level. Then cigarette smoking arrived with British troops, who'd seen it done during the Crimean War (1854–86) by their French and Turkish allies.

At first, cigarettes were of the roll-your-own sort and made from any type of paper. Then English manufacturers started turning out hand-made varieties consisting chiefly of Turkish and Egyptian leaves. By 1870 the 'bright' Virginian blends were coming over in bulk and London fashion transferred back across the Atlantic. Now also came the innovation that opened the way to the great tobacco empires that dominate in our own time: the 'Bonsack' automatic rolling machine. Patented in 1881, it could do the work of forty employees. The W. D. & H. O. Wills Company quickly secured 'absolute rights' in the UK, while in America a similar deal was struck by James Buchanan Duke, inexhaustible head of the American Tobacco Company (ATC). Within a few years 'Daddy' Duke had bought out every one of his US rivals. Then he came gunning for Wills and the other dozen leading British manufacturers. Uniting under the banner of Imperial, the family-owned British companies saw off the Duke's challenge, and even went for a chunk of the US market just to demonstrate that they weren't intimidated by the big man. As Peter Taylor notes in *Smoke Ring*,[34] a truce was declared. It was agreed, in 1902, that Imperial should confine itself to the British market and the American Tobacco Company to the US, while a new corporation would be formed, called British American Tobacco, to handle exports for both companies. The arrangement lasted nine years before the US Supreme Court, which was out hunting monopolies at the time, ordered that the American Tobacco Company be dismantled in the interests of greater consumer choice.

The rended segment that retained the ATC name later transmogrified into a multinational called American Brands.

As to Imperial, they stayed intact here in the UK where they concentrated future business.

The fate of the joint enterprise, British American Tobacco (BAT), was more fascinating: this was floated off as an independent corporation registered in London. Thereafter, through adroit licensing and diversification schemes, it was able to outstrip both its parents as well as all the new competition. Until the mid 1980s, it was the largest private-sector tobacco corporation in the world, operating in 180 countries and claiming brand leadership in thirty-six of them. Today, the number-one spot goes to Philip Morris.

Global and UK Brand Leaders

Marlboro, manufactured by **Philip Morris**, is estimated to be the world's most lucrative brand of any product, contributing the major part of the company's 1993 international tobacco profits of $5.2 billion. In fact, its tobacco income was substantially down on the previous year thanks to a merciless price war in the United States, fought out against the background of declining domestic sales. But Philip Morris – despite claiming around 11.6 per cent of the total world market – is about much more than tobacco. The group also owns the Miller Brewing company and the giant General Foods, a combination that produces total sales for the group of $51 billion. The multinational's origins lie in a small Bond Street, London tobacco shop opened by one Philip Morris in 1847.

The second biggest player on the world scene is **BAT Industries**, which in 1992 controlled more than 50 per cent of the cigarette market in thirty-one countries, produced over 570 billion cigarettes worldwide, claimed a 10.9 per cent global share, and racked up tobacco sales of £9.7 billion. In spring 1994, BAT bid £670 million for American Tobacco, owner of the Lucky Strike and Pall Mall brands within the US. The deal needed the OK of the American anti-trust authorities. If they give the nod, BAT's share of the US market would increase from around 11 to 18 per cent. In the UK (where very few of BAT's cigarettes are sold) its other main involvement is in financial services: the company owns Eagle Star and Allied Dunbar.

R. J. Reynolds claims third place in the world rankings: a 5 per cent global share, based on 1991 sales of $8.5 billion net. Headquartered in North Carolina, Reynolds' roots are in the tobacco belt of the US from where it peddled chewing and smoking tobaccos. Today, its main brands are Camel, Winston, Salem and More. In 1985 the company swallowed the Nabisco Foods conglomerate. Its share of the UK tobacco market is around 3 per cent.

Rothmans International originated, in 1890, with Ukrainian immigrant Louis Rothman's shop in London's Fleet Street. Principal shareholder is the Swiss firm Compagnie Financière Richemont AG, which, in turn, is owned by the South African corporation Rembrandt. Rothmans claims a 2 per cent global share and 1991 tobacco sales of £2.1 billion. Main brands are Rothmans King Size, Dunhill, Cartier, and Peter Stuyvesant. Also under the group's umbrella is the Vendome luxury goods company – notable for its Dunhill and Cartier product lines. None of Rothmans' tobacco brands feature in the UK's top-selling list, but the company still claims a more than 15 per cent share of the domestic market.

Gallaher is a UK rather than a world giant, with 42 per cent of the home market and the top three brands in its portfolio: namely, Benson and Hedges, Silk Cut, and Berkeley Superkings. Pre-tax profits in 1992 were £304.4 million. Its subsidiaries include the Prestige cookware company, Forbuoys newsagencies, and Whyte and Mackay whisky. Gallaher is, in turn, owned by the US tobacco firm American Brands.

Imperial Tobacco, now owned by Hanson plc, has a 34 per cent UK market share, second to Gallaher. Top sellers are Regal Kingsize, John Player Superkings, Embassy, Golden Virginia roll-your-owns, and Castella and Café Crème cigars. Trading profits in 1992 were £281 million. Hanson's other businesses include the Ever Ready battery company, Beazer Homes, The London Brick Co., and Seven Seas vitamins and fish oil.

The World Market

For the big London and New York companies the last thirty years have been a story of retrenchment at home – thanks to concerns about rising taxes and the impact on health – offset by massive expansion overseas. In the 1960s South America was the growth area. In the 1970s and 1980s Africa, the Middle East, and the Far East were the war zones. Where there was resistance – as in Japan, Taiwan, South Korea, and Thailand – the US government disposed of it by threatening trade sanctions. As a result, restrictions on 'imports and advertising were lifted and, in Taiwan especially, there followed dramatic rises in smoking (5 per cent in a single year), with marked increases among the young.

In Africa, sales climbed 33 per cent between 1970 and 1980. The line the companies pushed here was the one manufacturers of all manner of products habitually use – *our brand equals brain power, muscle power, and social success*. State Express was advertised in Malawi – one of the poorest countries in the world – by lining up a picture of the pack alongside a top-of-the-range Jaguar. In Kenya, examples of aspirational brand titles are Varsity and Sportsman. The quantities of cancer-causing tar per cigarette In 'poor South' countries such as these invariably exceed by some distance those that would be permitted in the rich North; all the better to hook the nascent consumer. And, in every other way, official restraints are usually more lax, with few if any curbs on advertising, limited health education, and no sign of the warnings to be routinely found on packs in richer countries.

In most of these virgin markets, the cultivators as well as the consumers get a punishing deal. Farmers, hooked on the help and advice that the tobacco companies lavish on them, end up growing a crop that is both inordinately labour-intensive and environmentally destructive. The sensitive tobacco plant, prone to a multitude of diseases, is fed up to sixteen applications of fertilizer, herbicide, and pesticide during its three-month growing period. And, during the curing process, an abundance of coal, oil, or timber is called for. Where wood is used (Brazil, Malawi, Tanzania, for example), a hectare of woodland must be cut for each hectare of tobacco grown. Around the world, some 10 per cent of all wood used is for tobacco curing – an arrangement that is subsidised and, thereby, legitimised by the United Nations Food and Agriculture Organisation.

The Battle for Eastern Europe

As these pages are being written, it is the newly deregulated countries of Eastern Europe and the former Soviet Union which are under the big hammer assault from the major New York and London companies. With a combined annual cigarette habit totalling 700 billion and an apparently insatiable demand for Western brands in these territories, the companies are sparing nothing. Initiatives include dropping multi-million-dollar sweeteners, downing gallons of vodka with heads of state, and staging some pretty tacky promotional stunts: e.g. dispensing free sunglasses at a Hungarian pop concert for anyone who took a cigarette and smoked it in front of the promo girl.

'It's trench warfare,' a Reynolds regional executive told a reporter for the *Observer*, 'hand to hand combat.'[35] Notionally, the Western companies are entering into 'joint ventures' with the formerly state-run enterprises. In reality, factories and whole industries are being bought up. Philip Morris purchased the entire Czech state industry of five plants in a $400 million deal – an investment, according to a beaming company spokesman, that represented the biggest American financial input of any description into central Europe. Morris also signed an important 'protocol' with Russia and did deals and buy-outs in Hungary, Poland, and Bulgaria.

Poland – annual consumption 100 billion cigarettes – was also a target for R.J. Reynolds and for Rothmans. 'We were hammering on the Berlin Wall longer than the American forces,' said a Rothmans International spokesman. 'Until recently, perhaps 40 per cent of the world's smokers were locked behind ideological walls. We've been itching to get at them.'

BAT Industries, late into the race, was targeting the Ukraine, Hungary and, most significantly, the central Asian republic of Uzbekistan, into which it was pouring a £133 million investment.

By 1994, Western companies controlled half the old Eastern Bloc tobacco market – up from 3 per cent just six years before. Consumption was booming, driven on by advertising, campaigns that, under communism, were prohibited; and the targets, it seemed, were women and adolescents.

Inevitably, such developments produced less than beneficial health outcomes for a population that was already suffering rapidly rising smoking-related illnesses. A fifteen-year-old boy in Eastern Europe was now twice as likely to die before reaching sixty than his Western counterpart, largely as a result of smoking.

After the former Eastern Bloc territories will come an assault on China, perhaps the last great frontier still relatively untraversed by the free-market tobacco giants. China possesses a state-run tobacco enterprise bigger than anything, public or private, seen anywhere in the world. Catering for 200 million domestic smokers, it turns out some 1,000 brands that are totally unknown outside her borders. Production, at around 750 billion cigarettes a year, is larger than Philip Morris's and the source for this enormous output is a domestic harvest that is also a world-beater – topping that which comes out of the USA's famed tobacco belt. But even in China the consumer is hungry for 'international' brands and so China is already entering into brand-sharing and other deals with Western companies that are winning her state-of-the-art assistance, in return for which she will have holes punched in the home market through which Marlboro, Camel *et al.* will enter.

The UK Market: Women and Children First

In the near-saturated home market the most receptive segments – the ones most likely to buck the twenty-year downward trend – are women and children. The latter are especially important because they represent the companies' futures. These days that future looks fairly promising, given that around 10 per cent of girls and 9 per cent of boys aged eleven to fifteen are already regular smokers – a pattern that barely changed between 1982 and 1993. Among fifteen-year-olds, almost one in four smoke regularly – again no change in more than a decade.[36] Altogether, more than one billion cigarettes a year are consumed by these eleven- to fifteen-year-olds, and they are shelling out around £120 million in the process.[37] If present trends continue, according to a World Health Organisation report,[38] smoking will kill one million of today's teenagers and children by the time they reach middle age.

Adults talk in terms of parental influence and peer pressure as reasons for children going on the fags. The young themselves will say it makes them feel grown-up and appealing. Warnings that smoking will shave X years off their life expectancy cut no ice with them; the young relish the sense of 'danger'. The brands they choose are the ones with the slickest, faddiest advertising and those that are locked into fast-sports sponsorship.

Women started smoking in a big way from the 1920s and, especially, after the Second World War. By 1972, 41 per cent of adult females were smokers, at which point the tobacco companies were identifying women's fondness for the weed as a mark of their emancipation. *You've come a long way baby*, ran one thoroughly condescending strapline. The products that are directed at women are often extremely long, sometimes mentholated, and invariably packaged in elegant, creamy colours with brand names like Kim, More, and Virginia Slims. But if 1972 marked a peak uptake, it's been downhill ever since, with the proportion of female smokers dipping from 41 per cent to a 1992 total of 28 per cent.[39] (The comparative numbers for men are 52 per cent smoking in 1972, 29 per cent in 1992.)

But though women in general are eschewing the habit, a number of surveys have shown that those under twenty five, and particularly the sixteen to nineteen age range, are more, not less, infatuated with the weed. Sex was a large factor in the explanation, together with the ever-appealing notion that smoking makes the flab float away. '. . . So long as thinness is equated with sexual attractiveness in women,' said a January 1993 *Harpers & Queen* article, 'they will continue to smoke whatever the risks. It is proven that people will risk death for sex.' And the act of smoking is itself sexy, according to the same author. 'Not sexy?' she asks rhetorically. 'Smoking? The flare of the match on the upturned face, the half-closed eyes, the little red-kindled tip, not sexy? Not sexy the face half-concealed in a deliquescence of lavender smoke? I can hardly go on . . .'

Yet despite several surveys pointing in the other direction, government figures published in January 1994[40] indicated that 'only' 25 per cent of sixteen- to nineteen-year-old females smoked – a smaller percentage than applies both to older women and to their male counterparts. There was, it seemed, still plenty of effort required from the tobacco companies.

Giving Up

There are a million schemes for easing people out of their smoking habit. The basis for any successful method is to get the preliminaries right, which means establishing rationally and emotionally that quitting is a positive, worthwhile goal, and that, far from something being 'given up', something will be gained: improved health and personal esteem. Schemes whereby smokers, as it were, jump out of the bushes and startle themselves out of the habit are almost bound to fail. Having got the mind correctly adjusted, it is then not a bad idea to let the prospect bubble for a while, maybe for months or even a year or two. The actual moment of quitting can be arranged to suit temperament and circumstances. It might be done on holiday, at the start of a new year, or as a birthday treat. Some people like to shout about it and have bets; others like to keep discreet to lessen the pressure. Some take to ritual – pinning the last pack to the wall; others want to make it no big deal. Remember, it's easier than most people think. It's probably best to avoid extremely elaborate substitution ploys: sucking four packs of mints a day is a constant reminder as to the ex-smoker's great 'sacrifice'. But increasing numbers swear by the various no-smoke aids now on the market: the gums, patches, nasal sprays, inhalers, lozenges, tablets, and capsules – some of which contain nicotine, while others are dosed with silver acetate to make cigarettes taste disgusting.

Anti-smoking patches used to be available on the cheap through the NHS but in October 1993 the government announced the end of the arrangement. The decision was driven exclusively by financial consideration (if people can afford to smoke, they should buy their own patches and not rely on taxpayers' subsidies, said Health Secretary Virginia Bottomley), but there was already something of a nicotine-patch boycott following revelations about the macabre history of some of the brands. According to the *Sunday Mirror* (22 August 1993), during the development of Nicorette, made by Swedish drug company Kabi Pharmacia, guinea pigs were injected with amounts of nicotine equal to a human being smoking five thousand cigarettes at once. And rabbits had their backs shaved and patches attached to them for twenty-four hours, which produced skin irritation and epileptic-type fits. Other animal tests were carried out by Ciba Pharmaceuticals, makers of Nicotinell.

Dummy cigarettes and special tar-trap filters are other devices for the reluctant smoker. There are also special cessation clinics and self-help groups, although their success rates are variable.

A little weight might be put on after quitting. This is because the body is able to absorb more of what's eaten through the newly uncongested gastro-intestinal machinery. With a little discipline, body weight should quickly settle down.

Another worry is that by quitting there will be a loss of mental and physical edge. This is a particular concern of people in 'creative' activities and was voiced by an Oxford professor of modern history, who told the London *Evening Standard* that for him life without smoking would probably mean 'long, slow hours hammering out leaden sentences.' In the same article a 'young beauty and author' also insisted that 'people who are smoking are thinking, while people who are not are just staring into space.' The statement betrayed third-rate thinking, since no psychoactive drug can deliver the goods over the long term. Also, the physically debilitating effects of tobacco smoke soon knock away any edge that nicotine might provide.

More bogeyman stories abound concerning an alleged nicotine starvation that is supposed to seize the smoker after two months, six months, one year, five years, and so forth. Except in a small, chain-smoking minority – and then for only a matter of weeks – there will be no real nicotine starvation because not enough of the drug is consumed to work up a substantial physical relationship. If a person continues to feel vulnerable to stray plumes of smoke, it means s/he is still concentrating on old, dead habits. That is why elaborate substitution ploys in the period after quitting are not necessarily a good idea. A case history:

'I smoked for some twenty years from the days of my early teens. I would alternate between rollies and manufactured cigarettes and get through at least twenty a day, sometimes forty. Having made the decision to stop I let the idea sit there for a couple of years, not knowing when the right moment would present itself. Finally it came at the beginning of a holiday in Wales which required a long car journey. My wife asked me if I'd mind not smoking to avoid clouding up an already clammy atmosphere. I agreed and decided to lay off for the rest of that day. After that I managed to desist for the first week, on the third day of which my lungs purged themselves of a putrid, sticky material that had me coughing and spluttering for half an hour. I was encouraged to keep off the fags for the second week.

'Abstaining in the hills and valleys of Wales was all very well, but I anticipated a much graver test back in London, faced with deadlines and telephone bills. I made no promise to myself and yet when it did come to writing my first article – which I considered the first big test – I actually forgot that I was ever a smoker. A couple of tremors of desire came in the following months, but nothing of consequence. Now I continually remind myself (nearly fifteen years later) how lucky I am to be free of such an idiotic habit.'

Notes

1 Alan Stewart, MP, 'The Right to Smoke: A Conservative View', FOREST, London, 1989.
2 T. Liddle, 'The Right to Smoke: A Socialist View', FOREST, London, 1989.
3 'US ruling turns smokers into junkies', in *New Scientist*, 13 August 1994, p. 10.
4 The Drug Abuse Advisory Committee. They were appointed to their task by David Kessler of the Food and Drug Administration.
5 *Hear the Other Side*, newsletter of the Tobacco Advisory Council, London, July 1993.
6 'Tories "returned election favour to tobacco firms"', in the *Guardian*, 11 February 1994.
7 I. Stolerman, 'Nicotine on the brain', in *New Scientist*, 3 November 1990, pp. 33–5. This is an examination of the latest laboratory research, most of it involving rats.
8 Ibid.
9 In M. Gossop, *Living with Drugs*, Temple Smith, London, 1982, p. 96.
10 'Family spending: A report on the 1990 Family Expenditure Survey', Central Statistical Office, HMSO, London, 1991.
11 Press release, Department of Health, 7 February 1994.
12 'The smoking epidemic – counting the cost in England and Wales', Health Education Authority, 1991.
13 'Smoking or Health?', Royal College of Physicians, Pitman, London, 1977.
14 In 1992 there were 6,300 fires. Sources: Home Office; Fire Statistics United Kingdom; Government Statistical Service, June 1994.
15 'Health or Smoking?', follow-up report of the Royal College of Physicians, Pitman, London, 1983, p. 3.
16 'Dangers of smoking – benefits of quitting', American Cancer Society, 1980, p. 8.
17 Commons Hansard Session 1988/89, 143 c764–5W, 16 December 1988.
18 *Deaths by Cause*, OPCS, General Register Offices, Belfast and Edinburgh, 1992.
19 J. L. Townsend and T. W. Meade, 'Ischaemic heart disease mortality risks for smokers and non-smokers', in the *Journal of Epidemiology and Community Health*, 1979, pp. 243–7.
20 'Smoking and health – a report of the US Surgeon General', USGPO, US Department of Health and Human Services, 1979, p. 1136.
21 Royal College of Physicians, 'Health or Smoking?', op. cit.

22 D. Baird and A. J. Wilcox, in the *Journal of the American Medical Association*, 253, 1985, pp. 2979–83.

23 R. J. Albin, in the *New York State Journal of Medicine*, 86, 1986, p. 108.

24 'Smokers' sperm spell trouble for future generations', in *New Scientist*, 6 March 1993.

25 J. Kline *et al.*, in the *New England Journal of Medicine*, Vol. 297, 1977, pp. 793–6.

26 N. Sidle, 'Smoking in pregnancy – a review', Spastics Society Hera Unit, London, 1982.

27 M. Meyer *et al*, in the *American Journal of Epidemiology*, 103, 1976, pp. 464–76.

28 This according to the then Health Minister, Dr Brian Mawhinney, at the February 1994 launch of a £12 million government anti-smoking campaign.

29 'Smoking and the Young', Royal College of Physicians, 1992.

30 Stolerman, op. cit.

31 *A History of the Tobacco Trade*, Imperial Group, London, 1979, p. 8.

32 In S. Gabb, 'Smoking and its enemies – a short history of 500 years of the use and prohibition of tobacco', FOREST, London, 1990. A fascinating, scholarly treatise, from the perspective of a liberty lobby zealot.

33 Imperial Group, op. cit.

34 P. Taylor, *Smoke Ring*, The Bodley Head, London, 1984, p. 24.

35 M. MacAlister Hall, 'The $225,000,000,000 habit', in the *Observer* magazine, 8 November 1992.

36 Office of Population, Censuses and Surveys survey of 3,140 pupils at 110 schools, reported in 'Renewed call for ban on tobacco advertising as campaigns fail', in the *Guardian*, 28 July 1994.

37 1991 Office of Population, Censuses and Surveys data, published in 'Protecting children from tobacco', a report by Parents Against Tobacco, Long Bennington, Notts., 1993.

38 'Smoking will kill 1m young people', in the *Guardian*, 20 September 1994.

39 *General Household Survey*, Office of Population, Censuses and Surveys, HMSO, February 1994.

40 Ibid.

TRANQUILLISERS

Intro

The term tranquilliser is used to refer to drugs from the class of chemicals known as benzodiazepines, which began pouring on to the market thirty-odd years ago with the launch of Librium. For most of that time they were regarded as sublimely innocuous substances – pacifiers of addled housewives, the means by which a busy doctor could speedily empty his surgery. It was said, only half jokingly, that the only way to suffer a lethal reaction to the benzodiazepines was to be buried under an avalanche of them.

Some people always knew better. The quest for a thoroughly safe, non-addictive substance capable of calming the human spirit is as futile as it is ancient. No psychoactive product, in all circumstances, can be hazard-free, and in this modern era of laboratory-produced, high-potency compounds we seem further away than ever from the foolproof elixir.

Concerns about the benzos took more than twenty years to surface in a conspicuous way. For the delay we can look to the extraordinary firepower of the drug companies' marketing efforts; also to the dim-wittedness (or is it plain moral corruption?) of those in the regulatory bodies and the specialist media who should have been properly scrutinising the companies' claims.

By the time the jig was up – in the mid to late 1980s – there were between 200,000 and 1.75 million licitly prescribed dependent users.[1] And benzos had also become a major item among the recreational set. The head of a South London street agency told me in 1993[2] that the most significant development of the past four years was the way the benzos – usually temazepam – had gone from a drug of little street repute to one that large numbers of her clients were chasing down in volumes of twenty, even sixty 20 mg capsules a day.

441

People, she said, 'were getting horribly strung out and very seriously dependent'.

The story elsewhere in the UK – Glasgow, Liverpool, the north-east – was comparable. As a cheap alternative to heroin or as a comedown from too much stimulant, temazepams were proving unbeatable. Major problems began when large amounts were taken together with other downers (central nervous system depressants), such as alcohol, heroin or methadone. The combination could pitch the user into a fatal coma.

Messy endings also came to some of those who injected temazepam capsules, especially the version containing a gel that was supposed to make the drug uninjectable. Abscesses turned to gangrene which often led to fingers, toes, or whole limbs being surgically amputated.

Thus, the benzodiazepine had, in the space of a few years, transformed itself from an innocuous substance of proven utility into a scourge that was responsible for the death and emasculation of large numbers of young people.

In this chapter I chart the part played in these developments by the manufacturers and the regulatory bodies, also by physicians, whose idiotically lax prescribing made possible the dual phenomenon of the licit and illicit benzo junkie.

Could anyone have guessed what was coming? Yes – anyone who'd bothered to examine the careers of benzodiazepines' chain of discredited predecessors, all of which had once been hailed as safe, effective and non-addictive. In order of appearance they were ethyl alcohol, chloral hydrate, paraldehyde, bromides, barbiturates, and methaqualone (brand names Quaaludes and Mandrax). The damage these drugs caused was known years before their distribution was controlled or banned, but such measures, as in the case of benzodiazepines themselves, were always delayed until the drug industry had a profitable new cure in the works.

As we'll see, there are now at least two strong candidates for that replacement role: buspirone and, more especially, Prozac. We're asked to believe that both are a beneficial and benign addition to the medical pharmacopeia . . . watch this space.

442

What are they?

The term tranquilliser is generally used to refer to a class of chemicals known as benzodiazepines, which are better known under brand names such as Librium, Valium, and Ativan. Their medically prescribed purpose is two-fold: to relieve daytime anxiety and/or to help insomniacs unwind at night so they can sleep.

The benzodiazepines are not the only kind of tranquilliser but they are the most popular in existence and still the most prescribed of all mood-altering agents. Nineteen million UK prescriptions were made out in 1991.

But first a little more on the terminology because it can be confusing. Two other words frequently crop up in relation to this class of drugs: *hypnotic* and *sedative*. The first is the term favoured by physicians to describe the sleep-inducing effects of the benzodiazepines. *Sedative*, though used in medical literature, is avoided by the pills' makers because it evokes memories of the drugs' predecessor -- the highly toxic barbiturates. To be 'tranquillised', the manufacturers believe, sounds less oppressively manipulative than to be 'sedated'.

Having got this far through the terminological thicket we must make another distinction between minor and major tranquillisers. Benzodiazepines are defined as minor tranquillisers, principally because the ailments they are set against are considered not especially severe. Major tranquillisers are used principally to manage severe forms of mental illness such as schizophrenia and mania. Important in this group is the compound chlorpromazine, marketed as Largactil. These majors are used to calm violent and hyperactive patients without, reputedly, any soporific action. But their nickname among inmates of prisons and mental institutions -- *liquid cosh* -- tells another story. It is because of the cosh effect that the majors have virtually no currency value among 'fun' users; at least, not at the time of writing.

So now we have isolated a class of drugs known chemically as the benzodiazepines and, because of their action, as minor tranquillisers. When administered at night they are further defined as hypnotics.

There are fifteen fairly well established benzodiazepine

derivatives being marketed at the time of writing, each one packaged under one or more brand names. While essentially the same in their chemical make-up, they are formulated in different potencies and to be effective over different time-spans – long- and short-acting. Long-acting benzos are the older drugs, such as Librium and Valium, which are more slowly metabolised (broken down by the body) and excreted. Their effects last up to twelve hours, which means that daytime use tends to lead to fatigue and, when taken as a sleeper, they produce a hangover the next day. Shorter-acting drugs were introduced to deal with these problems. More powerful but more rapidly secreted, they are designed to knock people asleep faster but without any grogginess upon waking. They are also given to people whose anxiety levels fluctuate and who are looking for a pill to dowse a sudden panic attack. The short-acting benzos have problems peculiar to themselves, not least a higher propensity to encourage dependence. See below.

Here is a list of commonly prescribed benzodiazepines.[3] Branded drug names – most of which are available officially only on private prescription – are given in brackets after the 'generic' title.

NAME	ACTION
alprazolam (Xanax)	Long
bromazepam (Lexotan)	Long
chlordiazepoxide (Tropium, Librium)	Long
clobazam (Clobazam, Frisium)	Long
clorazepate dipotassium (Tranxene)	Long
diazepam (Diazepam, Atensine, Tensium, Rimapam, Valium)	Long
flunitrazepam (Rohypnol)	Long
flurazepam (Dalmane)	Long
lorazepam (Lorazepam, Ativan)	Short
lormetazepam (Lormetazepam)	Short
medazepam (Nobrium)	Long
nitrazepam (Nitrazepam, Mogadon, Remnos, Unisomnia, Somnite)	Long
oxazepam (Oxazepam)	Short
temazepam (Temazepam, Normison)	Short

Sensations

The benzodiazepines produce feelings of tranquillity at low to moderate doses. They smother anxieties and relax muscular tension. They deliver 'Dutch courage' and, in street users, sometimes feelings of reckless invulnerability. A young Scottish woman told me she felt 'invisible' on the drug, and reports persist of users attempting to shoplift insanely large objects, believing no one can see them. At higher doses there will be drowsiness, a blurring of intellectual sharpness, wobbliness in the legs, and a decreased ability to perform mechanical tasks (for instance, driving suffers). Paradoxically, they can also release inhibitions so that people become talkative and over-excitable, prone to crazy mood swings and paranoid outbursts. Alcohol amplifies the effect (and greatly increases the risk of a fatal overdose) so that aggression is not uncommon – maybe borne out of the conviction that people all around are *deliberately misunderstanding me and trying to screw my head up*. Forgetfulness is part of the syndrome. The next day there might be no recollection of the night before's strange behaviour.

At higher dose levels, the simplest thing is to sleep. If this is resisted, brain performance becomes more and more erratic until stupor sets in. On awakening the size of the hangover will depend on the kind of benzodiazepine taken. Those classified as long-acting will still be chasing around the body, leading to sluggish limbs and a fat head.

Street names

Most of the slang terms active at the time of writing refer to the currently faddy product, the temazepam capsules. Because of their shape, they are known as *eggs, norries, rugby balls, jelly babies, goosies* or plain *temazzies*.

Typical patterns of use

The 'housewife junkie'

The state-authorised user is someone – twice as likely to be a woman – who receives a share of the millions of scripts written each year for dealing with insomnia, anxiety, the distress associated with menopause, the aftermath of a miscarriage or of a difficult childbirth. In 1991, 19 million prescriptions were made out; down from a 1979 peak of 31 million. Around one in four British adults have been prescribed this drug at one time or another[4] and a 1985 Mori poll found that 3.5 million individuals were using it habitually.

The trouble with tranquillisers is that, within a matter of days, they can stop working as intended; the insomniac once again has trouble sleeping and, during the daylight hours, the old anxieties return, together with additional horrors that are a feature of the drug itself. Some 'housewife users' up their dose or switch brands or top up on alcohol and other drugs in an ultimately futile effort to cope. More typically, long-term prescribed users subsist on an unchanging quantity that is no longer sufficient to alleviate withdrawal symptoms between each pill. In effect, they are constantly going in and out of withdrawal. Many endure this helter-skelter for years. Elderly users – and they account for around 70 per cent of the total number of benzodiazepine prescriptions[5] – have often been on the drugs for three or four decades. Theirs becomes the classic drug-centred existence more typically associated with heroin junkies.

Street users

Unauthorised use is a complex business with plenty of overlap between different scenes. But four fairly distinct categories of benzodiazepine user can be identified. At the time of writing temazepam was the clear street favourite, although Valium (once the preferred brand) was again beginning to figure more prominently.

The first user-category is the club habitué whose prime recreational buzz comes from stimulants and hallucinogens, such as amphetamine, cocaine, Ecstasy, and LSD. Benzodiazepines help bring them down and get them to sleep. In this role, it serves as an alternative to cannabis or booze.

446

The second is the more serious stimulant consumer who has been bingeing and used up his/her supplies. Again, temazepam will help bring them down, easing the crash.

The third is the heroin user whose cupboard is bare. Temazepam is not so much a substitute (it cannot directly alleviate heroin's withdrawal pangs) but a consolation. Those using the heroin substitute methadone also go for temazepam to enliven the meth experience.

The fourth group are those for whom temazepam is the drug of first choice, and since the late 1980s their numbers have been growing spectacularly in places like London, Scotland, and the north-east.

Beyond these four groups, we get into undefinable polydrug circles, where preferences are governed by availability and the demands of individual appetites. Combining stimulants with central nervous system depressants (downers) is as old as drug use itself. Where temazepam has proven to be particularly lethal is when it is taken with other depressants, notably alcohol and heroin – or heroin substitutes such as temgesic, methadone, and DF118s. Death from respiratory collapse – or from choking on vomit – is not unusual.

Injecting

That large numbers of street users would one day be jacking up these 'harmless' little pills was – we are asked to believe – contemplated by none of those responsible for making, licensing and dispensing them by the million.

Because of the format it came in (a capsule containing a liquid solution) temazepam was the first benzo to be injected illicitly on any scale. At the prompting of government, the manufacturers switched to a new gel formulation which was supposed to have rendered it abuse-proof. But while the new solution was uninjectable at room temperature, it could be heated to around 40°C and then pulled into a syringe. Big problems follow. Once inside the body the gel cools and solidifies, causing a high incidence of vein collapse and thrombosis (blood clots) which, in turn, lead to abscesses, gangrene, and loss of bits or of whole limbs. Hitting a vein can produce all these outcomes. Hitting an artery often requires major life-saving surgery.

Some temazepam injectors continued with the practice even when news of the damage the gel does was widely circulated. But the injection of any benzodiazepine in its pill form is also a messy business, given that they were not designed for that purpose. Impurities collect in the veins leading to some of the problems associated with the gel.

The sharing of injecting equipment (including spoons and filters) is no less a risk with benzodiazepines than with other drugs. The odds against a safe outcome can be said to be higher because the drug encourages forgetfulness and feelings of omnipotence in relation to the chances of picking up an infection.

Tolerance

Tolerance develops relatively easily to the anxiety-relieving and sleep-inducing properties of benzodiazepines – within three to fourteen days according to the standard medical and trade guide, the *British National Formulary*. This means the dose has to be steadily increased in order to maintain the desired effects. Without such an increase the pills/capsules become psychoactively useless. Even when the dose is repeatedly raised, a ceiling is reached beyond which no favourable response is possible. There is a high degree of cross-tolerance between benzodiazepines and other CNS depressants. This means that to recover the old sensitivity to the tranks, all other depressants must be cut out of the diet for several weeks. Conversely, using other CNS depressants on top of benzodiazepines amplifies the whole effect, with sometimes dire consequences.

Dependence

A person can be said to be dependent on a drug when tolerance has developed and when the pain of withdrawal overcomes the user when supplies are cut off. Another useful definition is that the person's drug consumption is drug-induced. The degree of dependence relates to how much is used and how often, as well as to the physical and mental make-up of the individual concerned. Not everyone who uses over a long period becomes dependent. It depends how they manage their habit.

The idea that benzodiazepines can produce physical and emotional dependence was resisted for years by the drugs' manufacturers and their handsomely paid 'independent' consultants. Yet as long ago as 1964, four years after the drugs' debut in America, the World Health Organisation warned that benzodiazepines caused the same kind of dependence as the now virtually blacklisted barbiturates.[6] The WHO document was ignored, as were one hundred other reports of dependence during the drugs' first fifteen years on the market. The strategy then – as today among many physicians – was to blame the patient: *They are 'addictive personalities', the symptoms that occur pre-date use of the drug and are not to be blamed on it.* The miseries endured during withdrawal are *simply a return of the symptoms for which the drug was prescribed in the first place.*

It was also argued that addiction reports were as nothing compared with the hundreds of millions of supposedly distress-free individuals worldwide who were regularly consuming the drugs. The bubble burst in 1979 following a US Senate Sub-Committee hearing that had been initiated by public demand. But it was not until 1988 that the UK's Committee on the Safety of Medicines (CSM) officially recognised the hidden addiction problem and issued new guidelines to prescribers. These say that the drug is 'indicated' for severe rather than mild anxiety and then only for a maximum of two to four weeks. In the case of insomnia, it should only be used where the problem is 'severe, disabling, or subjecting the individual to extreme distress'.

The pain of dependence and withdrawal

The sensations experienced during withdrawal from most mood-altering drugs are generally the exact opposite to those that were sought in the first place. Thus, whereas amphetamine withdrawal causes exhaustion and depression, and stopping long-term heroin use produces pain, the symptoms of benzodiazepine withdrawal include profound agitation and sleeplessness.

Such symptoms are invariably already present while regular use continues. That's because long-term consumers can rarely find a dose on which they can physically and emotionally stabilise themselves. When consumption does stop, the feelings of distress are amplified and some new symptoms often appear. Last-ditch defenders of benzodiazepine argue – as we've seen – that there is no withdrawal with the cessation of habitual pill use, merely a return of the old anxieties for which the drugs were originally prescribed. But research proves otherwise.[7] Symptoms not initially experienced manifest themselves, and there is the presence of a whole range of effects entirely untypical of anxiety states. They include hyper-sensitivity to sounds, light, and smells, and peculiar 'perceptual distortions' whereby floors and walls tilt and undulate. There is also what is known in the medical trade as 'formication' – a symptom familiar to dedicated users of amphetamine: what feel like insects trek up and down the skin and other 'bugs' infest the hair and scalp.

A typical journey from tranquillity to addiction and then withdrawal is as follows.[8] You feel anxious and fearful, maybe you can't sleep, so you start the pills, which instantly remedy the problem. Because they worked so miraculously, psychological attachment has already been forged. Things rub along nicely but gradually anxieties return, small problems become large, fears become terrors. The phone rings and you become breathless and panicky. You try to avoid using it. You have a panic attack while down the high street so you become fearful of going out alone in case it happens again, only with more catastrophic results. Your feelings have no source, they are inexplicable, especially to family and friends. You are now guilty about burdening others, as well as being enfeebled and agoraphobic (scared of open spaces).

Tensions develop with your partner; you split. Perhaps your fear of going out alone leads you to keep your child from school so that s/he can help with the shopping and other worldly chores. More guilt.

'The essence of tranquilliser suffering', says the Council for Involuntary Tranquilliser Addiction (CITA), 'is contained in one word: "fear". Life comes to consist of unexplained, irrational, uncontrollable fear. That fear is associated with a variety of physical symptoms: diarrhoea, irritable bowel syndrome, headaches, skin rashes, disturbed vision, queasy stomach, shaking and vague aches and pains.'[9]

Paradoxically, long-term use also leads to a muffling of the senses. The world is viewed through a veil. Normal emotional contact with friends and family is extinguished. It is this unresponsiveness which often kills relationships.

Protracted withdrawal symptoms

Experiences are personal but here are some relatively common symptoms which persist in the long term.[10]

Anxiety. This includes panic and agoraphobia. It's thought that use of the drug depresses people's ability to cope in stressful situations so that once it is withdrawn the person feels essentially helpless. Strategies for handling stress have to be relearnt.

Depression. This can be caused or aggravated by benzo-diazepine use and is also a feature of the withdrawal syndrome. It may be serious enough to qualify as a major depressive disorder for which doctors will often want to prescribe more drugs.

Tinnitus. This is ringing, whistling, and other noises in the ears. It comes and goes during drug use and also after withdrawal. It is thought to result from nerve-endings being hyper-sensitive to any kind of sensory stimulation. Usually resolves itself within a few weeks.

Pins and needles. The medical term is paresthesia. This can develop into burning sensations affecting fingers, feet, and legs.

The mechanism of addiction

While knowledge of how the brain works is still primitive, a theory has emerged as to how benzodiazepines might exert their malign effects during long-term use and subsequent withdrawal. The Council for Voluntary Addiction pulled the strands together for a booklet published in 1988.[11] It goes like this:

451

Sensory 'information' is carried through the nervous system by chemical messengers. The information is picked up by tiny receptors each of which recognises a particular type of message. Benzodiazepines block some of these receptors and possibly damage them, preventing information from getting through. The reason people initially feel on top of things when taking the drug is because it succeeds in blunting life's hard corners.

As drug use continues the receptors, including the damaged ones, fight to release the drug's blocking effect and, in so doing, become abnormally sensitive to stimuli. Hence the emotionally discordant responses to life's nine-to-five travails. When drug use stops and the receptors are suddenly freed, they drown under the incoming flood of information: sensory overload.

Physical symptoms/damage

The brain

Efforts have been made to test for structural brain damage, such as shrinkage of the layer of nerve cells on the surface (the cerebral cortex), but have so far drawn a blank. This could be because the tests are not sufficiently sensitive.[12] At least one leading benzodiazepine watcher feels that long-lasting withdrawal symptoms such as tinnitus could signal structural nerve damage caused by the drug.[13]

Other physical problems

The standard medical trade textbook, the *British National Formulary* (BNF), warns against prescribing benzodiazepine sleeping pills for elderly people because they make them confused, unsteady on their feet, and therefore prone to falls. Despite the advice, there were more than a million elderly consumers of these tablets in the early 1990s.

The BNF points to a range of other physical ailments associated with benzodiazepines. These include headache, disorders of the bowel and stomach, rashes, jaundice, blood disorders, and retention of urine. CITA report additional problems, including a worsening of arthritis, double vision, and sinus discomfort caused by inflamed mucous membranes. Pre-menstrual tension can be made worse and cystitis might be a problem during withdrawal, as might enlargement of the prostate gland – an important part of the male reproductive package situated immediately below the urinary bladder.

With other conditions

The BNF cautions against issuing these drugs where there is respiratory disease, muscle weakness, liver or kidney ailments, 'marked personality disorder', and to women who are pregnant or breast feeding. (Other reports show that babies born to regular users of benzodiazepines may experience withdrawal symptoms after their supply – through their mother's placenta – is cut off.) A stronger BNF warning relates to people with breathing difficulties or who are suffering various mental disorders such as phobias and obsessional states.

With other drugs

Benzodiazepines can interfere with the functioning of various drugs, such as those for epilepsy and bacterial infections. Check with your doctor – or get a copy of the BNF. An established hazard has been their use with other central nervous system depressants such as alcohol, heroin, and methadone. Each depresses breathing and other vital functions. Their combined effects are more than the sum of the parts and can prove fatal.

History

The great benzodiazepine glut dates back to 1960 when the Swiss multinational Hoffman–La Roche released Librium (chlordiazepoxide) on to the market following tests on mice, cats, various zoo-captive animals (including some 'vicious, agitated monkeys and dingo dogs'), and, for the clincher, a lion who was filmed co-existing peacefully with a lamb.[14]

Although chemically novel in many respects, the paren compound from which chlordiazepoxide was derived also gave birth to the *liquid cosh* major tranquillisers such as Largactil. The majority of early reports on the new drug looked good. Trials involving 800 doctors and some 16,000 patients demonstrated a sometimes 'miraculous' capacity to liberate hitherto strained and withdrawn individuals.

But already the process of gloss and wishful thinking was under way. As Charles Medawar reports, in his book *Power and Dependence*, those first trials failed to compare chlordiazepoxide with anything else – another drug or a placebo. And none was conducted 'blind', so investigators as well as patients knew they were testing an exciting new drug.

Warnings ignored

An early discordant note was struck by a California researcher Dr Leo Hollister of the Pala Alto Veterans Administration Hospital. In a series of punishing human trials, Hollister produced marked withdrawal reactions in ten out of eleven psychiatric patients who'd been treated with 'monumental doses' of Librium for between two and six months and then abruptly withdrawn. Two of the group suffered seizures.

The Hollister experiment was considered irrelevant to the general pattern of therapeutic prescribing and the band marched on, with early trade journal ads for the drug sometimes idiotically self-glorying. One showed a male hand feeling a female pulse together with the legend: 'Whatever the diagnosis . . . Librium'.

Three years after Librium's introduction the same company issued, with another bellow of pride, the more powerful Valium (diazepam). This was allegedly safer, it went to work quicker and in a more precise way on the central nervous system, and – best of all – the margin between the therapeutic dose and the one that killed was almost incalculably huge. But once again Hollister found addiction potential, this time using lower doses for a shorter period. Thirteen of his patients were given no more than twice the maximum dose of diazepam for six weeks before the drug was withdrawn. Six showed withdrawal reactions and one of these experienced a major seizure.

The findings were again buried under a welter of more favourable data, as was a 1964 World Health Organisation report that identified chlordiazepoxide as one of a range of drugs capable of producing 'dependence of the barbiturate type'. The newer product, diazepam, wasn't fingered by WHO, but only because they hadn't yet got round to scrutinising it. But by the mid-1960s there was good reason to think that any benzodiazepine would be liable to cause barb-type dependence.[15]

They hit the street

It was the barbiturates, together with amphetamines, which were the big worry in early-1960s America, and specifically the volumes that were washing out of surgeries and pharmaceutical warehouses on to the street. According to the Food & Drug Administration, approximately half the 9,000 million capsules and pills manufactured annually were being diverted to illegal use.[16] The response, in 1965, was new regulations requiring that the trade in all such products be properly documented, with clear record-keeping all down the line. A year later a US public inquiry recommended similar controls for benzos but Roche successfully resisted, making clear that it resented 'the libel of comparing Librium and Valium with the barbiturates'.[17]

Roche introduced a third product – Mogadon (nitrazepam) – promoting it exclusively for insomnia, even though sleep studies were providing increasingly good evidence as to the critical limitations of all so-called 'hypnotics'. The brands proliferated. Other companies entered the field. The scramble for market share got rougher. Roche found themselves under investigation by the UK Monopolies Commission, which was troubled by a pricing policy – made possible by the company's dominant market position – that for some years had 'produced profits on a very large scale'. There was also the suggestion that an inordinately large amount of UK income was being absorbed by the group operation to cover 'research and central administration' costs, thereby depriving the Inland Revenue of its statutory cut.

More troublingly, Roche had been supplying British hospitals with free Valium and Librium, which not only blocked competition but helped numerous patients on the road to habitual use. This stopped after the Monopolies Commission inquiry got under way. But the company was less pliant in other respects. The MC's final report called for a repayment to the government together with substantial price cuts. Roche made the reductions but fought the compensation order. In an out-of-court settlement it drove the amount down from £12 million to £3.75 million.

The bad news continued trickling in. A Belgian consultant psychiatrist reported in 1972 that two of his patients suffered convulsions after withdrawing from lorazepam (brand name Ativan; made by Wyeth), but the benzos continued to pour forth so that by the mid-1970s, in the UK alone, annual 'prescriptions were approaching 30 million. Most patients were on 'repeats' – the script being signed by the GP's receptionist with patient and doctor not seeing each other for months, even years. A 1980 survey revealed that some three-quarters of all mood-altering drugs were prescribed this way.[18]

The tide turns in the US

But America, at least, was beginning to rouse itself. Public pressure forced a Senate sub-committee hearing, headed by Ted Kennedy. Among the 500 pages of evidence was a 1979 Roche internal memo in which the US company's chairman acknowledged that Roche had neither conducted nor supported any studies on dependence or long-term effects of diazepam.[19]

Around the same time came an important review by the US Institute of Medicine which found that benzodiazepines when used by insomniacs 'appeared to lose their sleep-promoting properties within 3 to 14 days of continuous use.' The only exception seemed to be flurazepam, and that only worked for up to twenty-eight days. Back in the UK, the Committee on Review of Medicines (CRM) endorsed the IMO's findings, adding an additional warning for elderly users, in whom the drug more easily accumulated. But the CRM report went on to perform a serious pratfall: the number of individuals who developed dependence on benzos between 1960 and 1977, it declared, totalled all of twenty-eight. The figure had been arrived at by counting the number of adverse reaction Yellow Cards returned by prescribers to the Committee on Safety of

Medicines – which is like calculating how many people speed on motorways by the number of drivers who walk into police stations and confess their crime. Complacency, ignorance, idleness and guilt all contribute to the failure, then as now, of the Yellow Card scheme, and if the CRM didn't know this, then it should have been looking for other work.

Changes were recommended to the company data sheets that went out with the drug to doctors. Modest though these recommendations were, lack of cooperation from the manufacturers meant that it took five years for most of the alterations to be made.

A step forward in 1981 was a reconstituted *British National Formulary* (BNF), the guide to prescribed drugs jointly produced by the British Medical Association and the Pharmaceutical Society of Great Britain. Some sound information and warnings were communicated, but it took many more years for most doctors to lock on to the central message that tranks do nothing for patients in the long term except cause addiction and make them sicker than when they started.

Self-help

The public were quicker on the uptake and, ultimately, turned to each other for support. The first self-help group, called Tranx, was established by a recovering addict, Joan Jerome. I met seventeen of its members at a November 1984 meeting in Wealdstone, Middlesex. There were nine men and eight women present, in various states of pain and recovery. Among them was a young man who worked as a dance-hall bouncer; a grey-faced, middle-aged couple who came to Valium via a booze habit; a grey-haired woman who looked the sort they put on the front of cake-mix packets; a thin, blank-looking man alone at the back reading the *Financial Times*; a young woman who, in the middle of describing her unhappiness, became engulfed in tears and had to be led upstairs; and a dapper business executive who'd been using for twenty years and was there, he said, not because they'd caused him problems – far from it, he felt great – but because he'd heard about Tranx on the radio and thought he might as well drop in. The idea of quitting appealed to him.

'Do you get cold sweats?' a man asked a woman.

'No, I get hot flushes,' she answered to a peal of laughter.

457

Others got numb, wobbly mouths and panic attacks; or agoraphobia, feelings of unreality, floors shifting beneath their feet, and weird noises and lights. Tips for recovery were exchanged: avoid substituting alcohol for tranks ('the booze is a wet version of the pills') and remember that recovery means eating healthily and keeping busy . . .

By now the dam of public disfavour was about to burst. Media horror stories proliferated. A MORI poll suggested that about 3.5 million adults in the UK had taken the drugs for more than four months. Medical experts, such as GP-turned-campaigning-writer Dr Vernon Coleman, piled on the pressure. Sales of the benzodiazepines peaked and began to decline. When a decisive move was made against the drug companies it was, as always, with a view to the Exchequer's rather than the public's health. In November 1984 the Department of Health announced than it was fed up with the kind of unfettered 'clinical freedom' that allowed GPs to prescribe through the NHS whatever costly, useless, dangerous product drug company reps could swing them over to. A Limited List was introduced which excluded about 18,000 branded preparations, most of which were an essentially redundant assortment of cough syrups, antacids, and the like. The most controversial element concerned the seventeen benzodiazepines that were available through the Health Service. The government wanted only three on tap to NHS patients – diazepam, nitrazepam, and temazepam. The rest of the sizzling range would remain available but without a subsidy paid for by the taxpayer. Opponents read the move as yet another kick at the poor by the Tory government of Margaret Thatcher, an interpretation the industry was pleased to encourage through a £250,000 advertising campaign. The Labour Party, together with the British Medical Association, whined in tune with the drug companies and, within a year, a compromise was reached. Nine rather than three benzodiazepines would be available on the NHS.

A couple of years later, against the background of a growing media clamour, another squeeze was put on the benzos. They were controlled under the Misuse of Drugs Act. Then, in 1988, the Committee on Safety of Medicines at last broke its vow of silence by issuing guidelines to prescribers. The drugs were suitable only for short-term use (two to four weeks) in cases of severe disabling anxiety and, where insomnia was concerned, only when it was 'severe, disabling or subjecting the individual to extreme distress.'

Court action

In that same year, the benzos became the subject of what would turn out to be the biggest personal injury claim ever brought before the British courts when the first of 17,000 people came forward identifying themselves as victims of the drug. Neither the companies that made and marketed the drugs nor the doctors who prescribed them, they complained, offered a proper warning as to their addiction potential. The claimants joined with over 2,000 firms of solicitors, forty barristers, and dozens of psychiatrists. More than 13,000 of the alleged victims were granted legal aid.[20]

But in 1993, the legal aid was abruptly withdrawn for the claims relating to the Roche products – Valium, Mogadon, and Librium. And a year later, already facing a bill of between £25 and £30 million for the work so far done, the Legal Aid Board jettisoned 1,200 claims relating to Ativan. The board feared that the costs involved in yet more years of legal wrangling and then the lengthy trial itself would dwarf any damages that might ultimately be awarded. The chances of a British court finding a pharmaceutical company liable for injuries were, in any case, remote. It had never happened before for any class of drugs – the few cash awards to date all having been settled out of court.

An additional problem was that, unlike their US counterparts, British courts fail to recognise a 'group action', whereby people with a common complaint pool their resources and make a joint argument. In treating them as a collection of individual claims, the process becomes unbearably laborious as well as expensive.

All that remained after the Board had shed its load were a few hundred claims over Halcion (triazolam), a product that already had an exotic history. Once the world's best-selling sleeping pill because of its ultra-short half-life (the time taken for it to do its business and then vacate the body), it had long been associated with a high incidence of side effects such as memory loss, confusion, agitation, hallucinations, and bizarre behaviour.[21] The CSM investigated in 1989 but

took no action. Two years later came the most dramatic o
a series of court cases in which it was stated that the dru
provoked awesome violence. A Utah woman, Ilo Grundberg
claimed Upjohn's product had caused her to fire eight bullet
into the head of her eighty-three-year-old mother, a lapse fo
which she was now facing a charge of second-degree murder
Upjohn paid her a reputed $6 million in an out-of-court settle
ment – this after psychiatrists had argued that Ms Grundberg
had been 'involuntarily intoxicated'. As a result, the murde
charges were dropped.

It was during the Grundberg trial that Upjohn document
came to light revealing that reports of early clinical trials o
the drug had left out important details of adverse effects
The company blamed the omission on a 'transcription error'
but the growing anti-Halcion sentiment was sufficient t
prompt the CSM to suspend the drug's licence. 'If the
information had been presented completely and correctly,
the CSM apparently told Upjohn, 'it is highly unlikely that the
committee would have been able to recommend the grant o
a product licence.'[22]

Other countries followed the UK ban, although some late
retracted and the US never did join in the boycott. At the
time of writing, a lobby is growing in the UK, bolstered by
various heavyweight medics, to allow the product back on
the market. Upjohn, meanwhile, is taking on its most severe
critics by issuing writs for libel.

Though there will always be people eager to damage
themselves whatever rules are made to protect them, the
conduct of the UK regulatory authorities throughout the
thirty-five-year history of the benzodiazepines has been
marked by feeble-hearted, feeble-minded inaction. The evi
dence was there for years that hundreds of thousands o
individuals, most of them ignorant of the drug's pharmacology
and therefore reliant on the medical 'experts', were being
further damaged rather than cured of the anxieties they
imagined the tablets would magic away. Those who were
ready to fight for recompense were denied their day in
court, and the larger number who now look to the state for
support as they endure the protracted agonies of withdrawa
and rehabilitation find there is little in the way of services,
and those that do exist are dangerously cash-starved. The
problem for the 'housewife junkies' is that they lack the bite

of other drug-using constituencies. They seem to harm no one but themselves, to commit no crimes of violence or harbour anything in the way of incurable diseases.

The same is not uniformly true of the street users of tranks. Valium was the first to make it in recreational circles. But by 1987, in accordance with prescribing fads among GPs, temazepam was the top choice. Reports from as far afield as Plymouth and Glasgow suggested that the drugs were producing problems familiar from the barbiturate era of the late 1970s. Injecting was commonplace and, as with barbs, heavily dosed individuals were exhibiting both violence and severe withdrawal symptoms. While the drug was frequently used as an accompaniment to alcohol or as a substitute for opioids, for many it was the drug of first choice.

The problems of injecting are described elsewhere in this chapter, as is the risk of fatal overdose when the drug is combined with one or more other central nervous system depressants. In Glasgow between January 1992 and November 1993 at least 112 drug injectors died.[23] They perished in public toilets, on waste ground, at home with young children clinging to them. Temazepam, heroin, and the synthetic narcotic temgesic were – in one combination or another – invariably the lethal ingredients.

Glasgow lives

Glasgow is an instructive case, especially when compared with events forty-four miles to the east in Edinburgh. Glasgow, the insular town, more pervasively gloomy and run-down than its neighbour, looked on with bemused complacency as the capital went through an AIDS trauma in the late 1980s, landing itself with the soubriquet *HIV black spot of Europe*. But thanks to an adept voluntary street sector, a drugs treatment package was put in place which, after some resistance, included not only clean needles and syringes but the heroin substitute methadone. By mid-1993, the numbers were looking good. Overdose deaths were less than a quarter of those in Glasgow, and while there was no large-scale abandonment of drug use, one survey showed that three-quarters of injectors had eschewed the needle during the past six months. As a result, the HIV epidemic was being contained and crime was down 8 per cent in a year, almost certainly because methadone scripts had reduced the need to steal in order to make a score.

Glasgow – for reasons that are disputed (a more static population; plain luck?) – missed out on the kind of HIV infection rates seen in Edinburgh. That's despite having developed a pool of injecting users which, by 1993, had swollen to around 10,000 individuals.[24] The response to the injecting phenomenon by the drug treatment agencies was inflexible and heavily bureaucratised. Methadone was resisted as a matter of policy (prescribing it would have amounted to an explicit recognition that there was a major heroin problem which needed to be catered for). More by accident than design a heroin-substitute prescribing policy grew up around temazepam and temgesic, two drugs that were morally neutral compared with either heroin itself or methadone. Dependent heroin users who couldn't coax a benzodiazepine script out of their often ill-informed and always isolated GPs might seek to persuade a respectable-looking relative to call on the doctor with a bogus complaint about some vague pain or other and then hand over the bounty – an act of filial love and support. In this way the streets became awash with *tems* and *temazzies*, and Glasgow won a reputation to rival that of the AIDS city to its east: *the overdose capital of Europe*.

In March 1994, a decade after visiting the city to research the first edition of this book, I returned for a reassessment. The stone heart of the town centre looked as formidably austere as ever, the black metal statues of warriors and inventors gazing out from George Square with imperturbable self-confidence. There were some smart new clubs and deli shops. But in the neglected parts, such as Possilpark, or the giant housing estates on the city's periphery, my overwhelming impression was of a lugubrious, semi-defeated populace, many of whom (who can know how many?) had turned to heroin, sedatives and other downers to mask their defeat. These were the terms the people themselves often spoke in. I'd heard it a decade before and I was hearing it said again, only more insistently.

Possilpark, just a few minutes from the centre, is a complex of low-rise, yellowstone tenement blocks dating from the 1930s and 1940s. Once there was work, building and repairing railway coaches. Lots of it. That ended fifteen to twenty years ago and, these days, if you say *Possilpark* to a Glaswegian he's likely to wince and tell you what a sordid junkie hellhole it is. The people of Possil are no worse or better than those you'll find in any other place, but the vicinity is depressed. I visited a bar that was huge and empty like a urinal. A second one was narrow, crowded with men chain-smoking: racing was on the TV. Young male drug dealers stood plying their trade in shop doorways. Many of the tenements were crumbling and boarded-up. On waste ground garbage and rubble were piled high. I visited a new drug rehabilitation project, called PARC, and discussed temazepam and many other things with several of its clients as well as members of the young, committed staff. Temazepam, according to a veteran of the scene, came along about nine years ago, about the same time as temgesics. The media fuss had made it more difficult to screw a script out of GPs and now the main source was pharmacy robberies or by doing a deal with the genuinely prescribed. The press had recently found a new scapegoat – the old-age pensioner pusher who, motivated by greed and malice, was selling off his script to young junkies. The *Evening Times* found an exemplar of the 'vile' trade in cloth-capped Mick the Fix, who, looking bleary-eyed and nonplussed, was featured on its front page. At the PARC I heard that it was actually a quid pro quo arrangement these OAP dealers were engaged in: pills for booze or for cash, to make up a shortfall.

One of the temazepam aficionados at PARC was twenty-three-year-old Joe, who'd been 'jagging' (injecting) the stuff together with other items since he was eighteen. Using the needle, he said, gets you to that 'comfortably numb' place quicker.

The appeal for Diana was that it left you 'oozing with confidence. No one can touch you, it's like you're invisible.' But she recognised, in retrospect (at PARC everyone was trying to remain straight), that her drugs got her on to stealing, conning, cheating, and lying.

Tam, forty-three-years-old, a sweet, nervous man who's been round half a dozen times on life's big dipper, didn't personally use temazepam but plenty of users of his acquaintance 'became awfully aggressive . . . folk who were normally nice and placid, people you'd never see in a temper.'

'If you're on heroin,' said Dorothy, a senior staff member,

'you stand a better chance of staying clean. Temazepam users lapse that much more when trying to come off because some of the side effects are so terrifying – convulsions, hallucinations like you get with the DTs. You see a lot of it in prison where they don't have a chance to detox slowly. You see them fitting [convulsing], and getting really badly paranoid.'

The drug, she said, was particularly popular among the city's three or four hundred 'sex workers', a couple of dozen of whom operated in the city centre. For those of them who had children, it was a more secure occupation than stealing. Temazzies helped them get on with the job and it was not unusual, said Dorothy, for forty capsules to be chucked down in a day, each of them with a shell coating that, in such quantities, tore and burnt the stomach lining.

Twenty-five pounds was the going rate for straight sex, cheaper on the estates where the service providers were often in their young teens. Dorothy's own sister had been drawn into the life. Pregnant at fourteen and now, aged nineteen, with three children to raise, she tried waitressing for a while before slipping into a life of booze, heroin, temazepam, and prostitution. 'She's got a *what's the point* attitude,' says Dorothy; a frame of mind that's not altogether unusual. But Big Sister's not inclined to judge her, not publicly anyway. She counts herself lucky to have escaped slipping down the chute herself. Social services removed her from her trouble-addicted family when she was eleven and later put her in the keep of her old-fashioned granny, with her front and back garden and old-fashioned ways.

Drugs, in places like the Possil or the Easterhouse estate, can seem romantic and full of absorbing ritual. They are a diversion, a currency, and an excuse for failing to hack it in (perennially) uncomfortable times.

For all the miseries of habitual drug use, the biggest hurdle many of them face after they've passed through detoxification and withdrawal is, as Dorothy puts it, 'the utter boredom of being straight. "I'm straight, they'll say, what next?"'

Withdrawal Tips

Dependence generally builds more rapidly with the shorter-acting benzodiazepines and the advice is to switch to the long-acting type, as these are less traumatic to withdraw from. Withdrawal, in any case, should never be attempted abruptly because this can cause convulsions and other extreme reactions. Better to adjust the dose downwards in stages, over a period of weeks or even months.

The Campaign for Involuntary Tranquilliser Addicts offers detailed advice on how to come down and strategies to make the journey less painful – e.g. yoga, relaxation, physical exercise, and a sound diet that is free of (or low on) sugar, fats, stimulants (coffee, tea), and other junk items.

There is an immediate post-withdrawal crisis period lasting, perhaps, a few weeks. The lingering symptoms can go on for months or even years, though diminishing all the while (notwithstanding the odd setback). See above for details.

Watch consumption of alcohol and other drugs, both during and after withdrawal. Intake often goes up to compensate for the trank deprivation. In fact, users frequently step up alcohol consumption *prior* to withdrawal in order to juice up the drug's flagging effect.

Keep occupied, even with mundane chores. Don't dwell too much on personal misery and resist the desire to crawl back under the sheets. Tell family and friends what you're going through so that they can begin to understand the process and adapt to the changing you.

Remember that it takes time, so try to dispense with guilt over your rate of progress.

Buspirone

Benzodiazepines have been magnificently profitable for drug companies such as Roche these past several decades, which is why the in-house stress levels induced by the growing public disquiet can only be guessed at – especially because the task of finding a substitute that could even half credibly be presented as a 'safe, non-addictive' replacement has proven exceptionally difficult. A heroic effort has come from Bristol–Myers, who in March 1988 launched a novel chemical entity called buspirone (brand name Buspa), which was 320 times more expensive than diazepam.[25] Originally developed as a treatment for schizophrenia, its alleged anti-anxiety properties were discovered in the early 1970s when it was forced on laboratory monkeys. It has no cross-tolerance with benzodiazepines, which means it cannot be used to relieve the withdrawal symptoms of benzos, and it is said to produce no 'rebound' effects when use is stopped, or problems of dependency.

The data sheet made available in Britain lists various side effects including dizziness, nausea, headaches, nervousness, insomnia, light-headedness, and excitement. These symptoms have affected between 12 and 33 per cent of those participating in clinical trials. However, the US data sheet specified several reactions missing from the British list. Among them are claustrophobia, stupor, slurred speech, photosensitivity, pressure on the eye, and psychosis. The US sheet also warned that 'its central nervous system effects on any individual patient may not be predictable.' Manufacturers Bristol–Myers baulked at the suggestion that they were being miserly with their data. The decision about what goes on the British sheet, they said, is that of the Committee on Safety of Medicines. Nonetheless, at the 1988 British launch, Charles Medawar, director of the drugs industry watchdog Social Audit, asked the obvious question: 'How can we be sure this is not going to become another scandal like Opren or involuntary tranquilliser addiction?'[26]

But, incredibly, among Medawar's antagonists was Professor Malcolm Lader, a man who did much to bring the problems of benzodiazepine before the public but who was now lending his support to Bristol–Myers and buspirone.

'This drug will certainly expand the options available to practitioners in the treatment of anxiety,' he said at the launch. Trials for dependency, he noted, had been satisfactory and patients taken off the drugs had shown no 'rebound anxiety . . . If we are making a mistake, we are making a new mistake.'[27] No, Professor Lader, the same old mistake wearing a different hat.

Since the launch, Buspa-loyalists have stuck to the line

that the drug presents virtually no dependence hazard and that its side effects are modest and rare. 'The search for the ideal anxiolytic [anti-anxiety drug] has been a long one,' noted one American celebrant.[28] 'The azapirones in general, and buspirone specifically, represent a major advance in this search. Buspirone is the first anxiolytic drug that is simultaneously effective, safe for clinical use, and free of the liability for abuse or addiction.'

But, inevitably, there then followed the medical journal reports of buspirone-induced mania, cravings, users who were wildly escalating their intake, and withdrawal symptoms, including 'severe anxiety'.[29]

So far these reports are few in number and are invariably associated with people with prior histories of mental illness and/or liberal drug-taking. But this is a large category. Additionally, history teaches us that it can take literally decades (as in the case of barbiturates) for a drug's addiction potential and its poor performance to be properly recognised. This is because physicians invariably attribute untoward symptoms to a failure in the patient. Buspirone seems much like its predecessors in this regard, and although Lader continues to put up a valiant if cautious defence ('. . . on present evidence, the short-term use of buspirone is unlikely to be followed by rebound or long-term use through dependence; nor is abuse likely to be a problem . . .') we did find him asserting, in a 1988 medical paper, that 'high dose sporadic abuse of benzodiazepines usually for recreational purposes is not common . . .' This was precisely at the point when the current epidemic of street use was taking off.

Will buspirone become a big deal among the recreational set? When surveyed, most users describe the drug as boring, one they're unlikely to reach for if alternatives are around. But while, by the autumn of 1994, there was no evidence of major business through illicit channels, the picture is not unalterable. Benzos themselves took some twenty years before achieving mass street appeal. Factors that could trigger a buspirone fad include the following: shortages of other substances; and the discovery of more interesting methods of administration (i.e. taking handfuls of pills at once, perhaps together with other drugs, or use through a needle).

Prozac

If Bristol–Myers could manage one-fiftieth of the frothy media coverage attending Prozac they'd be in corporate nirvana. Prozac (chemical name fluoxetine; made by American drug company Eli Lilly) took fifteen years to develop and, aided by a best-selling book by Rhode Island psychiatrist Dr Peter Kramer called *Listening to Prozac* (Fourth Estate), has become the pharmaceutical star turn of the last twenty years. It has spawned several TV specials, radio talk shows, any number of major magazine articles, together with some not very stringent analysis from the medical-scientific fraternity. In headline-speak the drug is *bottled sunshine . . . an escape capsule . . . the happy drug.* This very 1990s product is, above all, being sold as a balm for the frazzled professional classes. It is said to help them become skinny and young-looking, to transform their lacklustre, nervy personalities into something evincing of faith and confidence. Most significantly, it is said to be able to change – at the root – a personality, rather than merely mask problems. Kramer, a freelance Prozac adept, has called the process 'cosmetic psychopharmacology', an alluring claim based on controlled trials by Eli Lilly lasting only a few weeks, while Kramer's own book rests principally on anecdotes detailing the experience of about a dozen of his patients. There has been no systematic study of the drug's potential for abuse, tolerance, or physical dependence.[30]

Prozac was introduced in December 1987 and, by 1992, had already been swallowed by more than 11 million people, half of them in the US, and around 500,000 in the UK.

The limited trials so far undertaken suggest it's no more or less effective than other types of anti-depressants that have been around for thirty years. But it is believed to be safer than its predecessors: the tricyclics and the monoamine oxidase inhibitors (MAOIs) The first sort can cause low blood pressure, heart disturbances, weight gain, tremors, blood sugar changes, and more. The MAOIs can be lethal in combination with many common foods such as aged cheese, wine, beer, pickled herrings, and beef extracts. Both types are reported to cause dependence,[31] despite insistent claims to the contrary by leading medical authorities. The common side effects of Prozac are, according to the current consensus, 'milder' but still none too appealing. The list given in the March 1994 *British National Formulary* includes nausea, vomiting, diarrhoea, anorexia, headache, nervousness, insomnia, anxiety, tremor, sexual dysfunction, vaginal bleeding on withdrawal, violent behaviour, and hair loss. (For 'sexual dysfunction' read failure to reach orgasm – a not inconsiderable price to pay for chemical bliss.)

In pre-marketing trials, one in seven patients had to quit because of adverse effects, most commonly of a psychiatric nature.[32] Social Audit's Charles Medawar has commented: 'The broad spectrum of these unwanted symptoms is worrying, with some people becoming badly agitated and hyped up and others brought right down; in extreme cases, manic psychoses and suicides have been mentioned as real risks [and have formed the basis of law suits against the drug's makers]. In a mass market there will certainly be many casualties and much more could be done to prevent them.'[33]

Prozac is not only 'broad-based' in its negative side effects but multifarious in the desired impact it is reported to have on users – being able to tackle everything from depressive disorders to bulimia and obesity.

This non-specificity is deeply ironic given that Prozac was specifically designed to be focused in its pharmacological effects. Its mission was to boost levels of a brain chemical known as serotonin, which is believed to be involved in regulating emotional behaviour, sleep, appetite, and sex. The older anti-depressants – the tricyclics and MAOs – also seemed to boost serotonin levels, but they also lashed out at other nervous system chemicals. Hence the multiplicity of side effects.

But even if Prozac is able to hit the serotonin button, can depression really be tied to a single brain chemical? Only in the sterile, reductionist, profit-seeking world of pharmaceutical research. Even loyalist journals like *New Scientist* are forced to acknowledge that, despite the flatulent boasts, neuroscience functions in a state of pervasive ignorance. Information-processing in the brain, noted a March 1994 article in the *NS*, depends on 'upwards of two dozen neurotransmitters interacting with scores if not hundreds of molecular receptors'. While research into this area 'is blossoming like never before, neuroscience remains almost totally ignorant about how neurotransmitters and networks of neurons [nerve cells] act together in the brain to produce complex mental states such as depression or anxiety.'[34] The 'answer', the article postulates, might actually lie with an altogether different class of body chemicals.

Prozac, the wonder drug, is already being prescribed for patients who are moderately miserable, especially in the US, where the natural human condition of unhappiness is seen by the pampered classes as intolerable. The habit there is to assign each species of discontent a new medical name, a trend that is likely to continue. The next two decades, according to the aforementioned NS article, 'will see a gradual expansion of psychiatric categories into the realms of normality as psychiatrists and pharmaceutical companies indulge their habit of defining as abnormal anything that responds to drug treatment.'

In other words, Prozac is the first in an inevitable torrent of purpose-built, specially targeted 'smart drugs' which will aspire to greater than ever safety and efficacy but will more accurately reflect the ignorance and ambitions that lay behind their development.

Even if we discount the more lurid accusations against Prozac – that it has precipitated suicide, self-mutilation, and mass murders – there still remains a mass of user testimonies declaring that the drug 'takes the edge off life' . . . numbs the emotions . . . messes up the sex life . . . creates paranoia and anxiety.

That it has addiction potential – despite the official line – will, I'd hazard a guess, be clearly demonstrated a few billion tabs down the line. 'Oh God, I'm like a total basket case when I'm off Prozac,' one user told the *Independent on Sunday* (30 January 1994). 'Hysterical, crying all the time. An absolute nightmare. On Prozac, I can deal, you know, get through the day, generally behave like a normal person. Prozac is, like, Mother's Humungous Helper.'

Perhaps the most ludicrous aspect of the Prozac debate is that those pundits who do have a niggling worry tend to talk in terms of the drug working *too well*, i.e. that it is so good at contenting the discontented that everyone will want to take it, and that way we'll all end up far too much like each other: the Huxleyite nightmare of uniform waves of hatched humanity. History shows that medical science is simply not that competent; science is more often dangerously inept than

470

excessively efficient. Nor is it disposed, logistically or morally, to finding such 'solutions'. Its major concerns are product marketing and the enhancement of personal reputations.

And so Prozac rather than buspirone will probably take the baton from the benzodiazepines. Although Prozac is classed as an anti-depressant rather than as an anxiolytic, the trend in recent times has been for anxiety to be redefined in the medical literature as depression. This paves the way, says the mental health charity Mind, 'for the apparently legitimate prescribing of antidepressant drugs for anxiety.'[35] Mind sees 'obvious benefits to the drug industry' in such a development, given that benzodiazepines are now supposed to be prescribed for no more than a few weeks whereas anti-depressants are given in courses lasting at least six months – with recommendations of indefinite prescribing for some elderly people.

We have, then, vast quantities of a heavily hyped miracle product circulating through licit channels. It is a near-certainty that a substantial proportion will reach the street where the innovative recreational user will discover innovative methods of administration (e.g. 30 pills or an armful at a time, alternated with coke, booze, etc.), and fall prey to all kinds of exotic ailments that the makers and regulatory authorities never believed could occur. In this way the Prozac miracle will be superseded by the Prozac nightmare, and those who have turned their faces from the history of lab-manufactured mind-altering drugs will wonder how it ever happened.

Notes

1 '"Minor" Tranquillisers: not such minor effects', Mind, London, February 1994, p. 3.
2 This was Lorraine Hewitt of the Stockwell Project.
3 Compiled from the *British National Formulary*, a joint publication of the British Medical Association and the Royal Pharmaceutical Society of Great Britain, No. 27, March 1994; *Back to Life: The Great Escape from Tranquilliser Addiction*, Pam Armstrong, The Council for Involuntary Tranquilliser Addiction, Liverpool; and from Mind, op. cit.
4 In Mind, op. cit.
5 Ibid, p. 4.
6 C. Medawar, *Power and Dependence, Social Audit on the safety of medicines*, Social Audit Ltd, 1992, p. 120. Medawar heads Social Audit, a highly effective monitoring group 'whose job is to ask timely questions about the organisations whose decisions and actions shape our lives'. Much of its best work has been done in the field of pharmaceuticals. *Power and Dependence* is a characteristically top-quality piece of work looking at benzodiazepines, their predecessor drugs, their likely successors, and associated shady politics and corporate manoeuvrings.
7 H. Ashton, 'Protracted withdrawal symptoms from benzodiazepines' in the *Journal of Substance Abuse Treatment*, Vol. 8, 1991, p. 20.
8 Drawn from, among other sources and contacts, Armstrong, op. cit.
9 Ibid, p. 12.
10 Drawn largely from Ashton, op. cit.
11 Armstrong, op. cit., p. 13.
12 Ashton, op. cit., p. 27.
13 Ibid, p. 27.
14 Medawar, op. cit., p. 82.
15 Ibid, p. 89.
16 Ibid, p. 91.
17 Ibid, p. 91.
18 R. N. Anderson, 'The use of repeatedly prescribed medicines', in the *Journal of the Royal College of General Practitioners*, October 1980, p. 609.
19 Medawar, op. cit., p. 136.
20 'Sad story of the happy pills', in the *Guardian*, tabloid section, 5 April 1994, p. 21.
21 Medawar, op. cit., p. 190.
22 Ibid, p. 194.
23 'Inquiry into city's heroin death toll', in the *Independent*, 2 November 1993, p. 4.

24 '"100 addicts" die in 14 months in Glasgow', in *Druglink*, ISDD, March 1993, p. 4.

25 *A Prescription for Improvement*, Audit Commission, HMSO, London, 1994, p. 30.

26 The *Observer*, 27 March 1988.

27 Ibid, 20 March 1988.

28 J. Steinberg, 'Anxiolytic Therapy and Addiction: Primary care concerns', in *International Medicine Certification*, Vol. 3, No. 2, September 1989.

29 Nicholas Rock, 'Possible adverse effects of Buspirone when used with other psychotropic drugs', *J. Clin. Psychopharmacol.*, Vol. 10, no. 5, October 1990, p. 380.

30 *Physicians' Desk Reference*, 4th edition, Medical Economics, Oradell, New Jersey, 1993, pp. 943–6.

31 The legal aid organisation Release are among a number of drug agencies who report anti-depressant users coming forward complaining of serious withdrawal symptoms when they tried to quit. The experience is much like that reported by people cutting out benzodiazepines: depression, shakiness, aches and pains brought on by tension. Despite this, doctors continue to insist (shades of benzodiazepines) that no such dependence/withdrawal syndrome exists.

32 C. Medawar, 'Through the doors of perception', in *Nature*, Vol. 368, 24 March 1994, p. 370.

33 Ibid.

34 D. Concar, 'Design you own personality', in *New Scientist*, 12 March 1994, pp. 22–6.

35 Mind, op. cit., p. 10.

APPENDIX I
DRUGS AND THE LAW

Misuse of Drugs Act

The Misuse of Drugs Act 1971 is the instrument by which the state prosecutes individuals for possession, supply or manufacture of 'controlled' substances. Consolidating numerous bits of legislation dating back to 1908, the MDA divides the substances into three categories of seriousness and awards penalties accordingly. It does not deal with those most ubiquitous of all recreational drugs – alcohol, tobacco and caffeine, nor does it incorporate amyl and butyl nitrite and, until Januay 1985, it also excluded barbiturates.

Class A

The materials drawing the most severe penalties are called Class A drugs. These include: cannabinol (except where contained in cannabis or cannabis resin), coca leaf, cocaine, dextromoramide (e.g. the product Palfium), diamorphine (heroin), dipipanone (Diconal), fentanyl and its derivatives, LSD, Ecstasy mescaline, methadone (Physeptone), morphine, opium, pethidine (Pamergan) and its derivatives, phencyclidine (PCP), poppy straw and concentrate of poppy straw (poppy straw means all parts except the seeds of the opium poppy after mowing. The advice agency Release notes that it is not an offence to possess, supply or produce a poppy straw, but it is one to smoke it. Concentrate of poppy straw means the material produced when the straw's alkaloids are concentrated. Possession, supply and production of this material *is* an offence), psilocin (as found in 'magic mushrooms'), n,n-dimethyltryptamine (DMT).

Class B

Class B drugs draw mid-range penalties. They include: amphetamine, barbiturates (e.g. Tuinal, Nembutal, Seconal, Soneryl, Amytal), cannabis and cannabis resin, codeine, dexamphetamine, dihydrocodeine (DF-118), methaqualone, methylamphetamine, methylphenidate (Ritalin), phenmet-razine (Filon). Class B drugs become Class A if prepared for injection.

Class C

Least severe category is Class C, which includes: Benzo-diazepine tranquillisers (e.g., Temazepaimg), dextropropo-xyphene (Distalgesic, Doloxene) plus other mild amphetamine-type stimulants.

Schedules

The MDA regulations divide controlled drugs into five 'sched-ules', relating to the handling of the substances by trade and professional people. Drugs in Schedule 1 (such as LSD and cannabis) are the most stringently controlled in that they can only be supplied, possessed or administered in accordance with a Home Office licence. They are not for medical prescription but more usually for research. Schedule 5 preparations are the most casually controlled. These are various dilute, small-dose, non-injectable products that can often be sold without prescription over a chemist's counter and all can be possessed with impunity. Technically, once bought, they cannot be supplied to someone else: an injunction that's rarely enforced. The products include cough medicines, anti-diarrhoea agents and mild painkillers. In between come Schedules 2 to 4, which cover the majority of controlled drugs. They are available for medical use but must generally be supplied or administered in accordance with a prescription. The exceptions are the benzodiazepine tranquillisers, in Schedule 4, which can be legally possessed without a doctor's authority so long as they are in the form of a medicinal product.

An offence is committed if a prescribed person passes on a part of the prescription to somebody else. The recipient, ironically, would be in the clear since s/he is merely in possession. The supplier, even if no money changed hands, would be liable to a trafficking prosecution, carrying a possible five-year prison term.

Offences

There are numerous charges brought under the various sections of the MDA, from simple possession to complex issues like 'assisting in the commission of an offence outside the UK.' The sentences available to the courts run from a modest fine to life imprisonment. In summary, with their maximum penalties indicated, the major offences are as follows.

Possession

The vast majority of offences are for possession, and the great majority of those relate to cannabis. 'Possession' means the smallest measurable trace, whether or not it is sufficient to cause a whisper of intoxication. In each case of alleged possession the prosecution must prove three major points – that the substance was in the defendant's possession or control (a verbal admission of past possession is sufficient if made in front of a police officer); that it is a controlled drug; and that the defendant knew s/he possessed the drug. If the evidence for possession results from a blood or urine test, this alone does not constitute possession. It is also possible for a defendant to get an acquittal when the drug is found in a container and where s/he can satisfy the court that s/he neither knew nor suspected what its contents were. This is difficult. There are other factors complicating the possession issue, such as: 'I had just taken it off another person and was on my way to the police to hand it in.' This would constitute a proper defence. The advice agency Release have produced an excellent brochure called *Drugs and The Law*, which gives more clarification. Release themselves can fill in the remaining blanks.

Sentencing: – possession charges can be brought in either

magistrates,' or crown court with far more severe penalties available to the latter authority. In reality the penalties fetched in are considerably less than the maximum available – unless, that is, the person has a history of serious offences, or the current charge involves a large quantity. Around 85 per cent of all drug offenders are convicted of unlawful possession and three-quarters of these will be fined £50 or less. Twenty per cent of the total, however, still receive a custodial sentence (although not all will actually go to prison).

The maximum penalties available to the courts for simple possession are: for Class A drugs dealt with in a magistrate's court – six months, £5,000 fine or both. Cases heard in crown court – seven years, unlimited fine or both. Class B drugs – three months, £500* fine or both (magistrates); five years, unlimited fine or both (crown). Class C – three months, £200 or both (magistrates); two years, unlimited fine or both (crown).

Possession with Intent to Supply

The amount in question is not relevant and it is possible that a small gift to a friend will render a person liable to this charge. A large amount for personal use might well be construed as proof of intent to supply, as might a smaller amount of, say, amphetamine sulphate that has been bagged up in half a dozen wraps.

Offering to Supply a Controlled Drug

The offence is complete once an offer is made, whether or not it is accepted. The prosecution can even succeed if the material turns out not to be a controlled drug (e.g. an attempt by person A to 'burn' person B).

Supplying/Producing a Controlled Drug

If one person buys on behalf of a group then this amounts to supplying. Cultivation of cannabis rates as production.

Maximum penalties for the above three 'supplying' offences

* Due to be raised to £2,500 under the 1994 Criminal Justice Act.

478

are: for Class A or B drugs dealt with in a magistrate's court – six months, £5,000 fine or both. For Class C before magistrates – three months, £500 fine or both. For Class A drugs before a crown court – life, unlimited fine or both. Class B – fourteen years, unlimited fine or both. Class C – five years, unlimited fine or both.

Supply of Steroids

In Novermber 1994 the Home Office announced a new offence, under the Misuse of Drugs Act, of supplying anabolic steroids. Proposed maximum penalties were a £2,500 fine and three months' imprisonment where the case came before magistrates, or five years in prison and an unlimited fine when heard in crown court.

Opium Offences

This is a residue from the turn-of-the-century paranoia over Chinese opium smokers. Coming in addition to the other offences applicable to opium as a controlled drug, the prosecution merely has to prove that the defendant smoked opium, frequented a place used for opium smoking, or that s/he possessed pipes or other gadgetry used for smoking. The defence can argue that s/he never knew or bothered to find out the place visited was a 'den', but turning a blind eye isn't good enough. Note the stiff crown court sentences as compared with those for possession of other Class A drugs.

Maximum penalties: six months, £5,000 or both (magistrates); fourteen years, unlimited fine or both (crown).

Allowing Premises to be Used

This could apply to the occupier or anyone concerned in the management of a private address, squat, pub, club, student hostel, etc. The prosecution must prove the defendant knowingly permitted or suffered production, supply, or the smoking of cannabis or opium (these giving off a detectable odour).

Maximum penalties: for Class A and B – six months, £5,000 or both (magistrates), fourteen years, unlimited fine or both (crown). For Class C – three months, £500 or both (magistrates); five years, unlimited fine or both (crown).

Obstruction

It is an offence to obstruct intentionally a police officer searching for drugs by swallowing or concealing them, or by concealing or failing to produce documents when asked, unless there is a reasonable excuse. But the police must show in court that the obstruction happened after the person learned the search was conducted under the MDA. In other words, a pill swallowed before the police announced they are doing an MDA search is not obstruction.

Maximum penalties: for all classes – six months, £5,000 or both (magistrates); two years, unlimited fine or both (crown).

Incitement, Conspiracy or Attempt to Commit an MDA Offence

In any of these three categories no offence need have been completed. For the first it simply has to be proved that persuasion or pressure was brought to bear. For conspiracy there merely has to be evidence of an agreement with one or more other persons; while for the third there has only to be the intention to commit an offence.

Maximum penalties: the same as those for the offence to which the incitement, conspiracy or attempt charge relates.

The Law and Needle Swap Schemes

Drug users turning in syringes containing traces of controlled drugs at syringe swap schemes are technically liable to prosecution for possession – the traces possibly being used as evidence of prior possession of the drug. Prosecution is considered unlikely but not impossible. Those people running the schemes – particularly government-sanctioned projects – are assumed to be safe.

Drug Trafficking Offences Act

Introduced in January 1987, its declared object is to prevent major-league traffickers from retaining their proceeds after being apprehended. In this respect, it provides new powers for tracing, freezing and then confiscating assets presumed to be drug-related. In the run-up to an arrest, bank managers, solicitors, accountants, etc. can be called upon to break their tradition of confidentiality and provide details of a customer's transactions. Once charged a defendant can be restrained from dealing with his/her property. Before sentencing, the court determines whether the accused has benefited from drug dealing in any way. That decision will generally rest on a written statement supplied by detectives (a feature that especially worries the legal advice agency Release, which regards such police evidence as invariably 'unreliable and ill-informed'). If profit is assumed to have been made then the court makes a confiscation order assessed as being equal to the proceeds from the defendant's entire trafficking career. This could include all the trafficker's current property and everything owned in the previous six years.

The onus is on the defendant to show such items are not from the proceeds of drug sales. A receiver may be appointed to recover the property confiscated and the Act provides for lengthy periods of imprisonment for non-payment. The Act includes two other new imprisonable offences: one is for 'laundering', aimed at persons who facilitate another's 'retention, control or investment' of proceeds. The other prohibits a person making any disclosure likely to prejudice an investigation. In both instances the burden of proof is on the defendants to establish their innocence. The editors of the *Criminal Law Review* have criticised the legislation for reversing three 'supposed principles' of English criminal justice: the presumption of innocence until guilt is proven; the principal requiring criminal intent or knowledge of wrong-doing before conviction for a serious offence, and the principle that offenders should be dealt with only for offences before the court.

Drug Kits

An additional offence under the Drug Trafficking Offences Act is the selling of cocaine kits and other drug paraphernalia, such as hash pipes and hookahs. Maximum sentence is six months' imprisonment. However, because such items have other uses – e.g. ornamental – and because a drug like cocaine is often ingested using ordinary household items such as a razor blade and mirror, the Crown will have difficulty in successfully prosecuting cases. A shop advertising 'coke kits for sale' would be a strong candidate for court action. Hypodermic needles and syringes are specifically exempt from the legislation, even if suppliers believe they are likely to be used in the administration of illegal drugs.

Intoxicating Substances (Supply) Act 1985

This prohibits the supply of solvents or other substances (e.g. glues, typewriter correction fluid) to people under eighteen years of age if there is reasonable cause to believe the substances or their fumes will be inhaled to cause intoxication. The actual inhaling or sniffing of volatile substances is not illegal.

Scottish common law provides for a similar offence of 'recklessly' selling solvents to children knowing they will inhale them.

Stop, Search and Arrest

Under the MDA the police have powers to stop, search and detain a person where there is 'reasonable suspicion' of possession of a controlled drug. They can also search a vehicle or vessel, but need a search warrant specifying the suspect's name and address to raid a home – unless they see an offence being committed (e.g. a cannabis plant in a window box or a joint being smoked). Warrants are valid for one month only, but during this time they can drop in as often as they choose and take whatever they think might serve as evidence of an MDA offence, or anything they think indicates any other crime. They may also search anyone on the premises concerned even though they occupy a separate apartment.

The Police and Criminal Evidence Act (PACE) considerably extends police powers to enter and search. They may now call in without a warrant to arrest a named person and can also stop people in the vicinity of a 'serious arrestable offence' and set up road blocks to undertake searches in areas judged by themselves to justify such action.

Detention and Questioning

Many people held in police stations are not actually under arrest but said to be 'helping police with their inquiries'. If they try to leave, however, they then find themselves officially arrested. This can be an advantage, says the advice agency Release, for once forcible detention starts, certain protection is forthcoming – notably, a time limit on how long the person can be held. It might also be possible, subsequently, to sue in cases of wrongful arrest.

Release also warn that the complexities of the drug laws are such that even a relatively innocent statement such as: 'I smoke cannabis sometimes, who doesn't?' can present quite serious problems. Once arrested, they report, you are under no obligation to say anything or to make a statement, and you should resist pressure to offer information about other drug users. You should immediately demand to see a solicitor and not sign the custody sheet waiving that right. Everything said can be used as evidence against you, from the moment you first meet up with the police – even before being formally cautioned. Once charged you have the right to inform someone of the arrest, unless the police want to invoke the Police and Criminal Evidence Act, arguing that you are being held in connection with a 'serious arrestable offence'. Drug trafficking constitutes such an offence. If access to a solicitor or relatives is delayed you can ask why and have the reason recorded on your custody sheet. Release advise that notes be kept throughout, since these can be used as evidence on your behalf. If you are held in connection with a 'serious' offence, you are entitled to access to a solicitor after thirty-six hours, although a magistrate may order your continued detention for up to ninety-six hours. Then you have the right to be released if not charged.

If you are not suspected of a 'serious' offence you must be released or charged within twenty-four hours of detention. Under PACE it is the duty of police officers to provide a doctor for a suspect if they 'know or suspect' that the suspect is dependent on drugs.

Notification

Only doctors with a special Home Office licence can issue opioids and cocaine for reasons other than to relieve pain caused by illness. Where prescriptions are issued to dependent individuals, that doctor must notify the Home Office which then adds the name to its central register. Even if the doctor refuses to take on as a patient a person who shows signs of dependency and even if s/he refuses to give a one-off prescription, s/he must still notify the Home Office or risk coming before a tribunal. The information the Home Office receives includes: name, address, date of birth, NHS number and 'name of drugs to which the person is addicted'. With such data maintained centrally on computer the physician need only phone up the Home Office to check whether the person before him/her is already logged and receiving scripts from someone else.

In addition to these checks, the police regularly look into double scripting and over-generous prescribing by calling in on chemists and examining what's being prescribed to whom and by which doctor.

Medicines Act 1968

The other important piece of legislation is the Medicines Act. This directs itself to all retail and wholesale dealings in therapeutic medicines, some of which are used recreationally. Like the MDA, it divides the substances under its control into three groups. The least stringently governed are in the General Sale List – laxatives, antacids and so on which can be sold anywhere. Secondly, there is the Pharmacy Medicines List, covering those products that don't require a prescription, but can be sold only by chemists. Then come the Prescription Only drugs, which require medical supervision. The Act also watches over doctors, specifying maximum dosages, as well as certain methods of writing, dating and repeating prescriptions. Other obligations fall upon pharmacists and drug companies. The latter's imports and exports are governed, as is the information they supply to doctors about their products.

Tobacco

In contrast to the welter of controls that apply to the MDA drugs, society's favourite intoxicants get a wide berth. The only restraints on tobacco are that a tobacco product must carry a fairly insipid health warning, a note of tar content, and that advertising must not step beyond certain limits. All these measures are voluntarily agreed to by the trade. Under the Children and Young Persons (Protection from Tobacco) Act 1991 it is illegal (maximum fine £1,000) to sell tobacco products to children under the age of sixteen. In addition, retailers must prominently display signs announcing that fact, and local authorities are obliged to monitor such outlets. It is, nonetheless, extremely rare for any tobacconist to be prosecuted for selling to minors, even though the government's own figures* indicate that eleven to fifteen-year-olds in all parts of the UK, barring Northern Ireland, are consuming more than one billion cigarettes a year – shelling out around £120 million in the process.

* 1991 Office of Population, Censuses and Surveys data, published in 'Protecting Children from Tobacco', a report by Parents Against Tobacco, Long Bennington, Notts., 1993.

Alcohol

Drinking regulations also set out, notionally, to protect minors, but again are largely ignored. Except with special authority it is an offence to give intoxicating liquor to any child under five years of age, even in the home. A long-standing ban on children entering pubs was relaxed in 1994, after which it became permissible for youngsters under fourteen to enter bars so long as they are accompanied by an adult. The establishments concerned must first have a 'children's certificate', issued by licensing justices when they are satisfied that the premises are suitable and that food and soft drinks, as well as alcohol, are on sale. Youngsters aged fourteen and over may be allowed unaccompanied into any part of licensed premises providing they do not drink. Those aged sixteen to eighteen may drink beer, cider or perry with a meal in a place specially designated for dining. In Scotland this age group can also drink wine in such a setting. No one under the age of eighteen can act as a 'messenger' for an adult unless they are paid to do so or are related to someone who is employed in selling drinks. The normal adult freedoms start applying after a person's eighteenth birthday. A publican is free to refuse admission to anyone so long as it's not on grounds of race or sex.

Drunkenness

Technically it is an offence to be plain drunk in a public place – including licensed premises – although an arrest is generally made only if there is some rowdy or anti-social behaviour going on.

The more serious drink-linked offences come under the Road Traffic Act (1967), a piece of legislation which also applies to persons in charge of bicycles, horses or children. Where there are 'reasonable grounds' for suspecting a driver is drunk the police may stop him/her and ask that they blow into a breathalyser bag. If it comes up positive a second test will be ordered at a police station. Only if the person is incapable of blowing into the breathalyser or if the readings are marginal will that person have the right to ask for a blood urine test, to be conducted by a doctor. A prosecution will follow if the breath reading exceeds 35 mg per 100 ml, or if the blood or urine samples tops 80 mg of alcohol per 100 ml of blood or urine.

APPENDIX II: ADDRESSES

Introduction

Until funding cuts in the early 1990s, the number and range of drug treatment services had grown virtually without pause over the previous twenty-five years. Educational, research and reference material had also expanded, almost beyond comprehension.

The Institute for the Study of Drug Dependence (ISDD) is the key library and publisher of drug-related material in the UK – an enterprise probably without peer anywhere in the world. The Standing Conference on Drug Abuse (SCODA) is the national co-ordinating and representative body for drug services in the UK. I am greatly indebted to them for allowing me to publish the following paragraphs which explain who's offering what in the field of drug treatment and support.

Type of services

Day-Time Services

The categories of day-time services include street agencies, drug dependency units, community drug teams, self-help and volunteer services; all will refer to other services as appropriate.

Street Agencies – almost all are non-statutory, based in the community and provide a drop in service. The remit of these services includes: information, advice, counselling, home visits, outreach/detached, aftercare, group work, needle/syringe provision, condoms and advice on safer injecting and safer sexual practices. An increasing number of street agencies work with GPs to provide primary health care and where appropriate, a prescribing service which can range from detoxification through to stabilisation. The prescribing component is often confined to opioids although some services include stimulants in their remit.

Drug Dependency Units – these are statutory services usually situated within a hospital or hospital grounds and in most instances appointments are necessary. Some have waiting lists. The range of service provision usually includes information, advice, counselling, home visits, group work, aftercare, condoms, advice on safer sexual practices and in some instances needle/syringe provision and advice on safer injecting practices. Psychiatric and psychological treatment is also provided. The type of prescribing service is variable from short/medium-term detoxification through to longer term stabilisation; a few do not offer a prescribing service. Most prescribing relates to opioids although some services include stimulants in their remit. See section on in-patient detoxification.

Community Drug Teams – these are statutory services, frequently based in the community although some are hospital-based. The range of provision is similar to that of many street agencies although some do not offer a drop in service. Community Drug Teams are often linked to psychiatric and psychological services.

Self-help – most self-help for drug users and families is provided through Narcotics Anonymous and Families Anonymous. However, some drug services facilitate self-help groups and many self-help groups meet at drug services. ADFAM have information about support for families throughout the country.

Volunteer Services – these vary from telephone, advice and information through to counselling and referral.

Needle/Syringe Exchange Scheme – most day-time services provide needles, syringes and condoms as well as information on safer injecting and sexual practices. There are a few autonomous exchange schemes. Many pharmacists provide needle and syringe exchange or sell needles/ syringes and information about this can be obtained from local drug services.

In-patient Detoxification

There are a few specialist detoxification units; almost all operate a catchment area but it is worth telephoning to check this. The majority of in-patient detoxification is provided in general psychiatric or medical wards and information about this and specialist units is available through local drug services.

Residential Services

Almost all residential houses require residents to be drug-free on entry, but usually only for a very short time. Some houses will accept residents on court conditions or directions of residence. Some projects operate a catchment area, but this can be flexible.

Cost Most services are non-fee-paying with the cost being met by the DSS and the differential coming from the local authority, probation service or charitable sources. Practically all fee paying services take some residents on DSS, known as 'assisted places'.

Residential services broadly operate under the following five categories:

General House. These vary in their philosophical approach, but in all cases group and individual support is provided. Residents are encouraged to take a positive part in determining their therapy.

Minnesota Method. This treatment method was devised at the Hazelden Hospital in Minnesota, and is commonly referred to as the 'Minnesota Method'. It is based on the twelve steps of the Fellowship of Alcoholics Anonymous/Narcotics Anonymous and the belief that addiction/chemical dependency is a disease. Many of these services may require a financial contribution from the resident or their family, dependent on their disposable income.

Christian House. The nature of these houses varies: their common factor is an emphasis (in varying degrees) on the importance of a resident's acceptance of Jesus as Lord, and to trust in Him for their healing. The majority of these services will not accept lesbians and gay men.

House with Christian Staff. Group and individual work is provided and residents are encouraged to take a positive part in determining their therapy. Staff do not try to coerce residents into adopting Christianity. Will accept lesbians and gay men unconditionally.

Therapeutic Community. Have a hierarchical structure and residents, in working through the programme, work their way through the hierarchy. The structure is operated in conjunction with intensive group therapy sessions in which all members of the community are equal.

National services

Standing Conference on Drug Abuse
Waterbridge House
32 Loman Street
London SE1 0EE.
Tel. 071–928 9500
SCODA is the national co-ordinating and representative body for drug services and those working with drug users. Bi-monthly newsletter. Directories and county lists of services as well as needle exchange lists. Freephone Drug Problems provides a recorded message giving telephone contact numbers throughout England as well as contact numbers in Wales, Scotland and Northern Ireland. Dial 100 and ask for Freephone Drug Problems.

Open: M-F 9.30a.m.–5.15p.m.

Library, Information and Research

Institute for the Study of Drug Dependence
Waterbridge House
32 Loman Street
London SE1 0EE.
Tel. 071–928 1211
The Institute publishes up-to-date material on various aspects of the use and misuse of drugs. It provides a comprehensive library service for interested individuals and professionals. Also has a research department.

Open: M-F 9.30a.m–5.30p.m.

Centre for Research on Drugs and Health Behaviour
200 Seagrave Road
London SW6 1RQ
Tel. 081–846 6565

The National Addiction Centre
(The Addiction Research Unit) Addiction Sciences Building
4 Windsor Walk
London SE5 8AF
Tel. 071–703 5411

Education and Training

TACADE (The Advisory Council on Alcohol and Drug Education)
1 Hulme Place
The Crescent
Salford M5 4QA
Tel. 061–745 8925
Catchment Area: National
Education and training, resources, information, consultancy project. Management for all professionals working with young people and the community.

Family support and self-help

ADFAM National
First Floor
Chapel House
18 Hatton Place
London ECIN
Tel. 071–405 3923
Information, advice, counselling. National helpline for the
families and friends of drug users; also provides training and
project support for professionals and volunteers working with
the families of users.

Open: M-F 10a.m.–5p.m.
Self referals accepted
Disabled access

Families Anonymous
The Doddington & Rollo Community Assoc.
Charlotte Despard Avenue
Battersea SW11 5JE
Tel. 071-498 4680
Advice and support groups for families and friends of drug
users. Meetings throughout the country.

Open: M-F 1p.m–4.30p.m.

Parentline
(Formerly OPUS)
Rayfa House
57 Hart Road
Thunderley
Essex SS7 3PD
Tel. 0268 757077
Telephone advice and counselling service for parents under
stress twenty-four branches.

Self-Help Organisations For Drug Users

Narcotics Anonymous
UK Service Office
PO Box 1980
London N19 3LS
Tel. Helpline 071–351 6794. Recorded meeting list Tel. 071–351 6066. Publications Tel. 071–272 9040.
Self-help fellowship. Groups throughout the UK.

Counselling Services

NAYPCAS (National Association of Young People's Counselling and Advisory Services)
17–23 Albion Street
Leicester LE1 6GD
Tel. 0533 554775
Information on counselling and advisory services for young people throughout the country. Letter service only.

BAC (British Association for Counselling)
37a Sheep Street
Rugby CV21 3BX
Tel. 0788 78328/9
Information and referral to individual counsellors and counselling agencies throughout the country. Telephone M-F 8.45a.m–5p.m., or write enclosing a SAE.

Crisis Counselling

The Samaritans
10 The Grove
Slough
Berkshire SL1 1QP
Tel. 0753 532713
Telephone counselling service for people in crisis. Branches throughout the country.

Drugs, legal, welfare

Release
388 Old Street
London EC1V 9LT
Tel. 071–729 9904
Open: M-F 10a.m.–6p.m.
24-hour emergency helpline
Tel. 071–603 8654
Twenty-four-hour telephone advice for legal emergencies and drug information/advice. Training on drugs and the law. Publications.

Alcohol

Alcohol Concern
305 Grays Inn Road
London WC1X 8QF
Tel. 071–833 3471
Seeks to raise awareness at local and national level of the problems alcohol can cause and improve services for people with drink related problems.

Alcoholics Anonymous
PO Box 514
11 Redcliffe Gardens
London SW10 9BQ
Tel: 071–352 9779/5493
Branches throughout the country

Drinkwatchers
200 Seagrove Road,
London SW6 1RQ
Tel: 071–381 3155
Branches throughout the country

HIV/AIDS

Terrence Higgins Trust
52–54 Grays Inn Road
London WC1X 8LT
Helpline Tel. 242 1010
Office Tel. 071–831 0330
Buddying service, advice, information and counselling on the
law, welfare, housing and insurance for people affected by
HIV/AIDS. Does work on drug use.

National AIDS Helpline
Tel. 0800 567123 – 24 hour confidential freephone helpline.
Free leaflets on HIV infection and AIDS.

National AIDS Trust
Tel. 071–972 2845
Open: M-F 9a.m.–5p.m.
Grant-making trust for HIV-related services. Co-ordinating
function for HIV services, also respond to policy issues.

Positively Women
5 Sebastian Street
London EC1V 0HE
Tel. 071–490 5515
Health Authority: Bloomsbury and Islington
Open: M-F 10a.m.–5p.m.
Self-referrals accepted
Age: Any
Information, advice and support for and from women who
have HIV infection, AIDS or a condition connected with HIV
infection and AIDS. Meets in Central London.

Solvents

Re-Solv
30a High Street
Stone
Staffordshire ST15 8AW
Tel. 0785 817885
Open: M-F 9a.m.–5p.m.
Directory, information, advice, teaching materials, research,
grants.

Solvent Misuse Project–National Children's Bureau
8 Wakley Street
London EC1V 7QE
Tel. 071–278 9441
Produce a directory of residential services which accept young solvent users.

Tranquillisers

MIND (National Association for Mental Health)
22 Harley Street
London W1N 2ED
Tel. 071–637 0741
National organisation for mental health with a comprehensive number of offices throughout England and Wales. Many of their offices provide support for tranquilliser users and facilitate self-help groups. The information unit at MIND can provide further details.

Council for Involuntary Tranquilliser Addiction (CITA)
Cavendish House
Brighton Road
Waterloo
Liverpool L22 5NG
Tel. 051–949 0102
Health Authority: South Sefton
Open: M-F 9.30a.m.–5.30p.m.
National telephone advice, information and counselling for people with tranquilliser problems. Drop-in and appointments for local people.

Co-ordinating Services

Festival Welfare Service (FWS)
61b Hornsey Road
Islington
London N7 6DG
Tel. 071–700 5754
Co-ordinates welfare provision, including information and assistance for drug users, at festivals and events.

Association of Community Health Councils for England and Wales
30 Drayton Park
London N5 1PB
Tel. 071–609 8405
Information, advisory service for CHCs. Represents the users of health services at a national level.

Head Offices

Cranstoun Projects
148–150 Penwith Road
Earlsfield
London SW18 4QB
Tel. 081–877 0211
Residential services in London and Surrey.

Richmond Fellowship
8 Addison Road
London W14 8DL
Tel. 071–603 6373
Residential services in London and Surrey.

Turning Point
New Loom House
101 Back Church Lane
London E1 1LU
Tel. 071–702 2300
Extensive range of counselling, advice and support centres for users, families and friends.

Phoenix House
Head Office
47–49 Borough High Street
London SE1 1NB
Tel. 071–407 2789
Residential houses in different parts of the country.

Life for the World Trust
Wakefield Building
Gomm Road
High Wycombe HP13 7DJ
Tel. 0494 462008
Residential services in Norwich and Dorset.

Drugs and Sport

Sports Council
Doping and Control Unit
Walkden House
3–10 Melton Street
London NW1 2EB
Tel. 071–383 5667
Information about anabolic steroids.

Home Office

Drugs Inspectorate
Home Office Drugs Inspectorate
50 Queen Anne's Gate
London SW1H 9AT
Tel. 071–273 3727, 273 3765, 273 3815, 273 3856
Tel. 071–273 2213 – index – enquiries from doctors

Regional offices at:
10th Floor
Dudley House
133 Albion Street
Leeds LS2 8PB
Tel. 0532 429941

PO Box 26
Bristol BS99 7HQ
Tel. 0272 276736/293714
Responsible for Home Office Index (Notifications). Advice for doctors and other professionals on issues relating to drugs.

Home Office Index

Its Main Purpose is to eliminate duplicate prescribing. All doctors who come into contact with or treat people who they know, or suspect, are addicted to one or more of fourteen notifiable drugs (certain opioids and cocaine) are required to notify the Chief Medical Officer at the Home Office, giving limited details about the individual as laid down in the Misuse of Drugs (Notification of and Supply to Addicts) Regulations. Doctors wishing to make an enquiry with respect to the index should telephone 071–273 2213.

Drugs Prevention Initiative
Central Drugs Prevention Unit
Home Office
Horseferry House
Dean Ryle Street
London SW1P 2AW
Tel. 071–217 8713
Focus is on the prevention of drugs misuse at local and national levels. Branches throughout England.

Department of Health (DOH)

Child Health, Maternity and Prevention Division
Wellington House
133–155 Waterloo Road
London SE1 8UG
Tel. 071–972 2000
Remit for national funding. Advice, information on government policy.

Regional Services

Youthlink Wales
Ty Siriol
49 St Martins Road
Caerphilly CF8 1EG
Tel. 0222 885711
Open: M-F 8.30a.m.–4.30p.m.
Supports and develops young people's initiatives throughout
Wales in the primary prevention of substance misuse and the
spread of HIV.

Drugaid: All Wales Drugline
1 Neville Street
Cardiff CF1 8LP
Tel. 0222 383313 – 24-hour helpline

Alcohol

Alcohol Concern Wales and Health Promotion Authority for Wales
Floor 8
Brunel House
2 Fitzalan Road
Cardiff CF2 1ER
Tel. 0222 472472 (HPA for Wales)
0222 488000 (AC Wales)

Northern Ireland

Belfast

Northern Ireland Regional Unit
Shaftesbury Square Hospital
116–122 Great Victoria Street
Belfast BT2 7BG
Tel. 0232 329808
Individual and general counselling.
Health education and promotion.
Information on facilities throughout Northern Ireland.

Alcohol

Council on Alcohol Related Problems
12 Lombard Street
Belfast BT1 1RD
Tel. 0232 324176

Northern Ireland Council on Alcohol
40 Elmwood Avenue
Belfast BT9 6AZ
Tel. 0232 664434

Northlands Centre
68 Northland Road
Londonderry BT48 0AL
Tel. 0504 363011

Scotland

Scottish Drugs Forum
5 Oswald Street
Glasgow G1 5QR
Tel. 041–221 1175
Open: M-F 9.30a.m.–4.30p.m.
The Forum is the umbrella organisation for those concerned with drug problems in Scotland.

Scottish Drugs Forum (Edinburgh Office)
40 Shandwick Place
Edinburgh EH2 4RT
Tel. 031–220 2584
Open:-T, Th 9.30a.m.–4.30p.m.

Scottish Drugs Forum (Dundee Office)
84 Commercial Street
Dundee

Health Education Board for Scotland
Formerly the Scottish Health Education
Group
Woodburn House
Canaan Lane
Edinburgh EH10 4SG
Tel. 031–447 8044
Undertakes health education programmes within Scotland on drug misuse and HIV/AIDS.

Drugs Training Project
University of Stirling
Stirling
Tel. 0786 73171 ext. 2775 or 2774
Open: M-F 9a.m.–5p.m.
Offers training, information, advice and support to statutory and voluntary drug projects throughout Scotland. This service is also offered to other professional organisations and individuals outside the Health Service.

HIV/AIDS

Scottish AIDS Monitor
PO Box 48
Edinburgh EH1 3SA
Office Tel. 031–557 3885
Helpline Tel. 0345 090966 7.30a.m.–1a.m. weekdays
Support and assistance to people with AIDS and their families.
Welfare benefit service, hardship fund, buddy support, prison
counselling, various support groups.

Alcohol

Alcoholics Anonymous, Scottish Service Office
Baltic Chamber
50 Wellington Street
Glasgow G2 6HJ
Tel. 041–221 9027

Industrial Alcoholism Unit
Company and Employee Counselling Service
82 West Regent Street
Glasgow G2 2QF
Tel. 041–332 7936

Scottish Council on Alcohol
137–145 Sauchiehall Street
Glasgow G2 3EW
Tel. 041–333 9677

Residential services

Based in Scotland

Aberlour Child Care Trust
5 Scarrel Road
Castlemilk
Glasgow GH5 0DE
Tel. 041–631 1504
Women and their children. 6 bed spaces for women, 12 children. Age: women – no limit, children 0–11. Do not need to be drug-free on admission. Solvent/tranquilliser users accepted. Catchment: Strathclyde.

Brenda House
(Aberlour Child Care Trust)
9 Hay Road
Niddrie
Edinburgh
Tel. 031–669 6676
Women and their children. 6 bed spaces for women, 12 for children. Age: women – no limit, children 0–11. Do not need to be drug-free on admission. All illegal/legal drug use accepted. Priority given to Lothian Region.

Castle Craig Clinic
West Linton
Pebbleshire EH46 7DH
Tel. 0721–52625
Mixed. 69 bed spaces (47 primary treatment, 22 secondary). Age: Any. Fees and some DSS.

The Place
200 Balmore Road
Possilpark
Glasgow G22 6LJ
Tel. 041–336 8147
Mixed. 6 bed spaces. Age: 16+. Drug-free 24 hours before admission. Tranquilliser users accepted.

Roberton House
1 Lancaster Crescent
Glasgow G12 0RR
Tel. 041–334 1118
Mixed. 12 bed spaces. Age: 16+. Not necessary to be drug-free on admission. Married couples may refer. Solvent users accepted if part of wider drug use problem. Tranquilliser users taken but may have to undergo medical detox. Catchment: Strathclyde.

Channel Islands

Guernsey

Guernsey Alcohol and Drug Abuse Council
Brackside
The Grange
St Peter Port
Guernsey GX1 1RQ
Health Authority: States of Guernsey
Board of Health
Catchment Area: Bailiwick of Guernsey
Open: M-F 9a.m.–12.30p.m. and 2p.m.–5p.m.
Self-referrals accepted
Information, advice, counselling, home visits, outreach/detached, aftercare, group work. Alcohol service, but provide information/support for drug users.

Prevention Service
Guernsey Health Promotion Unit
Rosaire Avenue
St Peter Port
Guernsey
Tel. 0481 711161
Health Authority: States of Guernsey
Board of Health
Catchment Area: Guernsey
Open: M-F 9a.m.–12.30p.m. and 2p.m.–5p.m.
Information on drugs.

Jersey

Alcohol and Drug Service
Catherine Quirke House
2 Newgate Street
St Helier
Jersey
Tel. 0534 59000 ext. 2297
Health Authority: States of Jersey
Board of Health
Catchment Area: Bailiwick of Jersey
Open: M-F 9a.m.–5p.m.
Self-referrals accepted
Information, advice, counselling, primary health care, home visits, aftercare, psychological treatment.

INDEX

A1 allele gene 289–90
acid see LSD
Acid house *see* dance scene
addiction
  alcohol 50–1
  amphetamines 77–8, 85, 86
  anabolic steroids 395–6
  barbiturates 109, 111, 112
  caffeine 128
  cannabis 154–5
  crack 189, 196, 218–221
  hallucinogens 261, 262, 267
  heroin 287–8, 289, 290–3,
    315–19
  nicotine 425–6
  nitrous oxide link 85
  notification 30, 484
  poppers 349
  steroids 395–6
  tranquillisers 441, 446, 448–52
  volatile substances 369
  vulnerability 85, 287, 289–91
adhesives 360–1, 366
adulterants
  amphetamines 71
  cannabis 148
  cocaine 187
  Ecstasy 236, 258–9
  heroin 278, 320–1
  poppers 348
aerosols, sniffing 362–3
aggression
  amphetamines 82–3
  barbiturates 106
  caffeine 125
  steroids 392–4, 406–7
AIDS *see* HIV/AIDS
alcohol 35–67
  addiction 50–1
  controls 486–7
  deaths 30, 31, 42, 46, 48, 53
  measurement 40–1

  with other drugs 83, 115, 442
  treatment services 496,
    502, 503–4
  UK consumption 7, 60
  withdrawal 51–2, 63–5
Alcohol Treatment Units (ATUs)
  64
alkyl nitrites 347–56
alprazolam 444
Amanita muscaria see Fly Agaric
Amanita phalloides (Death
  Cap) 245
amphetamines 69–102
  addiction 77–8, 85, 86
  athletes 389
  barbiturate link 113–14
  history 87–90
  legal 73
  medical uses 91
  with other drugs 83, 86–7
  physical effects 84–7
  production 71–2
  psychosis 81–2
  Purple Hearts 71, 89, 113, 171
  sensations 76–7
  withdrawal 97–9, 86
amyl nitrite 347–8
  see also poppers
amylobarbitone 105, 106
Amytal 106
anabolic steroids 383–410
  brands 386
  dependence 395–6
  history 396–405
  legal status 405–6
  Misuse of Drugs Act 1971 479
  physical effects 389–96
  rave scene 250–1
  withdrawal 393, 395–6
anaemia 109, 349
anaesthetics
  barbiturates 104

509

513

514

515

517